STRUCTURE AND PHYSIOLOGY OF THE SLOW INWARD CALCIUM CHANNEL

RECEPTOR BIOCHEMISTRY AND METHODOLOGY

SERIES EDITORS

J. Craig Venter
Section of Receptor Biochemistry
and Molecular Biology
National Institute of Neurological and
Communicative Disorders and Stroke
National Institutes of Health
Bethesda, Maryland

Len C. Harrison
Department of Diabetes and
Endocrinology
The Royal Melbourne Hospital
Victoria, Australia

STRUCTURE AND PHYSIOLOGY OF THE SLOW INWARD CALCIUM CHANNEL

Editors

J. Craig Venter
Section of Receptor Biochemistry
and Molecular Biology
National Institute of
Neurological and Communicative
Disorders and Stroke
National Institutes of Health
Bethesda, Maryland

David Triggle
School of Pharmacy
State University of New York at Buffalo
Buffalo, New York

ALAN R. LISS, INC., NEW YORK

Address all Inquiries to the Publisher
Alan R. Liss, Inc., 41 East 11th St, New York, NY 10003

Copyright © 1987 Alan R. Liss, Inc.

Printed in the United States of America.

Library of Congress Cataloging-in-Publication Data

Structure and physiology of the slow inward calcium channel.

(Receptor biochemistry and methodology ; v. 9)
Includes bibliographies and index.
1. Calcium channels. I. Venter, J. Craig.
II. Triggle, D. J. III. Series. [DNLM: 1. Calcium—
physiology. 2. Electrophysiology. 3. Ion Channels—
physiology. W1 RE107KE v.9 / QV 276 S927]
QP535.C2S77 1987   599'.019'214   87-2951
ISBN 0-8451-3708-5

Contents

Contributors

P.F. Baker, MRC Secretory Mechanisms Group, Department of Physiology, King's College London, Strand, London, England **[247]**

G.N. Beaty, Department of Physiology, Biophysics, and Neurosciences, Centro de Investigación y de Estudios Avanzados del Instituto Politécnico Nacional, 07000 Mexico **[123]**

G. Cota, Department of Physiology, Biophysics, and Neurosciences, Centro de Investigación y de Estudios Avanzados del Instituto Politécnico Nacional, 07000 Mexico **[123]**

Michel Fosset, Centre de Biochimie du Centre National de la Recherche Scientifique, Parc Valrose, 06034 Nice Cedex, France **[141]**

Leo G. Herbette, Biomolecular Structure Analysis Center, University of Connecticut Health Center, Farmington, CT 06032 **[89]**

R.A. Janis, Miles Institute for Preclinical Pharmacology, New Haven, CT 06509 **[29]**

Robert S. Kass, Department of Physiology, University of Rochester, Rochester, NY 14642 **[71]**

Arnold M. Katz, Cardiology Division, University of Connecticut Health Center, Farmington, CT 06032 **[89]**

Douglas S. Krafte, University of Rochester, Department of Physiology, Rochester, NY 14642 **[71]**

Michel Lazdunski, Centre de Biochimie du Centre National de la Recherche Scientifique, Parc Valrose, 06034 Nice Cedex, France **[141]**

Richard J. Miller, Department of Pharmacological and Physiological Sciences, University of Chicago, Chicago, IL 60637 **[161]**

J.A. Sánchez, Department of Physiology, Biophysics, and Neurosciences, Centro de Investigación y de Estudios Avanzados del Instituto Politécnico Nacional, 07000 Mexico **[123]**

A. Scriabine, Miles Institute for Preclinical Pharmacology, New Haven, CT 06509 **[51]**

S. Martin Shreeve, Department of Pharmacology, College of Medicine, University of Vermont, Burlington, VT 05405 **[109]**

L. Nicola Siri, Department of Physiology, Biophysics, and Neurosciences, Centro de Investigación y de Estudios Avanzados del Instituto Politécnico Nacional, 07000 Mexico **[123]**

E. Stefani, Department of Physiology, Biophysics, and Neurosciences, Centro de Investigación y de Estudios Avanzados del Instituto Politécnico Nacional, 07000 Mexico **[123]**

David Triggle, School of Pharmacy, State University of New York at Buffalo, Buffalo, NY 14260 **[ix,29]**

J. Craig Venter, Section of Receptor Biochemistry and Molecular Biology, NINCDS, National Institutes of Health, Bethesda, MD 20892 **[ix,109]**

Egbert Wehinger, Bayer AG, Wuppertal, Federal Republic of Germany **[1]**

The number in brackets is the opening page number of the contributor's article.

Preface

Over one hundred years ago Sidney Ringer's article entitled, "A Future Contribution Regarding the Influence of the Different Constituents of the Blood on the Contraction of the Heart", was published in the Journal of Physiology (1). This work described the fundamental significance of Ca^{2+} to the maintenance of cardiac contractility. Although an accidental finding, this work may be regarded as an important base from which much of the subsequent focus on Ca^{2+} as an intracellular messenger linking cellular excitation to biological response has originated.

That Ca^{2+} functions as such an intracellular messenger stems from a set of comparatively simple observations:

1. The concentration of ionized intracellular Ca^{2+} in the resting (non-stimulated) state of the cell is normally very low $\leqslant 10^{-7} - 10^{-8}$ M;

2. During excitation the concentration of intracellular ionized Ca^{2+} rises to approximately 10^{-6} M;

3. Ca^{2+} interacts with a group of intracellular homologous Ca^{2+} binding proteins, including the ubiquitous calmodulin, whose affinities match the level of intracellular Ca^{2+};

4. The interactions of Ca^{2+} with these intracellular binding proteins, or Ca^{2+} receptors, initiates the Ca^{2+}-dependent cellular responses.

The informational role of Ca^{2+} thus depends upon its chemistry, which determines the nature of the complexes formed, and upon the existence of specific cellular processes that control the influx, efflux and sequestration of Ca^{2+} at both plasmalemmal and intracellular loci (2-7). This role of Ca^{2+} is played out through the life of the cell from the initial fertilization response to the finality of death from calcium overload.

The existence of these discrete processes that regulate Ca^{2+} movements make possible the concept of specific drugs that interact at one or other of these discrete steps. The Ca^{2+} channel antagonists, represented by the clinically available verapamil, nifedipine and diltiazem, are the best known examples of such drugs (8-10). These agents have not only proved to be substantial therapeutic tools in the control of a number of cardiovascular diseases but have subsequently proved to be major molecular tools with which to probe the properties of Ca^{2+} channels in excitable cells.

The past five years have seen an explosion of knowledge concerning the properties and functions of Ca^{2+} channels. The Ca^{2+} channel ligands, antagonist and activator, have proved to be valuable accomplices in the electrophysiological and biochemical assaults on the Ca^{2+} channel. As a consequence of such studies a great deal of information is now available detailing the properties, constitution, localization and classification of Ca^{2+} channels. This volume details some of this progress and attempts to record the properties of Ca^{2+} channels in major excitable cell systems. Much remains to be done, but progress is becoming dramatically swift. Contributions by molecular biology to defining the structures of Ca^{2+} channels are being made currently and will permit comparison of this system to other excitable cell constituents including the Na^+ channel and the nicotinic and muscarinic acetylcholine receptors.

The century following Ringer's original work has seen dramatic progress. The next decade is likely to exceed in its achievements all of the contributions of that first century. It is our hope that this volume will contribute to these achievements.

References

1. Ringer S (1883): J Physiol 4:29–42.
2. Campbell AK (1983): Intracellular Calcium. Its Universal Role as Regulator. New York: Wiley.
3. Sigel H (eds) (1984): Metal Ions in Biological Systems. Vol. 17. Calcium and the Role in Biology. New York: Dekker.
4. Rubin RP, Weiss GB, Putney JW (eds) (1985): Calcium in Biological Systems. New York: Plenum.
5. Parratt JR (ed) (1986): Control and Manipulation of Calcium Movements. New York: Raven Press.
6. Dalgarno D, Klevit RE, Levin BA, Williams RJP (1984): Trends Pharmacol Sci 6, 266.
7. Triggle DJ (1986): In Proceedings of Chemrawn V Conference, Heidelberg. Gesellschaft Deutscher Chemiker, in press.
8. Fleckenstein A (1983): Calcium Antagonism in Heart and Smooth Muscle. Experimental Facts and Therapeutic Prospects. New York: Wiley.
9. Janis RA, Silver P, Triggle DJ (1987): Adv Drug Res, in press.
10. Triggle DJ, Janis RA (1987): Ann Rev Pharmacol Toxicol, in press.

D.J. Triggle
J.C. Venter

Structure and Physiology of the Slow Inward Calcium Channel, pages 1–27
© 1987 Alan R. Liss, Inc.

1

Ca²⁺ Channel Ligands: Synthetic Approaches

Egbert Wehinger

Bayer AG, Wuppertal, Federal Republic of Germany

INTRODUCTION

Since their discovery in the sixties, calcium antagonists have become increasingly important in pure pharmacological research and in the clinical therapy of cardiovascular diseases [1–3]. Although a number of substances were credited with calcium-antagonistic properties, interest focused largely on three chemically different, clinically tested active substances, namely verapamil [4], nifedipine [5], and diltiazem [6], which at low doses are all able to selectively inhibit the transmembrane influx of Ca^{2+} ions through potential-dependent calcium channels. In the meantime, several derivatives, e.g., gallopamil [7], nicardipine [8], nitrendipine [9], and nimodipine [10], have been introduced onto the drug market, in addition to the prototypes. There are also numerous development products—particularly of the nifedipine type—in various stages of clinical testing.

The discovery of 1,4-dihydropyridine derivatives that stimulate the influx of Ca^{2+} ions in cardiac as well as in smooth muscle, represented an important advance in the understanding of the physiology of the calcium channel [11]. The observation that the properties of inhibiting and stimulating the flow of calcium can be included in the same dihydropyridine molecule shows that these compounds should really be regarded as calcium modulators [12].

The aim of this chapter is to give an overview of the synthetic aspects.

THE VERAPAMIL GROUP

The verapamil group comprises the derivatives in Table I. Verapamil (*1*) was introduced in 1962 as a coronary vasodilator and was first characterized as a β-blocker [13]. Through electrophysiological studies, verapamil was among the first drugs in which the principle of calcium antagonism was recognized [14].

Syntheses of Verapamil and Analogues

The syntheses of verapamil (*1*) [15], gallopamil (*2*) [15], and anipamil (*4*) [16] are analogous in that appropriately substituted CH-acidic phenylacetonitriles (*8*) are made to react with 6-aryl-1-chloro-4-methylazahexanes (*9*) after deprotonation by sodamide in toluene (Fig. 1).

Studies of structure-activity relationships within the verapamil group led to the development of tiapamil (*3*) [17,18]. In the synthesis of this compound, the 1,3-dithiane of 3,4-dimethoxybenzaldehyde (*11*) is first oxidized to the disulphone (*12*) with peracetic acid. This can be easily ionized with sodium in dioxane and converted into the free base of tiapamil by treatment with 1-chloro-6-(3,4-dimethoxyphenyl)-4-methylazahexane (9, Z = OCH_3) (Fig. 2).

TABLE I. The Verapamil Group

1	Verapamil: R=H
2	Gallopamil: R=OCH₃ (D 600)
3	Tiapamil (RO 11-1781)
4	Anipamil
5	Falipamil (AQA-39)
6	AQ-AH 208: n=0
7	UL-FS-49 : n=1

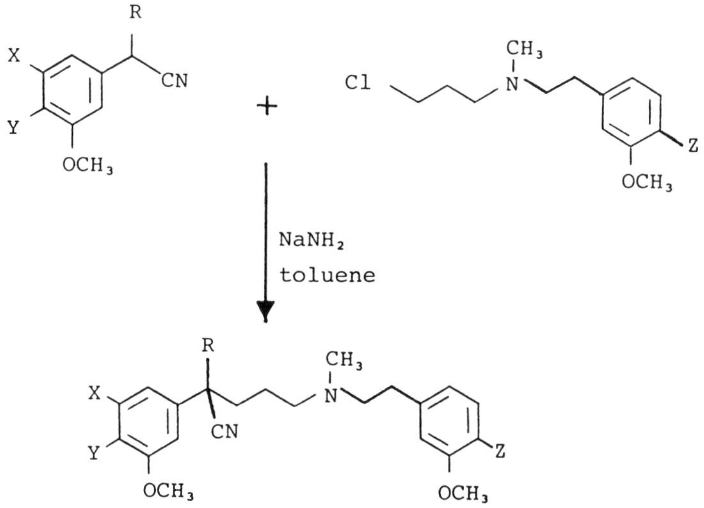

1 Verapamil : $R = CH(CH_3)_2$, $X = H$, $Y = Z = OCH_3$

2 Gallopamil : $R = CH(CH_3)_2$, $X,Y,Z = OCH_3$

4 Anipamil : $R = C_{12}H_{25}$, $X,Y,Z = H$

Fig. 1. *Synthesis of verapamil, gallopamil, and anipamil.*

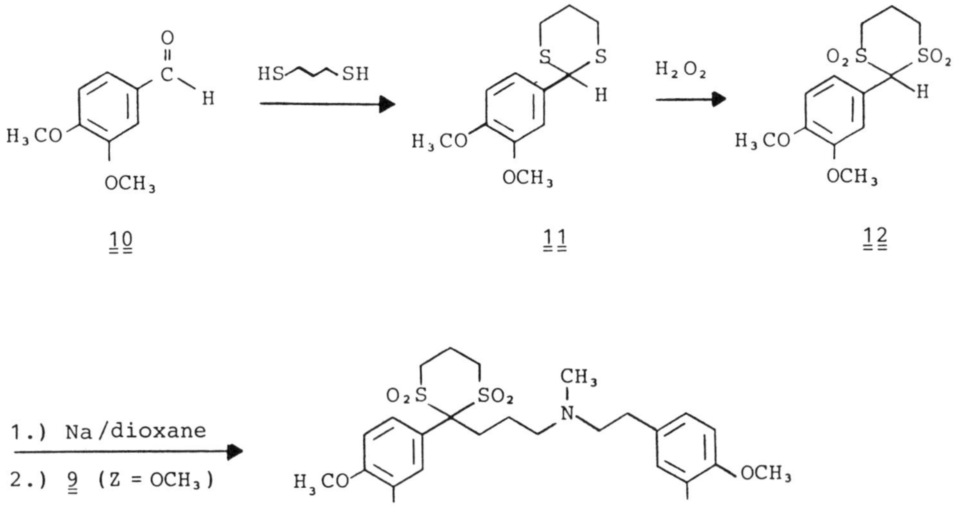

Tiapamil

Fig. 2. *Synthesis of tiapamil.*

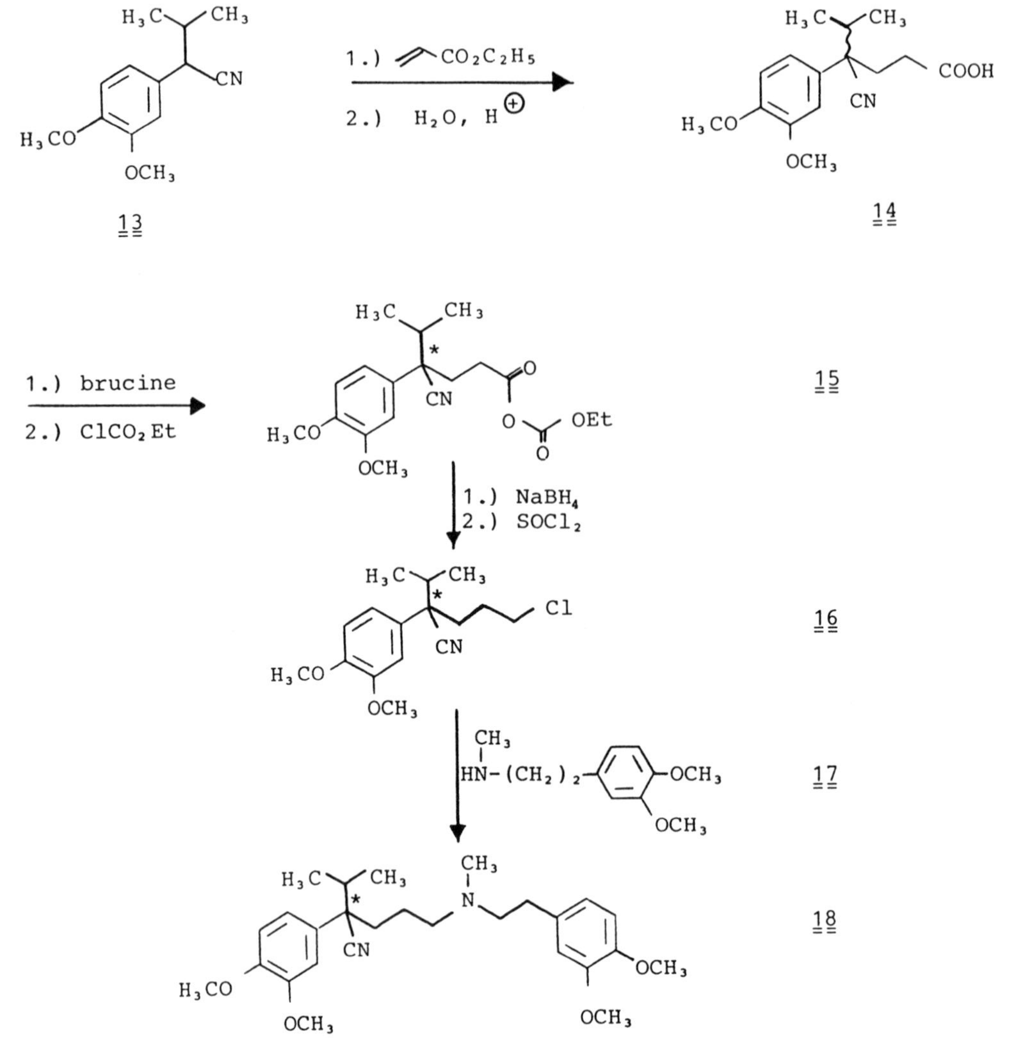

(S)-Verapamil: $[\alpha]_D^{20} = -25.5°$ (C = 100 mg/ml, benzene)

Fig. 3. *Synthesis of the enantiomers of verapamil.* * = optically pure.

The syntheses of falipamil (5) [19], AQ-AH 208 (6) [20], and UL-FS 49 (7) [21] have been described elsewhere.

Enantiomers of Verapamil

Verapamil, gallopamil, and anipamil are racemic forms of chiral compounds. Their structures permit the existence of two stereoisomers in each case, related like mirror images (enantiomers, optical antipodes).

Two pathways have been followed in the preparation of the antipodes of verapamil, both of which include a classic racemate resolution of a carboxylic acid via its diastereomeric alkaloid salts. In the first case (Fig. 3), the carboxylic acid (14) obtained by the addition of 3,4-dimethoxyphenyl-substituted isovaleric acid nitrile (13) to an acrylic acid ester and subsequent selective hydrolysis, is resolved via the brucine salts into the antipodes,

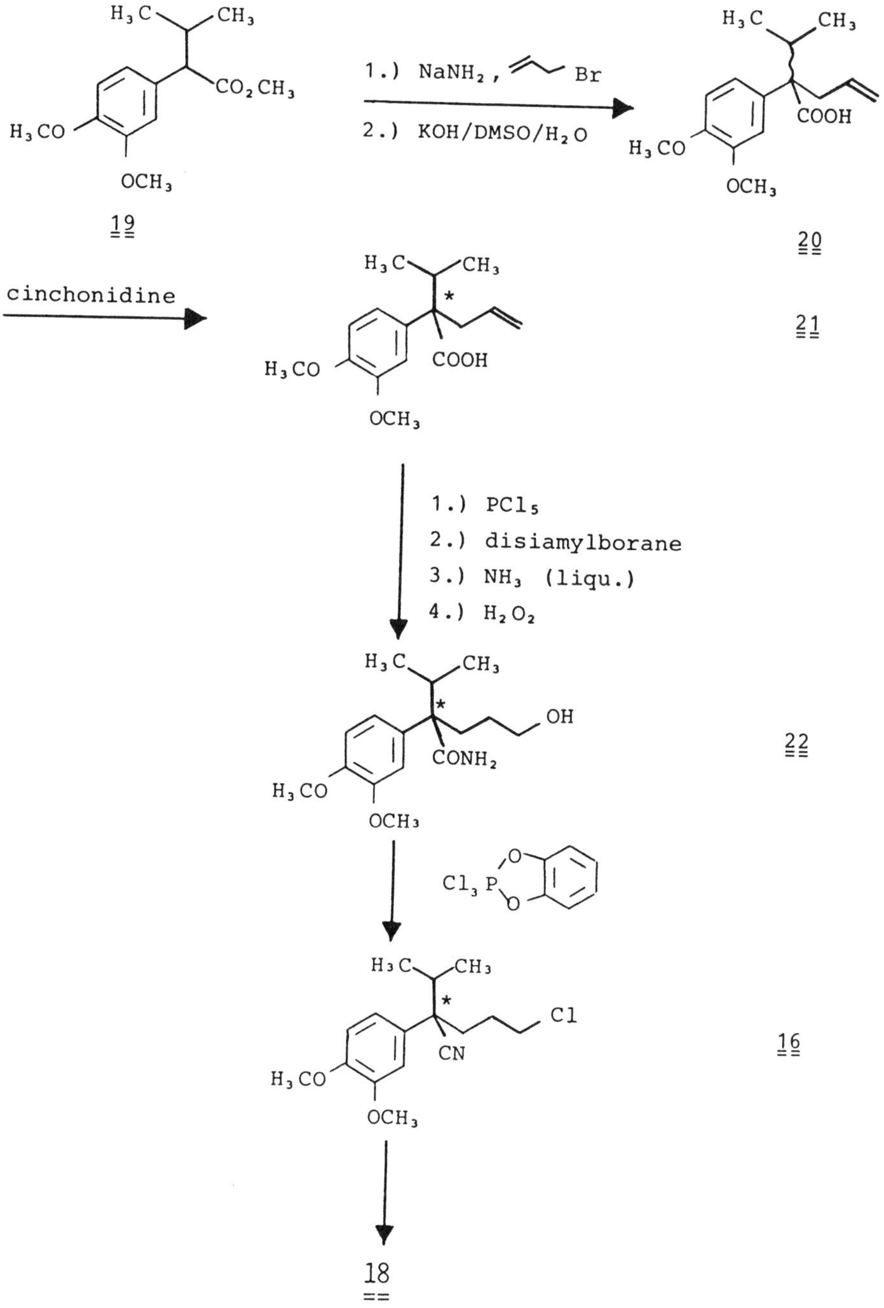

Fig. 4. *Reaction scheme of the alternative enantiomer synthesis of verapamil.* * = *optically pure.*

which are each converted into the optically active mixed anhydrides (*15*) with ethyl chloroformate [22]. The subsequent reduction with sodium borohydride, substitution of the resulting alcohol function with chlorine (*16*), and alkylation of the N-methylhomoveratry-

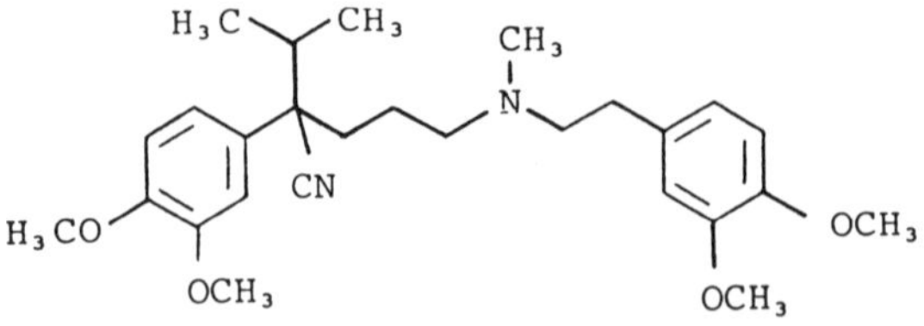

Fig. 5. *Some metabolites of verapamil. The percentages shown represent the percentage of the dose excreted in urine within 48 hours [27].*

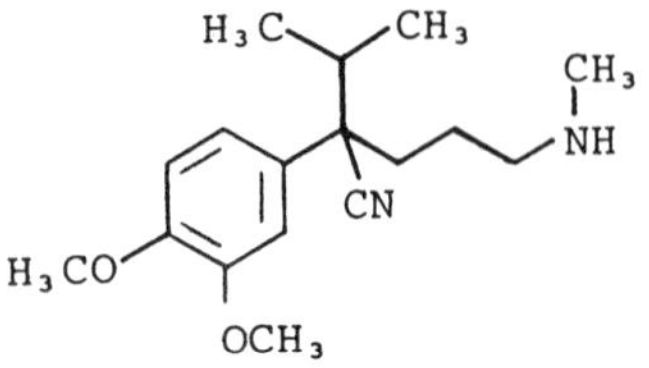

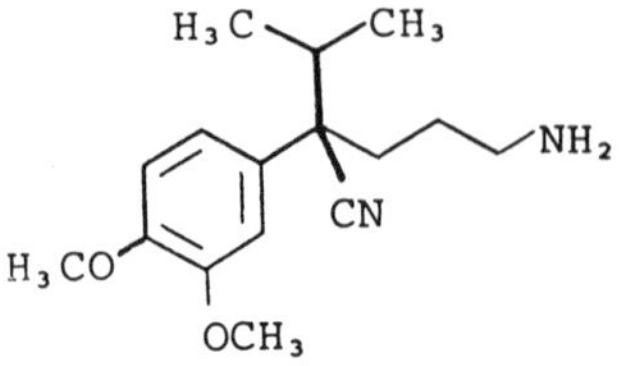

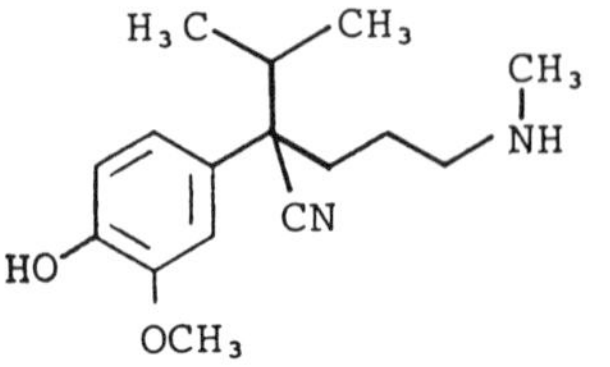

lamine (*17*) lead to the enantiomers of verapamil (*18*), with the relevant configuration at the quaternary carbon atom being maintained.

An analogous procedure was pursued in the synthesis of the dextrorotatory verapamil enantiomer—dideuterated at C5—which was used in the detailed study of the pharmacokinetics of the active substance [23].

The alternative preparation of the optical antipodes of verapamil starts with the allylation of the isopropyl-homoveratryl-carboxylic acid ester (*19*) in the α-position [24] (Fig. 4). Subsequent saponification of the sterically hindered ester with potassium hydroxide in aqueous dimethyl sulphoxide yields the acid (*20*), which can be separated into the antipodes (*21*) with cinchonidine. Further reaction via the optically active acid chlorides, hydroboration of the double bond with disiamylborane, ammonolysis of the acid chloride, and the oxidative introduction of the terminal hydroxy group yields the ω-hydroxycarboxylic acid amide (*22*), which is converted in one step to the ω-chloronitrile (*16*) with trich-

loro-2-benzodioxa-1,3-phosphol. Alkylation of the N-methylhomoveratrylamine as described above finally yields the enantiomers of verapamil (*18*). Determination of the absolute configurations of the optically active acids (*21*) allowed the configurations of the verapamil stereoisomers to be classified as (+)(R) or (−)(S).

The laevorotatory (S)-isomers of verapamil and gallopamil are the more potent antipodes in each case [25].

Biotransformation of Verapamil

Verapamil undergoes extensive biotransformation in dogs, rats [26], and man [27]. After oral administration to healthy volunteers, the drug has been shown (by a stable-isotope technique) to exhibit a stereoselective first-pass metabolism in the liver, with the more potent (−) isomer being eliminated preferentially [23].

The metabolic pathway of the drug has been studied in detail using [^{14}C]-verapamil (labelled in the nitrile group) [27]. In man, 12

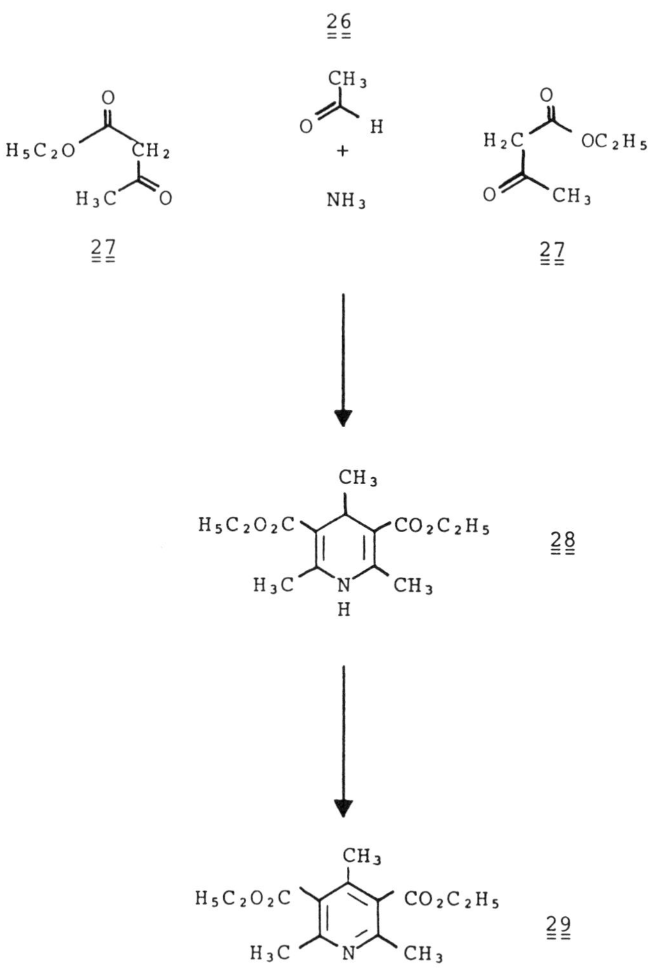

Fig. 6. *The Hantzsch pyridine synthesis.*

metabolites have been isolated from urine [27,28]. The most important reaction is the cleavage of the C–N–C bonds, mainly at the carbon atom that belongs to the shorter side chain (Fig. 5). In contrast to the general rule that in tertiary amines bearing an N-methyl group, the methyl is removed first, the N-demethylated metabolites constitute only 20 to 25% of the urinary biotransformation products, whereas 65% still contain the N-methyl group regardless of whether or not the C–N–C bond is already split.

The metabolic pathway of the N-dealkylated metabolites and of verapamil itself pro-

ceeds further via O-dealkylation, resulting in pharmacologically inactive derivatives which are excreted exclusively as conjugates.

There is only a quantitative difference between the metabolic patterns of verapamil in man, dogs, and rats.

1,4-DIHYDROPYRIDINES: STRUCTURES AND SYNTHESES

The chemist Arthur Hantzsch reported the first preparation of a 1,4-dihydropyridine derivative in 1882 [29]. Upon reacting one mole of acetaldehyde (26) with two moles of ethyl

TABLE II. Calcium Antagonistic 4-Dihydropyridines (DHP)

No.	DHP	R^1	R^2	R^3	R^4	R^5
30	Nifedipine	$2\text{-NO}_2\text{-C}_6\text{H}_4$	CH_3	H	CH_3	CH_3
31	Nicardipine	$3\text{-NO}_2\text{-C}_6\text{H}_4$	CH_3	H	CH_3	$CH_2CH_2N(CH_2Ph)(CH_3)$
32	Nitrendipine	$3\text{-NO}_2\text{-C}_6\text{H}_4$	CH_3	H	CH_3	C_2H_5
33	Nimodipine	$3\text{-NO}_2\text{-C}_6\text{H}_4$	$CH(CH_3)_2$	H	CH_3	$CH_2CH_2OCH_3$
34	Nisoldipine	$2\text{-NO}_2\text{-C}_6\text{H}_4$	CH_3	H	CH_3	$CH_2CH(CH_3)_2$
35	Felodipine	$2,3\text{-Cl}_2\text{-C}_6\text{H}_3$	CH_3	H	CH_3	C_2H_5
36	FR 7534	$3\text{-NO}_2\text{-C}_6\text{H}_4$	C_2H_5	H	CH_2OH	C_2H_5
37	Nilvadipine	$3\text{-NO}_2\text{-C}_6\text{H}_4$	$CH(CH_3)_2$	H	CN	CH_3
38	Darodipine	(benzoxadiazolyl)	C_2H_5	H	CH_3	C_2H_5
39	Isrodipine	(benzoxadiazolyl)	CH_3	H	CH_3	$CH(CH_3)_2$
40	Flordipine	$2\text{-CF}_3\text{-C}_6\text{H}_4$	C_2H_5	$-CH_2CH_2\text{-}N\text{(morpholino)}$	CH_3	C_2H_5
41	PO 219	$3\text{-NO}_2\text{-C}_6\text{H}_4$	CH_3	H	CH_3	$CH_2CH_2N\text{(piperazinyl)}N\text{-Ph}$
42	Ryodipine	$2\text{-OCHF}_2\text{-C}_6\text{H}_4$	CH_3	H	CH_3	CH_3
43	Amlodipine	$2\text{-Cl-C}_6\text{H}_4$	CH_3	H	$CH_2OCH_2CH_2NH_2$	C_2H_5
44	^{125}I-Iodipine	$2\text{-CF}_3\text{-C}_6\text{H}_4$	C_2H_5	H	CH_3	$CH_2CH_2N\text{-}\overset{O}{\overset{\|}{C}}\text{-}(CH_2)_2\text{-(3-}^{125}\text{I-4-OH-phenyl)}$
45	Azidopine	$2\text{-CF}_3\text{-C}_6\text{H}_4$	C_2H_5	H	CH_3	$CH_2CH_2N\text{-}\overset{O}{\overset{\|}{C}}\text{-(}C_6H_4\text{-}N_3\text{)}$

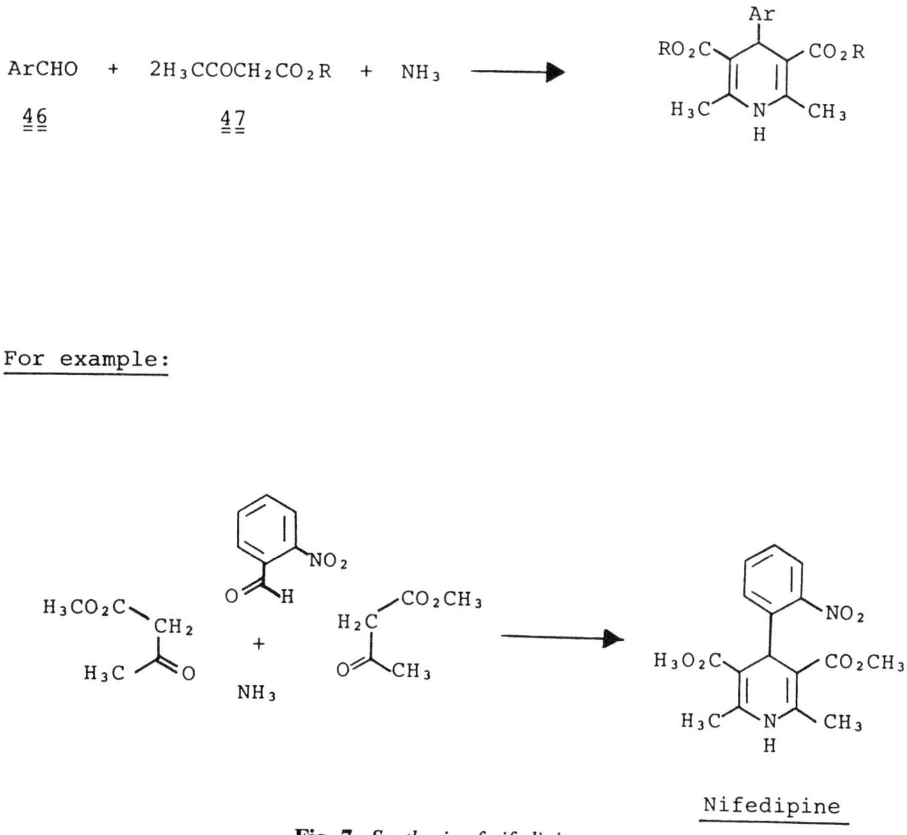

ArCHO + 2H$_3$CCOCH$_2$CO$_2$R + NH$_3$ ⟶

$\underline{\underline{46}}$ $\underline{\underline{47}}$

For example:

Nifedipine

Fig. 7. *Synthesis of nifedipine.*

acetoacetate (*27*) and one mole of ammonia, he obtained a crystalline compound which he was able to convert into the 2,4,6-trimethyl-pyridine-3,5-dicarboxylic acid diethyl ester (*29*) with nitric acid (Fig. 6).

Based on analytical investigations, he assigned the structure of a 1,4-dihydropyridine to that compound (*28*), which has since become well known as a stable intermediate in the Hantzsch pyridine synthesis. Hantzsch and other research groups were later able to show that the synthetic scope of the original reaction with respect to the components aldehyde, β-dicarbonyl compound and amine has wide limits [30–32], so that for the first time a source of pyridine derivatives was available that did not depend on coal tar.

Interest in the dihydropyridines was reawakened when it was discovered that the 1,4-dihydropyridine-pyridinium system is a unit

of the nicotinamide-adenine dinucleotide (NAD$^+$ ⇌ NADH) and, hence, acts as a co-substrate of numerous dehydrogenases [33]. Despite this key biochemical role and the relative ease with which 1,4-dihydropyridines could be obtained, the pharmacological potential and the therapeutic importance of this class of compounds have only been recognized in the last 20 years [34–37]. The rapid development achieved in recent times has led to a number of active substances, of which nifedipine (*30*), nicardipine (*31*), nitrendipine (*32*), and nimodipine (*33*) have been clinically tested and are available commercially (Table II).

Calcium-Antagonistic 1,4-Dihydropyridines

The synthesis of the calcium-antagonistic 4-aryl-1,4-dihydropyridine derivatives, which are presently in an advanced stage of devel-

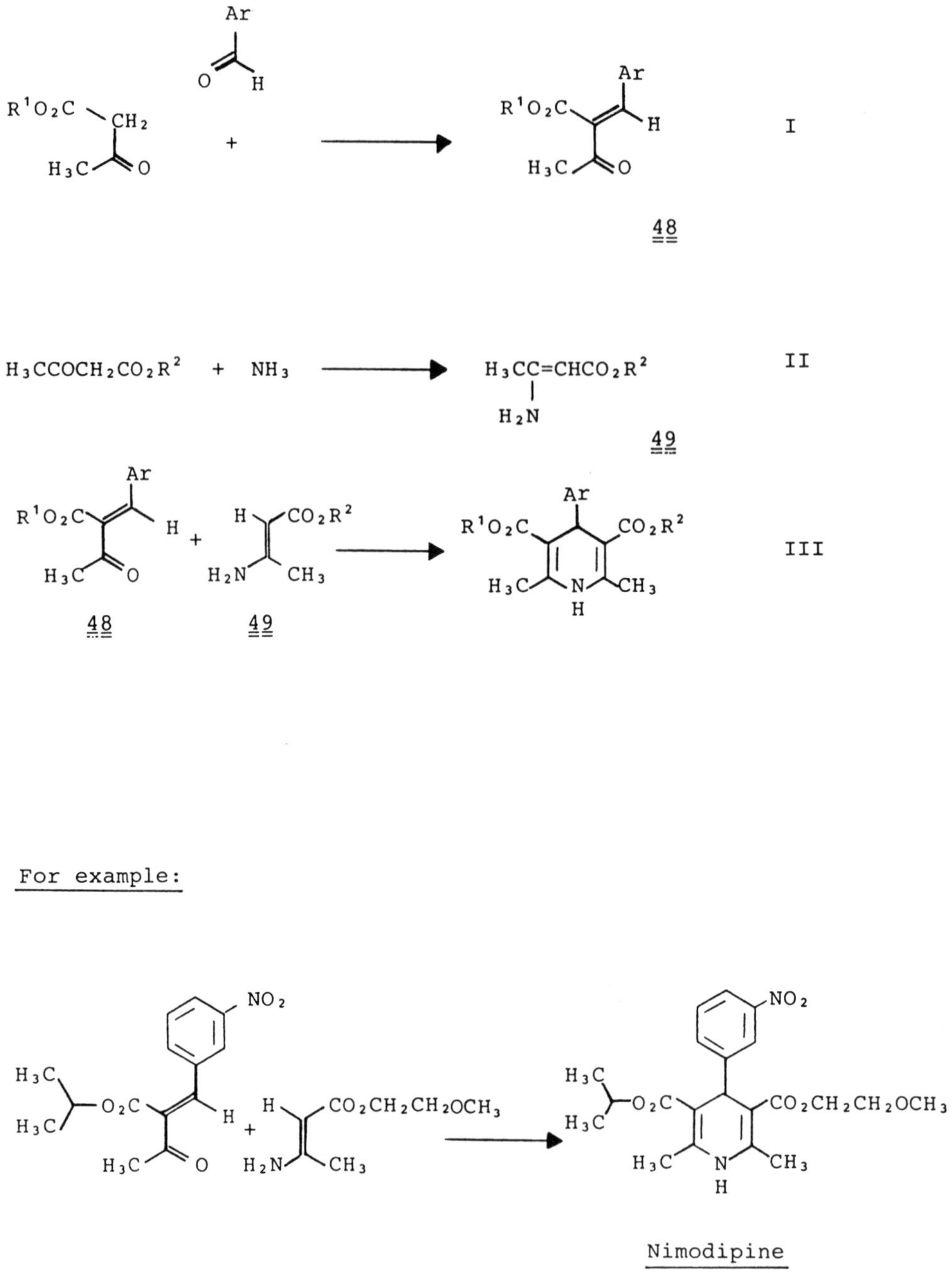

I

II

III

For example:

Nimodipine

Fig. 8. *Synthesis of nimodipine.*

opment (see Table II), is based on the Hantzsch condensation reaction, i.e., the re-action of one mole of aldehyde (46) with two moles of acetoacetic acid ester (47) and one mole of ammonia [29,38] (Fig. 7).

This three-component reaction, with which achiral products such as nifedipine (30) [39], darodipine (38) [40], and ryodipine (42) [41] can be prepared, is the more easily under-stood if one postulates as the primary step the

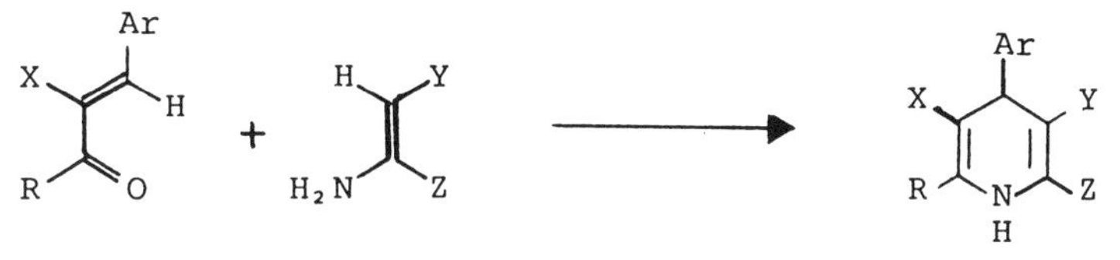

X,Y = CO$_2$R^1, COR^1, CN, SO$_2$R^1, NO$_2$, PO(OR^1)$_2$

Z   = alkyl, alkoxyalkyl, amino etc.

Fig. 9. *General scheme of the cyclizing Michael addition.*

Knoevenagel condensation from the aldehyde and the acetoacetic acid ester (reaction I) and the formation of the enaminocarbonyl compound from the acetoacetic ester and ammonia (reaction II) (Fig. 8). The subsequent reaction is then the conversion of the resulting 2-aralkylidene acetoacetic ester (*48*) and a 3-aminocrotonic acid ester (*49*) into the 1,4-dihydropyridine by a type of cyclizing Michael addition (reaction III).

If the intermediate products are synthesized separately, the two-component reaction (*48*) + (*49*) permits not only the specific preparation of derivatives with different ester groups in positions 3 and 5 of the dihydropyridine like nicardipine (*31*) [42], nitrendipine (*32*) [43,44], nimodipine (*33*) [43,45], nisoldipine (*34*) [46], felodipine (*35*) [47], isrodipine (*39*) [48], and PO 219 (*41*) [49], but also the introduction of various functional groups X, Y, and Z into the 3,5 and 2,6 positions of the heterocycle (*52*) (Fig. 9). An example of the exploitation of these possibilities is provided by the syntheses of FR 7534 (*36*) and nilvadipine (*37*) [50] (Fig. 10). The intermediate product for both compounds is the 2-formyl-1,4-dihydropyridine (*55*), which is obtained by reaction of the 4,4-dimethoxy-2-(3-nitrobenzylidene)-acetoacetic ester (*53*) and the 3-aminocrotonic acid ester (*49*) with ring clo-

sure (*54*) and subsequent hydrolysis of the acetal function.

If R^1 = R^2 = C$_2$H$_5$, the formyl group is reduced to the hydroxymethyl group (FR 7534) by sodium borohydride, whereas if R^1 = isopropyl and R^2 = methyl in formula (*55*), the aldehyde function is converted into the 2-cyano-1,4-dihydropyridine derivative (nilvadipine) via the oxime and subsequent dehydration.

The key reaction in the preparation of amlodipine (*43*) [51] is the cyclizing Michael addition of the 3-amino-4-(2-phthalimidoethoxy)-crotonic acid ethyl ester (*57*) to 2-(2-chlorobenzylidene)-acetoacetic acid methyl ester (*56*) with the formation of the expected 1,4-dihydropyridine (*58*), which yields the desired active substance on hydrazinolysis (Fig. 11).

Flordipine (*40*) [52] is finally obtained by the alkylation of the N-unsubstituted dihydropyridine (*59*) (which can be prepared by the Hantzsch method) with 2-(N-morpholino)-ethyl chloride (Fig. 12).

Calcium-Agonistic 1,4-Dihydropyridines

Calcium-agonistic 1,4-dihyropyridines (see Table III) are characterized primarily by a 3-nitro group in the dihydropyridine ring [BAY K 8644 (*60*), substance 202-791 (*61*)] or by a

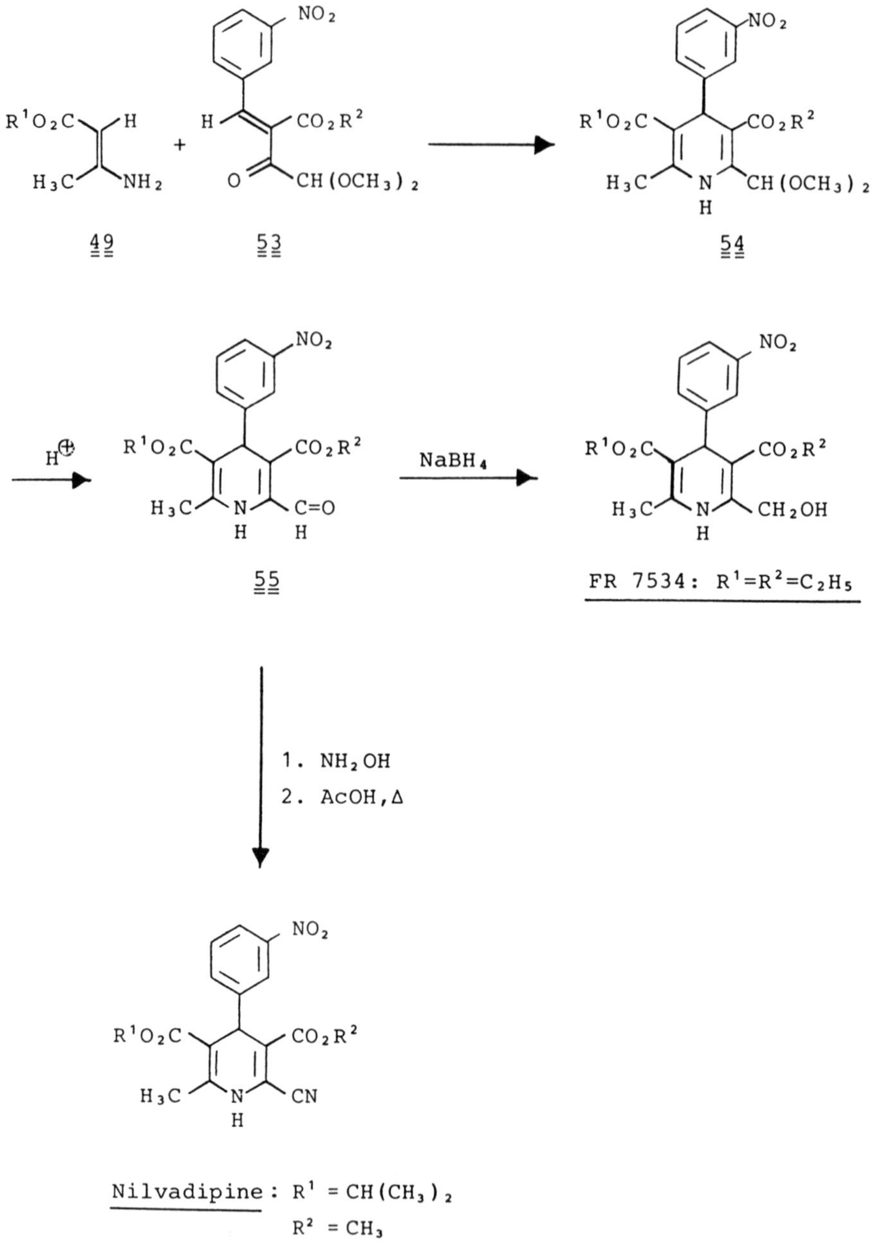

Fig. 10. *Synthesis of FR 7534 and nilvadipine.*

lactone ring [CGP 28 392 (*62*)]. The pharmacological Ca^{2+} channel-activating properties of H 160/51 (*64*) have recently been reported [53], and a weak vasoconstrictive effect has been shown for YC-170 [54].

The synthesis of BAY K 8644 [55] from 2-nitro-1-(trifluoromethylphenyl) -1,2-buten-3-one (*65*) and 3-aminocrotonic acid methyl ester (*66*) demonstrates in turn the broad spectrum of applications of the cyclizing Michael

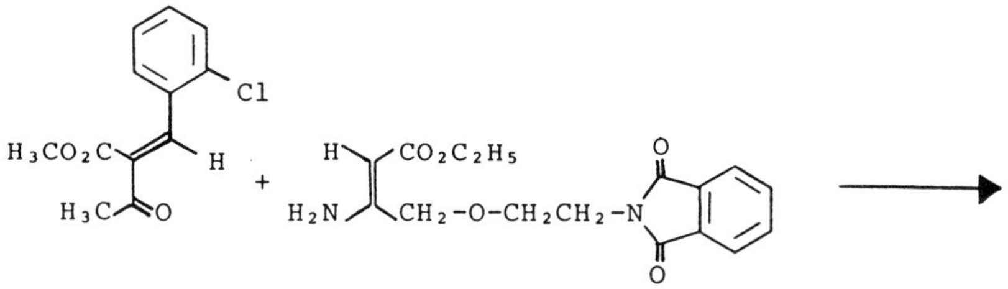

56 57

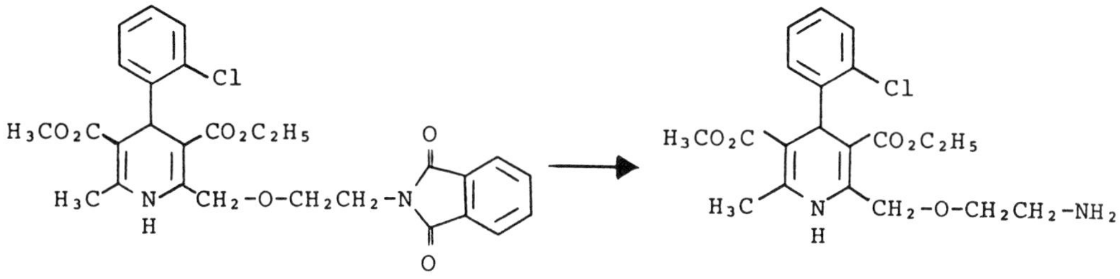

58 Amlodipine

Fig. 11. *Synthesis of amlodipine.*

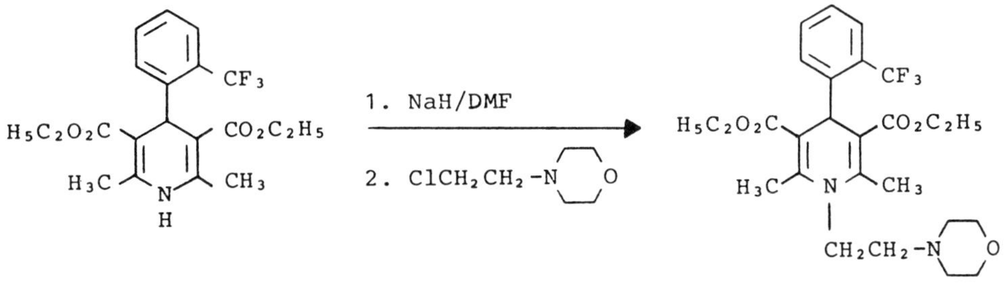

59 Flordipine

Fig. 12. *Synthesis of flordipine.*

TABLE III. Calcium-Agonistic 1,4- Dihydropyridines

$\underline{\underline{60}}$: BAY K 8644

$\underline{\underline{61}}$: 202-791

$\underline{\underline{62}}$: CGP 28 392

$\underline{\underline{63}}$: YC 170

$\underline{\underline{64}}$: H 160/51

addition in preparative chemistry (Fig. 13). 202-791 has been obtained in an analogous way.

The manufacture of CGP 28 392 [56,57] is unusual in that starting from 2-difluoromethoxybenzaldehyde (67), 3-aminocrotonic acid ethyl ester (68), and 4-chloroacetoacetic acid ethyl ester (69), intramolecular ring closure

after conversion into the dihydropyridine in situ yields the lactone with the splitting off of chloroethane (Fig. 14).

Enantiomeric 1,4-Dihydropyridines

The majority of the 1,4-dihydropyridine products at the development stage or on the market contain different ester groups in the

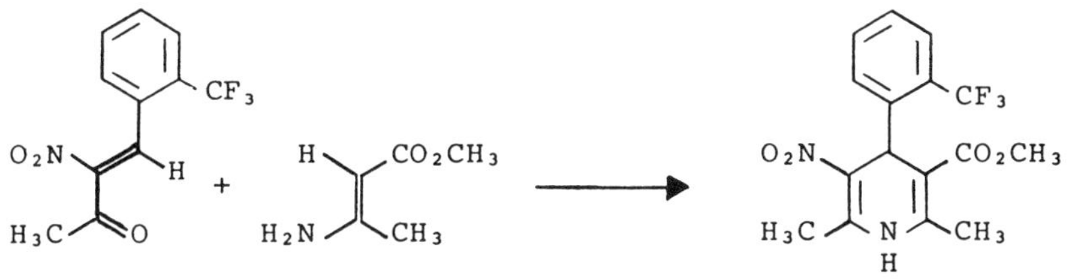

65 66 BAY K 8644

Fig. 13. *Synthesis of BAY K 8644.*

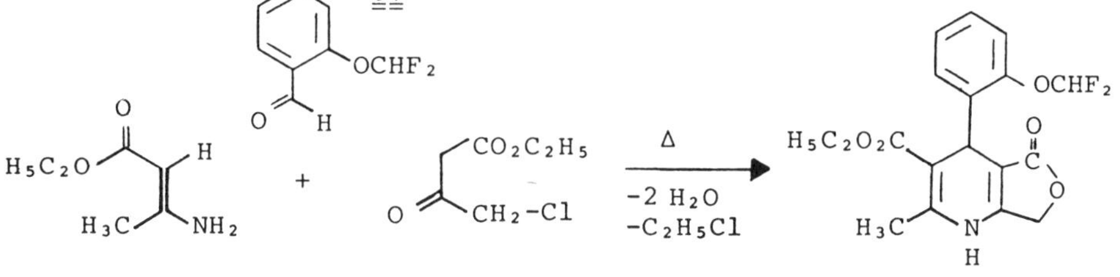

68 69 CGP 28 392

Fig. 14. *Synthesis of CGP 28 392.*

Mirror plane

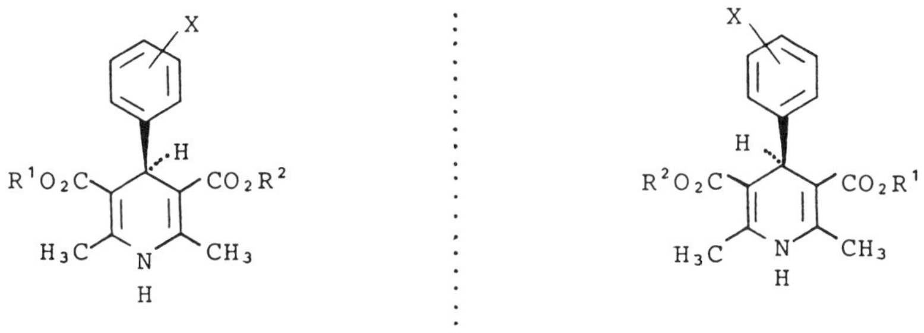

70 71

Fig. 15. *Enantiomers.*

3,5-positions of the dihydropyridine. This means that the compounds are chiral, i.e., they exist in two stereoisomeric forms (*70*) and (*71*) which relate to each other as if one were the mirror image of the other (optical antipodes, enantiomers) (Fig. 15). Several methods are known for preparing one or the other of the dihydropyridine enantiomers. The

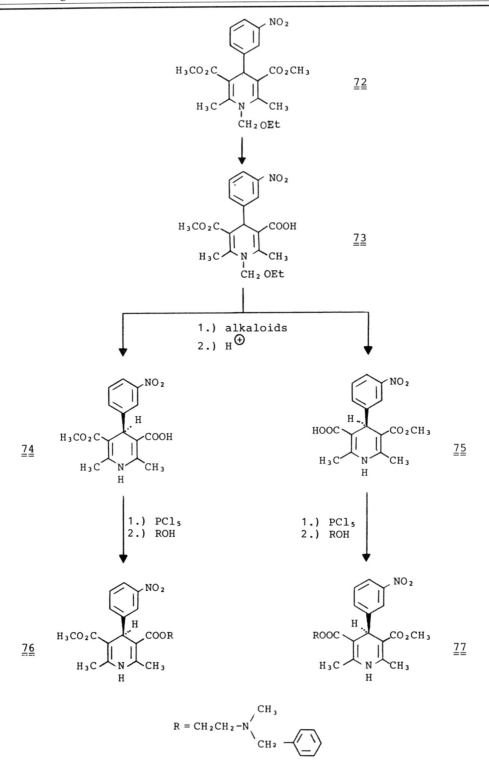

Fig. 16. *Synthesis of the enantiomers of nicardipine.*

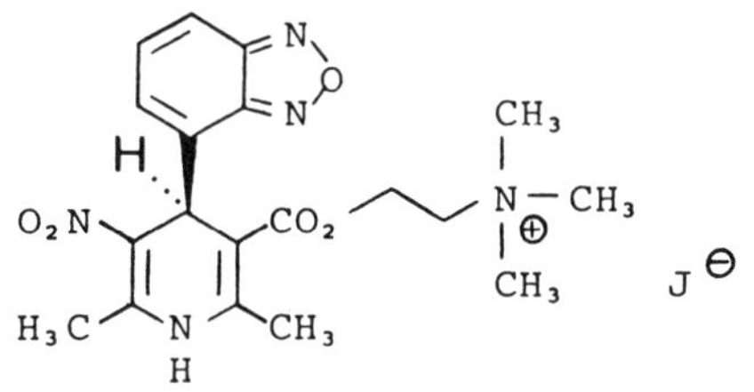

Fig. 17. *Intermediate in the optical resolution of racemic 202-791.*

classical route was followed by a Japanese group in the preparation of the nicardipine antipodes [58] (Fig. 16).

The central step is the resolution of the racemic, ¹N-protected 1,4-dihydropyridine-monocarboxylic acid (73) with optically active alkaloid bases like cinchonidine or cinchonine. Removal of the protective group yields the optically active acids (74) and (75) which can be re-esterified via the acid chloride to the enantiomers (76) and (77) of nicardipine.

The separation of the racemic 202–791 was also done by a classical route via the quaternization of a basic ester chain by means of optically active O,O′-di-p-toluoyl-(L)-tartaric acid [59], the absolute configuration being determined by x-ray structural analysis of the 1,4-dihydropyridine ester-ammonium iodine (78), which contains a heavy atom and in which the configuration is preserved [60] (Fig. 17).

An alternative route, which yields information about the absolute configuration about the C4 atom of the dihydropyridine and which was used, for example, in the preparation of the enantiomers of nitrendipine [61], nimodipine [61], and BAY K 8644 [62], was discovered in a diastereoselective 1,4-dihydropyridine synthesis (Fig. 18).

The asymmetric inductor used in each case was the relevant antipode (79,80) of the chiral 3-aminocrotonic acid 2-methoxy-2-phenylethyl ester, the antipodes being easily obtained

from the enantiomers of mandelic acid by standard reactions. The diastereoselective addition of these uniformly configurated enamino components to the prochiral benzal carbon atom of the aralkylidene acetoacetic acid ester (81) yields the two 1,4-dihydropyridine intermediates (82) and (83), which are related like mirror images and, thus, have the desired configuration about the C4 atom. Selective alkanolysis of the chiral ester group finally yields the enantiomerically pure target molecules (84) and (85), whose absolute configurations were determined by x-ray structural analysis of the intermediate dihydropyridine derivatives (82) and (83).

Labelled 1,4-Dihydropyridines

1,4-Dihydropyridine-3,5-diesters can be formally interpreted as vinylogous carbamic acid derivatives, which would explain the slowness of the reaction of the alkyl esters with solvolytic agents. From the point of view of preparative chemistry, the observation that 1,4-dihydropyridine 2-cyanoethyl esters (86) can undergo alkaline hydrolysis even under mild conditions [63] has proved particularly valuable (Fig. 19).

The dihydropyridinemono - or dicarboxylic acids (87) which can be produced easily by this route can in turn be converted into diesters (88) via variously activated intermediates, such as the acid chloride, the imidazolide, or the isourea. This reaction sequence has advantages over the classical procedure if

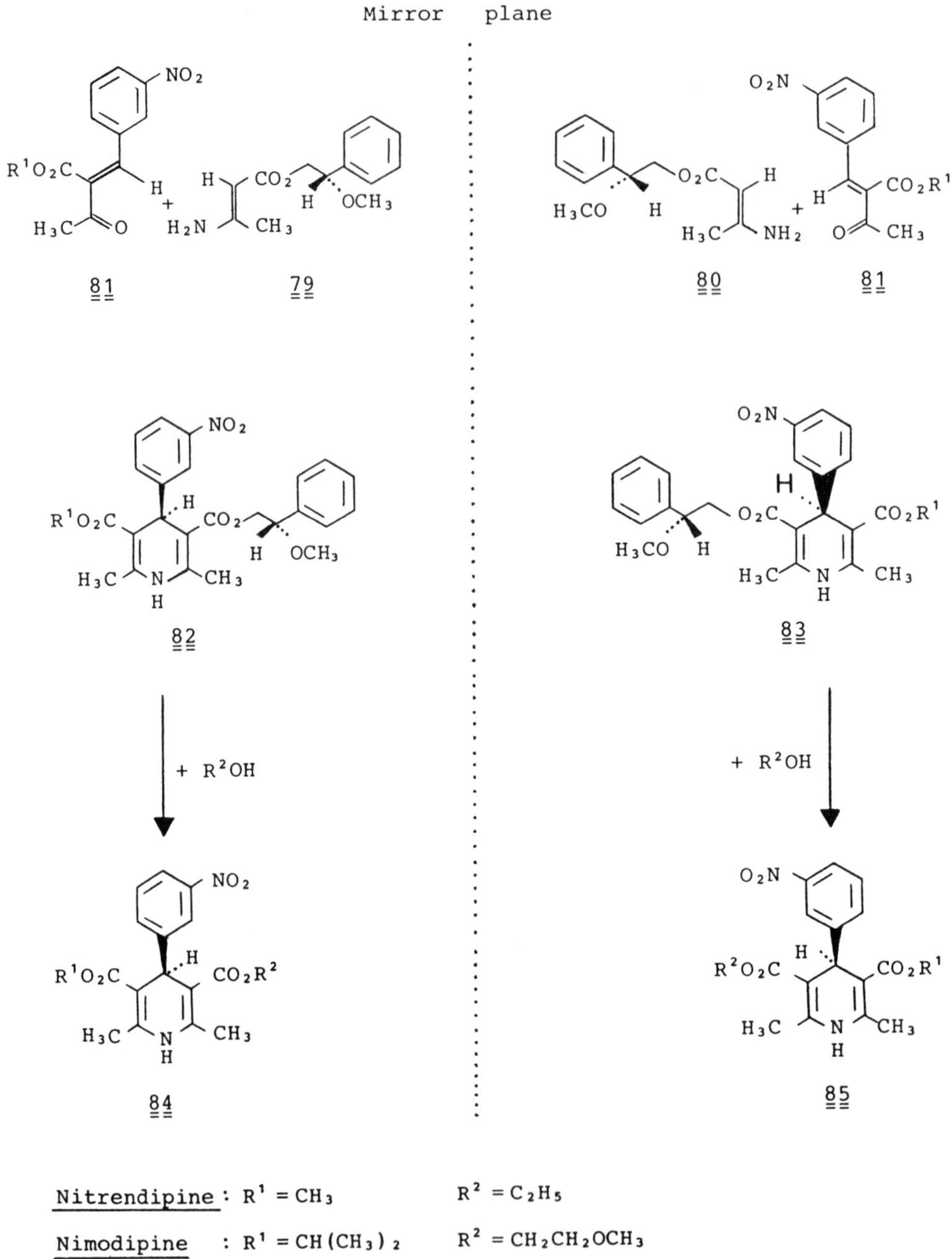

Mirror   plane

81   79   80   81

82   83

+ R²OH   + R²OH

84   85

Nitrendipine: R¹ = CH₃   R² = C₂H₅

Nimodipine : R¹ = CH(CH₃)₂   R² = CH₂CH₂OCH₃

Fig. 18. *Synthesis of the enantiomers of nitrendipine and nimodipine.*

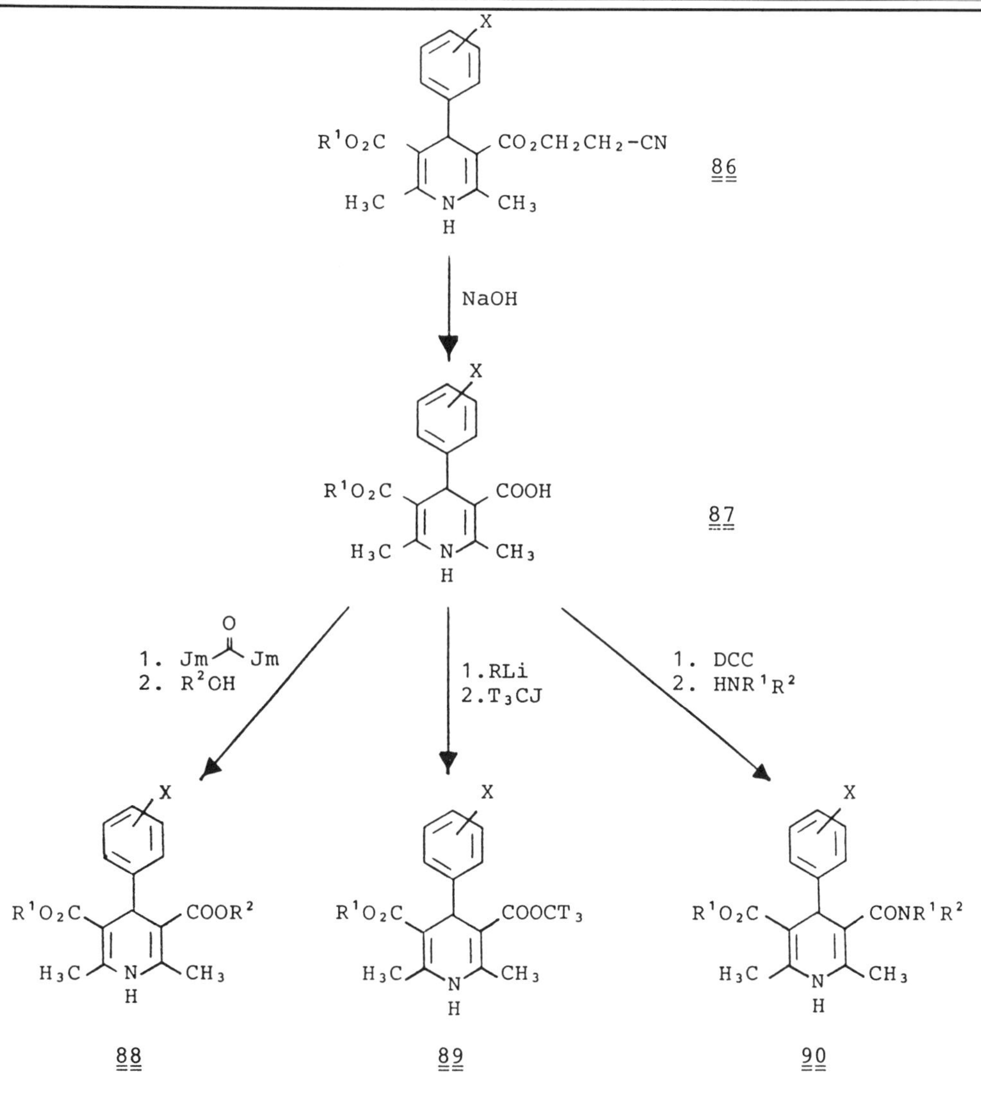

Fig. 19. *Reactions of 1,4-dihydropyridine-monocarboxylic acids.*

it is necessary to introduce an expensive alcohol component into the molecule, or one that is difficult to obtain.

An example of this route is the tritium labelling of nifedipine, nitrendipine, nimodipine, nisoldipine, isrodipine, and BAY K 8644 carried out within the framework of receptor-binding studies [64–67], by converting the lithium salts of the corresponding dihydropyridinemonocarboxylic acids into the labelled esters (*89*) with tritiated alkyl iodides [68].

The common starting material for the preparation of the ligands [^{3}H]azidopine (*45*) [69] and ^{125}I-iodipine (*44*) [70,71] is 1,4-dihydro-2,6-dimethyl-4-(2-trifluoromethylphenyl)-pyridine-3,5-dicarboxylic acid 2-aminoethyl ethyl ester (*91*), whose treatment with tritiated N-(4-azidobenzoyloxy)-succinimide (*92*) yields the [^{3}H]azidopine, and with N-(3-(4-hydroxy-3-^{125}iodophenyl) -propionyloxy)-succinimide (*93*) yields the ^{125}I-iodipine (Fig. 20).

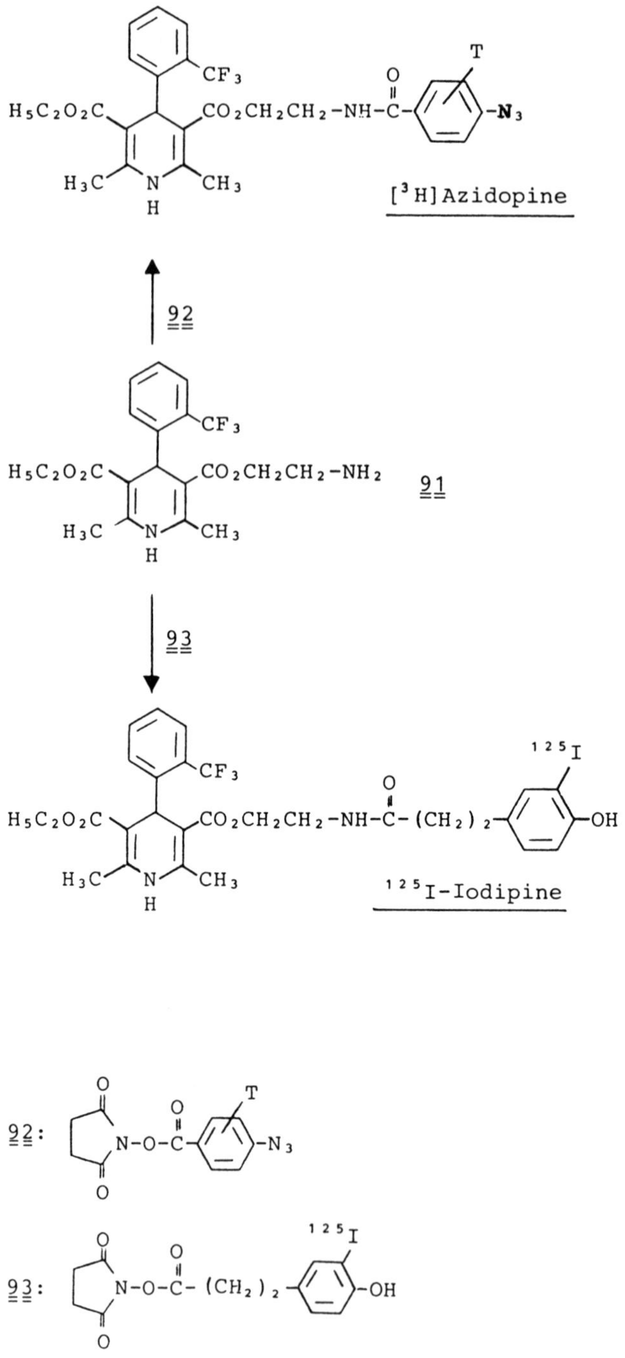

Fig. 20. *Synthesis of [³H]azidopine and ¹²⁵I-iodipine.*

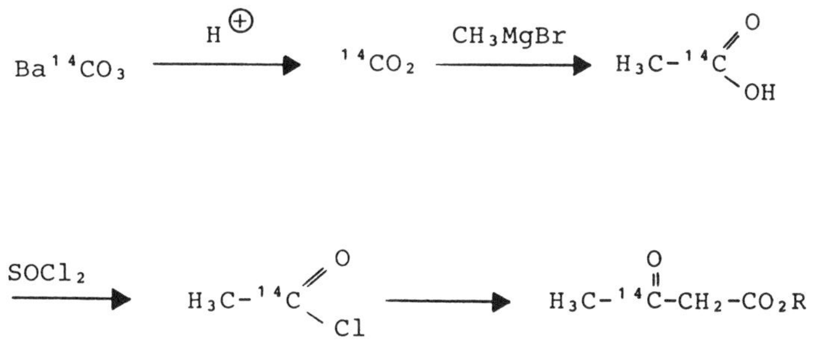

Fig. 21. *Synthesis of ^{14}C-labelled acetoacetates.*

For the purposes of biotransformation studies the ^{14}C-labelled 1,4-dihydropyridines nifedipine [72], nitrendipine [73], nimodipine [74], nicardipine [75,85], felodipine [76], and ryodipine [77,78] were prepared according to the classical scheme of dihydropyridine synthesis. Key compounds in the reaction sequence are the relevant 3-^{14}C-acetoacetic esters (*94*), which were obtained from barium ^{14}C-carbonate via the steps carbon dioxide, acetic acid, and acetyl chloride using standard reactions (Fig. 21).

Biotransformation of 1,4-Dihydropyridines

The biotransformation of the 1,4-dihydropyridines follows the general principle that the hydrophilicity of the metabolic products increases with increasing metabolization. Studies have been published on the metabolism of nifedipine [79–82], nicardipine [75,83–85], nitrendipine [73], nimodipine [74], felodipine [76], and ryodipine [77,78].

The metabolic degradation of nitrendipine can be used as a representative example (Fig. 22). Oxidation to the corresponding pyridine derivative (*95*) is taken as the initial step. Subsequent hydrolysis of the ester groups leads to the two possible pyridinemonocarboxylic acids (*96*) and (*97*), which are converted into the hydroxymethylpyridinemonocarboxylic acids (*98*) and (*99*) by oxidation of their adjacent methyl group. These were characterized as pyridine lactones (*100*) and (*101*) after the addition of acid.

DILTIAZEM

Diltiazem (*102*) was discovered in Japan in the late sixties and can be regarded—along with verapamil and the 1,4-dihydropyridines—as one of the prototypes of the calcium antagonists employed clinically [86]. Diltiazem is a weak base with a pKa of 7.70 [87]. Its structure contains two chiral centres in positions 2 and 3 of the benzothiazepinone ring, giving rise to four stereoisomeric compounds. Diltiazem (CRD 401) is the enantiomerically pure (+)-cis-isomer with the absolute configuration 2S,3S [88] (Fig. 23).

Synthesis of Diltiazem

The "classic" diltiazem synthesis [89–91] begins under achiral conditions with the stereoselective conversion of 2-nitrothiophenol (*103*) into the threo form of 2-hydroxy-3-(4-methoxyphenyl)-3-(2-nitrophenylthio)- propionic acid ethyl ester (*105*) with trans-(4-methoxyphenyl)-glycidic acid ethyl ester (*104*) [92,93] (Fig. 24). Reduction of the nitro group with iron(II)sulphate to an amino group and subsequent cyclization yield the racemic cis-3-hydroxy-2-(4-methoxyphenyl)-2,3-dihydro-1,5-benzothiazepine-4(5H)-one (*106*). Basic dimethylaminoethylation of the amide nitrogen after deprotonation in dimethyl sulphoxide, and the acetylation of the free hydroxy group with acetic anhydride, lead to the end product which is finally converted into the hydrochloride with hydrochloric acid. Chirality is introduced either by

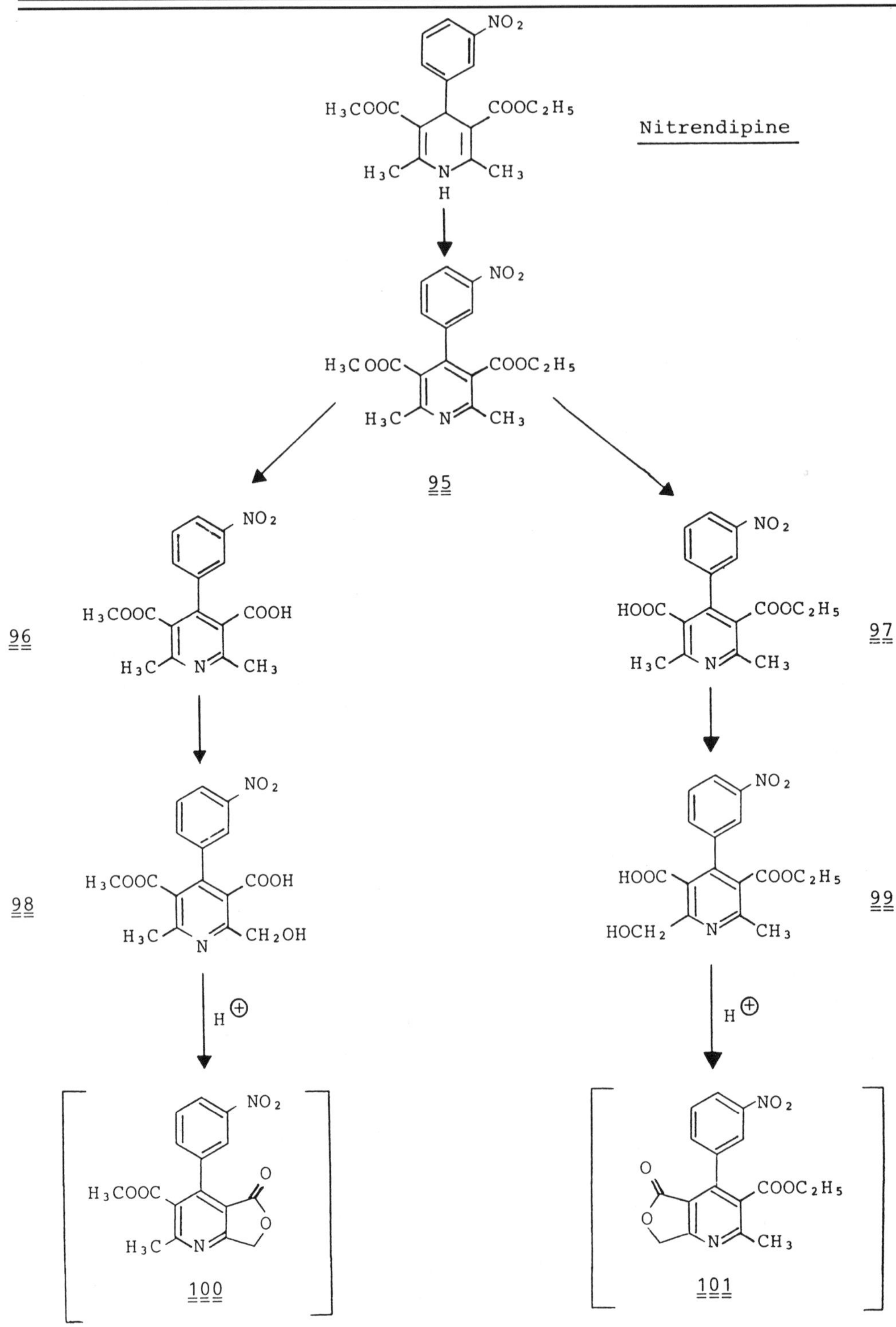

Fig. 22. *Biotransformation of nitrendipine.*

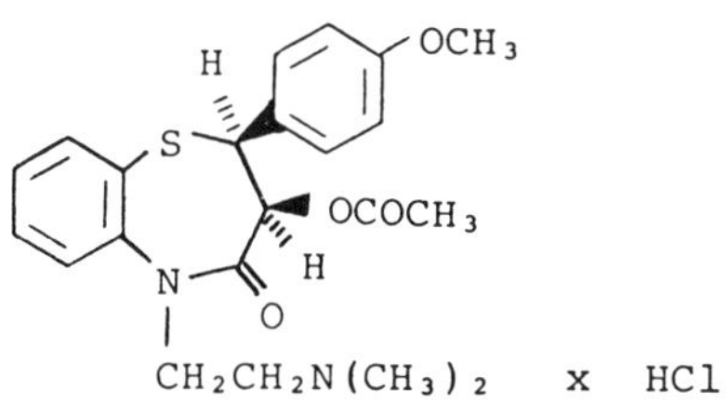

Fig. 23. *Diltiazem.*

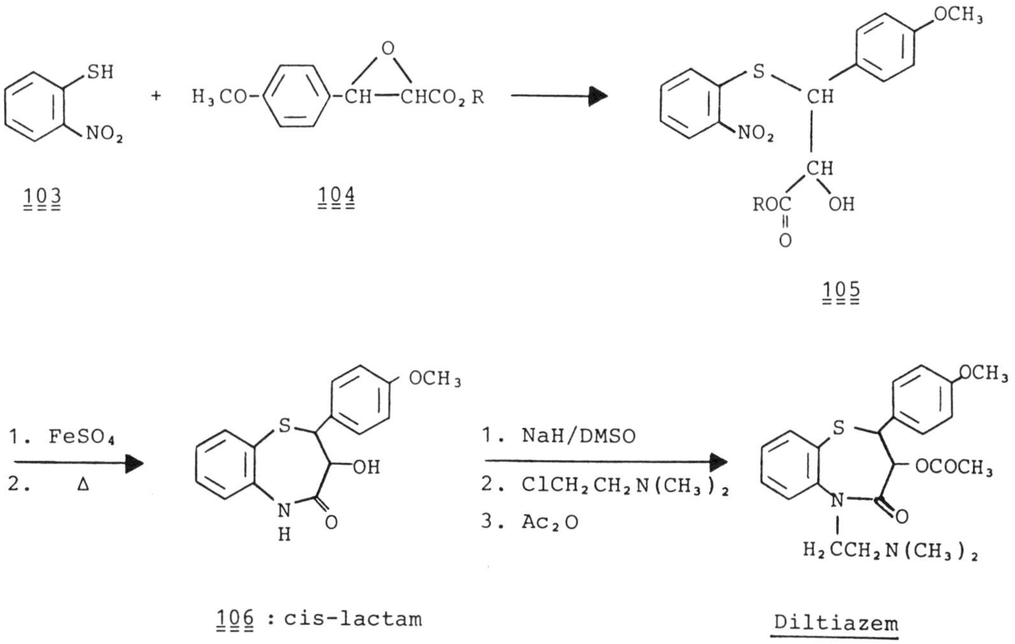

Fig. 24. *Reaction scheme for the synthesis of diltiazem without resolution.*

optical separation of the racemic intermediate product (*105*, R = H) with cinchonidine or lysine [94], or at the end of the synthesis sequence by resolution of the basic diltiazem with the aid of (−) camphorsulphonic acid [95].

An alternative method (Fig. 25) consists in the direct introduction of chirality at the start of the synthesis by the asymmetric epoxidation of the trans-cinnamyl alcohol (*107*) as per Sharpless [96], with the formation of the optically active (2S, 3S)-3-arylk-2,3-epoxypropanol (*108*) [97]. After oxidation of the

primary alcohol function to carboxylic acid and subsequent esterification to (*109*), the oxirane ring is opened by the addition of hydrochloric acid to yield the chlorohydrin (*110*), which is converted with a change in configuration with 2-nitro-thiophenol into the (2S,3S) -3-aryl-2-hydroxy-3- (2-nitrothiophenyl) -propionic acid ester (*111*). This optically active intermediate product (*111*) can be converted into the enantiomerically pure diltiazem by a route analogous to that described above by using an appropriate protective-group technique [97].

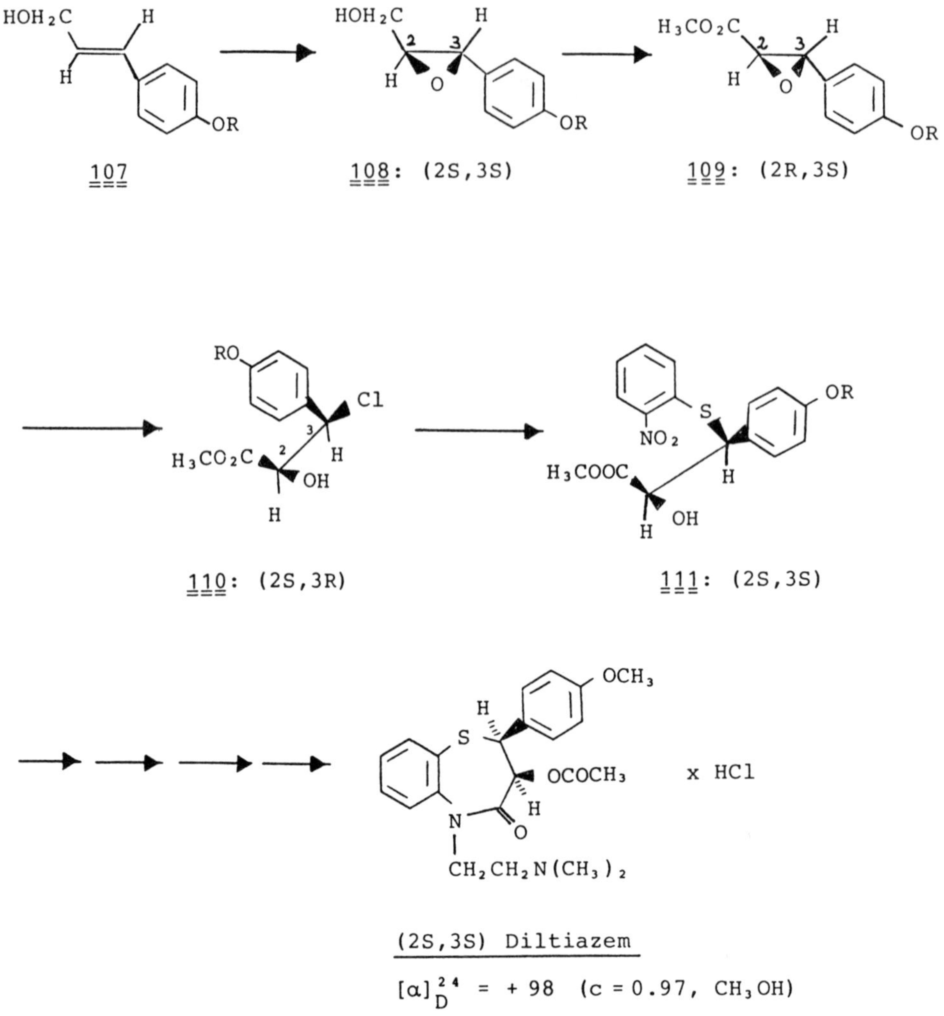

107   108: (2S,3S)   109: (2R,3S)

110: (2S,3R)   111: (2S,3S)

(2S,3S) Diltiazem

$[\alpha]_D^{24} = +98$ (c = 0.97, CH$_3$OH)

Fig. 25. *Asymmetric synthesis of diltiazem.*

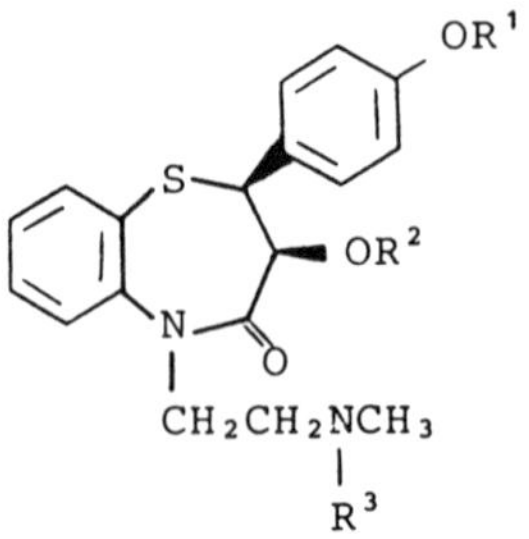

MA: R^1 = CH$_3$, R^2 = $\overset{\overset{\text{O}}{\|}}{\text{C}}CH_3$, R^3 = H

M$_1$: R^1 = CH$_3$, R^2 = H, R^3 = CH$_3$

M$_2$: R^1 = CH$_3$, R^2 = H, R^3 = H

Fig. 26. *Some metabolites of diltiazem.*

The derivatization of diltiazem necessary for the establishment of the structure-activity relationships was carried out mainly by making various substitutions in the aromatic ring, by changing the basic residue, or by varying the oxygen function in position 3 of the seven-membered ring [98].

Biotransformation of Diltiazem

Using ^{14}C-diltiazem with two ^{14}C-labels in the basic side chain, the absorption, excretion, and metabolism of the drug have been studied in various animal species [88,99,100] and in man [101]. The metabolic fate of diltiazem following oral administration consists of deacylation, N-demethylation, O-demethylation, hydroxylation, and oxidation. The metabolites are then converted into glucuronide and/or sulphate conjugates. In rats, only 0.1% of an oral dose of diltiazem was recovered unchanged from urine and bile. At least seven metabolites have been obtained and characterized by comparison with synthetic references (Fig. 26). In human urine, N-monodemethyl-diltiazem (MA) was identified as a new major biotransformation product in addition to deacetyl-diltiazem (M1), deacetyl-N-monodemethyl-diltiazem(M2),deacetyl-O-demethyl-diltiazem (M4), and deacetyl-N,O-demethyl-diltiazem (M6), which were already known as rat urinary metabolites.

REFERENCES

1. Fleckenstein A, (1983): Calcium Antagonism in Heart and Smooth Muscle. New York: John Wiley & Sons.
2. Stone PH, Antman EM (eds) (1983): Calcium Channel Blocking Agents in the Treatment of Cardiovascular Disorders. Mount Kisco, New York: Futura Publishing Company.
3. Opie LH (ed) (1984): Calcium antagonists and Cardiovascular disease. In Katz AM (ed): "Perspectives in Cardiovascular Research," Vol. 9. New York: Raven Press.
4. Baky S, (1984): Verapamil. In Scriabine A (ed): "New Drugs Annual: Cardiovascular Drugs," Vol 2. New York: Raven Press.
5. Sorkin EM, Clissold SP, Brogden RN (1985): Drugs 30:182.
6. Chaffman M, Brogden RN (1985): Drugs 29:387.
7. Kaltenbach M, Hopf R (eds) (1983): "Gallopamil, Pharmakologisches und klinisches Wirkprofil eines Kalziumantagonisten." Berlin: Springer Verlag.
8. Takenaka T, Miyazaki I, Higuchi S, Maeno H (1982): Jpn J Pharmacol 32:665.
9. Scriabine A, Vanov S, Deck K (eds) (1984): "Nitrendipine." Baltimore: Urban & Schwarzenberg.
10. Betz E, Deck K, Hoffmeister F (eds) (1985): "Nimodipine: Pharmacological and Clinical Properties." Stuttgart, New York: F.K. Schattauer Verlag.
11. Schramm M, Thomas G, Towart R, Franckowiak G (1983): Nature 303:535.
12. Thomas G, Gross R, Schramm M (1984): J Cardiovasc Pharmacol 6:1170.
13. Haas H, Busch E, (1967): Arzneim Forsch 17:257.
14. Fleckenstein A (1983): Circ Res 52 (Suppl I):3.
15. Ger. 1 154 810 (Knoll; Prior. 28.4.1961).
16. Eur. Pat. Appl. 64 158 (BASF; DE Prior. 10.4.1981).
17. Ger.Offen. 2 460 593 (Hoffman-La Roche; CH Prior. 21.12.1973).
18. Ramuz H (1978): Arzneim Forsch: Drug Res 28:2048.
19. Ger.Offen. 2 558 273 (Dr. Karl Thomae; DE Prior. 23.12.1975).
20. Ger.Offen. 2 639 718 (Dr. Karl Thomae, DE Prior. 3.9.1976).
21. Eur.Pat.Appl. 65 229 (Dr. Karl Thomae; DE Prior. 19.5.1981).
22. Ger.Offen.2 059 923 (Knoll; DE Prior. 5.12.1970).
23. Vogelgesang B, Echizen H, Schmidt E, Eichelbaum M (1984): Br J Clin Pharmacol 18: 733.
24. Ramuz H (1975): Helv Chim Acta 58: 2050.
25. Triggle DJ (1982): Biochemical pharmacology of calcium blockers. In Flaim SF, Zelis R (eds): "Calcium Blockers: Mechanisms of Action and Clinical Applications." Baltimore: Urban & Schwarzenberg, p 121.
26. McIlhenny HM (1971): J Med Chem 14: 1178.
27. Eichelbaum M, Ende M, Remberg G, Schomerus M, Dengler HJ (1979): Drug Met Disp 7: 145.
28. Remberg G, Ende M, Eichelbaum M, Schomerus M (1980): Arzneim Forsch / Drug Res 30: 398.
29. Hantzsch A (1882): Justus Liebigs Ann Chem 215: 1.
30. Eisner U, Kuthan J (1972): Chem Rev 72: 1.
31. Kuthan J, Kurfürst A (1982): Ind Eng Chem Prod Res Dev 21: 191.
32. Stout DM, Meyers AI (1982): Chem Rev 82: 223.
33. Stryer L (1983): Biochemie, 2nd ed. Braunschweig, Wiesbaden: Friedr. Vieweg & Sohn, p 191.
34. Bossert F, Vater W (1971): Naturwissenschaften 58: 578.
35. Vater W, Kroneberg G, Hoffmeister F, Kaller H, Meng K, Oberdorf A, Puls W, Schlossmann, Stoepel K (1972): Arzneim Forsch: Drug Res 22: 1.
36. Loev B, Goodman MM, Snader KM, Tedeschi R, Macko E (1914): J Med Chem 17: 956.

37. Fleckenstein A, Van Breemen C, Gross R, Hoff-meister F (eds) (1985): "Cardiovascular Effects of Dihydropyridine-Type Calcium Antagonists and Agonists." Berlin: Springer-Verlag.

38. Bosssert F, Meyer H, Wehinger E (1981): Ang Chem Intern Ed 20: 762.

39. Ger. Offen. 1 670 827 (Bayer; DE Prior. 20.3.1967).

40. Eur.Pat.Appl. 0150 (Sandoz; CH Prior. 20.6.1977).

41. Ger. Offen. 2 900 537 (Institute of Organic Synthesis, Latvian SSR Academy of Sciences; SU Prior. 11.1.1978).

42. Ger. Offen. 2 407 115 (Yamanouchi; JP Prior. 20.2.1973).

43. Ger. Offen. 2 117 571 (Bayer; DE Prior. 10.4.1971).

44. Meyer H, Bossert F, Wehinger E, Stoepel K, Vater W (1981): Arzneim Forsch/Drug Res 31: 407.

45. Meyer H, Wehinger E, Bossert F, Scherling D, (1983): Arzneim Forsch/Drug Res 33: 106.

46. Ger. Offen. 2 549 568 (Bayer; DE Prior. 5.11.1975).

47. Eur. Pat. Appl. 7 293 (Hässle; SE Prior. 30.6.1978).

48. Ger. Offen. 2 949 491 (Sandoz; CH Prior. 18.12.1978).

49. Eur. Pat. Appl. 97 821 (Pierrel; IT Prior. 3.6.1982).

50. U.S. 4 284 634 (Fujisawa; GB Prior. 2.7.1975).

51. Eur. Pat. Appl. 89 167 (Pfizer; GB Prior. 11.3.1982).

52. Ger. Offen. 3 109 794 (USV Pharmaceutical; US Prior. 11.4.1980).

53. Gjörstrupp P (1985): Cardiovascular Pharmacotherapy, International Symposium, Genf, 22.-25.4.1985, Abstr. 127.

54. Takenaka T, Maeno H (1982): Jpn J Pharmacol 32: P139.

55. Franckowiak G, Schramm M, Thomas G, Towart R (1984): 188th ACS National Meeting, Philadelphia, 26.-31.8.1984, Abstr. MEDI 8.

56. Eur. Pat. Appl. 111 453 (Ciba-Geigy; CH Prior. 10.12.1982).

57. Eur. Pat. Appl. 111 455 (Ciba-Geigy; CH Prior. 10.12.1982).

58. Shibanuma T, Iwanami M, Okuda K, Takenaka T, Murakami M: (1980):Chem Pharm Bull 28: 2809.

59. Ger Offen. 3 320 616 (Sandoz; CH Prior. 15 .1982).

60. Hof RP, Rüegg UT, Hof A, Vogel A (1985): J Cardiovasc Pharmacol 7: 689.

61. Ger. Offen. 2 935 451 (Bayer; DE Prior. 1.9.1979).

62. Franckowiak G, Bechem M, Schramm M, Thomas G (1985): Eur J Pharmacol 114: 223.

63. Ger. Offen. 2 847 237 (Bayer; DE Prior. 31.10.1978).

64. Bellemann P, Ferry D, Lübbecke F, Glossman H (1981): Arzneim Forsch/Drug Res 31: 2064.

65. Bolger GT, Gengo P, Klockowski R, Luchowski E, Siegel H, Janis RA, Triggle AM, Triggle DJ (1983): J Pharmacol Exp Ther 225: 291.

66. Bellemann P, Schade A, Towart R (1983): Proc Natl Acad Sci USA 80: 2356.

67. Ferry DR, Goll A, Glossman H (1983): Naunyn-Schmiedeberg's Arch Pharmacol 323: 276.

68. Ger. Offen. 2 921 429 (Bayer; DE Prior 26.05.1979).

69. Ferry DR, Rombusch M, Goll A, Glossman H (1984): FEBS Lett 169: 112.

70. Ger. Offen. 3 341 806 (H. Glossman; DE Prior. 19.11.1983).

71. Ferry DR, Glossmann H (1984): Naunyn-Schmiedeberg's Arch Pharmacol 325: 186.

72. Duhm B, Maul W, Medenwald H, Patzschke K, Wegner LA (1972): Arzneim Forsch/Drug Res 22: 42.

73. Meyer H, Scherling D, Karl W (1983): Arzneim-Forsch/Drug Res 33: 1528.

74. Meyer H, Wehinger E, Bossert F, Scherling D (1983): Arzneim Forsch/Drug Res 33: 106.

75. Higuchi S, Sasaki H, Shiobara Y, Sado T (1977): Xenobiotica 7: 469.

76. Weidolf L, Borg KO, Hoffman KJ (1984): Xenobiotica 14: 657.

77. Parinov VJ, Odinec AG, Gilev AP, Dubur GJ, Muceniece DH, Ozol JJ, Shatz VD, Gavars MP, Vigante BA (1985): Arzneim Forsch/Drug Res 35: 808.

78. Inoue Y, Nakayama K, Wachi M, Kumakura K, Matsumoto T, Iwamoto M, Motoyoshi Y, Aikawa K (1985): Arzneim Forsch Drug Res 35: 813.

79. Medenwald H, Schlossmann K, Wünsche C (1972): Arzneim Forsch/Drug Res 22: 53.

80. Kondo S, Kuchiki A, Yamamoto K, Akimoto K, Takahashi K, Awata N, Sugimoto I (1980): Chem Pharm Bull 28: 1.

81. Raemsch KD, Sommer J (1983): Hypertension 5 (Suppl. II) II-18.

82. Kleinbloesem CH, van Harten J, van Brummelen P, Breimer DD, J Chromatog 308: 209.

83. Shibanuma T, Iwanami M, Fujimoto M, Takenaka T, Murakami M (1980): Chem Pharm Bull 28: 2609.

84. Higuchi S, Shiobara Y (1980): Xenobiotica 10: 889.

85. Rush WR, Alexander O, Hall DJ, Cairncross L, Dow RJ, Graham DJG (1986): Xenobiotica 16: 341.

86. Ger. Offen. 1 805 714 (Tanabe Seiyaku; JP Prior. 28.10.1967).

87. Flaim SF (1984): Diltiazem. In Scriabine A (ed) "New Drugs Annual: Cardiovascular Drugs," Vol 2. New York: Raven Press, p 123.

88. Miyazaki M, Iwakuma T, Tanaka T (1978): Chem Pharm Bull 26: 2889.
89. Kugita H, Inoue H, Ikezaki M, Takeo S (1970): Chem Pharm Bull 18: 2028.
90. Kugita H, Inoue H, Ikezaki M, Konda M, Takeo S (1970): Chem Pharm Bull 18: 2284.
91. Kugita H, Inoue H, Ikezaki M, Konda M, Takeo S (1971): Chem Pharm Bull 19: 595.
92. Eur.Pat.Appl. 59 335 (Tanabe Seiyaku; JP Prior. 27.2.1981).
93. Hashiyama T, Inoue H, Konda M, Takeda M (1984): J Chem Soc, Perkin Trans I, 1725.
94. Ger. Offen. 3 337 176 (Istituto Luso Farmaco d'Italia; IT Prior. 15.10.1982).
95. JP 5 920 273 (Tanebe Seiyaku; Prior. 27.7.1982).
96. Katsuki T, Sharpless KB (1980) J Am Chem Soc 102: 5974.
97. Ger. Offen. 3 415 035 (Shionogi; JP Prior. 21.4.1983).
98. Nagao T, Sato M, Nakajima H, Kiyomoto A (1973): Chem Pharm Bull 21: 92.
99. Sakuma M, Yoshikawa M, Sato Y (1971): Chem Pharm Bull 19: 995.
100. Meshi T, Sugihara J, Sato Y (1971): Chem Pharm Bull 19: 1546.
101. Sugihara J, Sugawara Y, Ando H, Harigaya S, Etoh A, Kohno K (1984): J. Pharmacobiodyn 7: 24.

Structure and Physiology of the Slow Inward Calcium Channel, pages 29–50
© 1987 Alan R. Liss, Inc.

2

Calcium Channel Ligands: Structure-Function Relationships

D.J. Triggle and R.A. Janis

*School of Pharmacy, State University of New York, Buffalo,
New York 14260 (D.J.T.) and Miles Institute for Preclinical
Pharmacology, New Haven, Connecticut 06509 (R.A.J.)*

INTRODUCTION

The fundamental role of Ca^{2+} as an intracellular messenger, coupling membrane excitation to a variety of cellular events, is embraced by the term "stimulus-response coupling," includes cellular contractile and secretory events, and demands that calcium movements and storage within the cell be subject to a number of regulating processes. A schematic representation of such regulation is depicted in Figure 1. An understanding of the locations and mechanisms of these several processes together with appropriate test systems will, in principle, generate discrete classes of drugs with which to modulate each of these processes. Although this desirable state has not yet been achieved, analysis of cellular Ca^{+2} function is moving with sufficient rapidity that it will probably be attained within the next few years. At the present time, one well-defined group of drugs, the Ca^{2+} channel antagonists, has achieved both pharmacologic and clinical significance.

This defined group of drugs includes diverse structures, notably the 1,4-dihydropyridine nifedipine, the phenylalkylamines verapamil and D 600, and the benzothiazepine diltiazem (Fig. 2) [for reviews, see Fleckenstein, 1977, 1983; Weiss, 1978, 1981; Janis and Triggle, 1983; Schwartz and Taira, 1983; Opie, 1984; Flaim and Zelis, 1982; Rahwan and Witiak, 1982; Godfraind et al., 1985; Fleckenstein et al., 1986]. These agents have been defined by biochemical, electrophysiologic, and pharmacologic techniques to serve as antagonists at voltage-dependent Ca^{2+} channels. Their chemical heterogeneity suggests that they likely accomplish any common action by interacting at different sites by different mechanisms. This is supported very strongly by the pharmacologic and therapeutic nonequivalence of these agents. Nifedipine and other 1,4-dihydropyridines have preferential effects on smooth muscle, both vascular and nonvascular, while verapamil and diltiazem also affect cardiac Ca^{2+} currents in nodal regions.

Our definition of this class of drugs is now expanded because of the recent discovery that the 1,4-dihydropyridine structure embraces both antagonist and activator structures (Fig. 3) [Takenaka and Maeno, 1982; Schramm et al., 1983; Preuss et al., 1985; Fleckenstein et al., 1986]. Although at present the Ca^{2+} channel activators have no therapeutic roles, they are proving to be immensely valuable tools with which to probe Ca^{2+} channel structure and function.

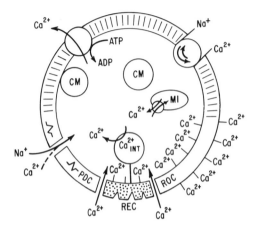

Fig. 1. *Schematic representation of cellular Ca^{2+} regulation. Ca^{2+} influx is depicted as occurring through the Na^+ channel (minor component), through potential-dependent and receptor-operated Ca^{2+} channels (PDC, ROC), and through a $Na^+:Ca^{2+}$ exchange process. Ca^{2+} efflux is depicted as occurring through a Ca^{2+} ATPase and through $Na^+:Ca^{2+}$ exchange. Intracellular sequestration and release is depicted in endoplasmic reticulum (Ca_{INT}^{2+}) and mitochondria (MI). Ca^{2+} binding proteins are depicted as calmodulin (CM).*

Although the greatest pharmacologic and clinical attention has been paid to the compounds of Figure 2, there is a very large number of other agents of generally related structure which are in clinical use or in some stage of development (Table I). Additionally, very diverse structures have been reported to act as Ca^{2+} channel antagonists in one or another preparation (Fig. 4). Often this activity is secondary to other and better-defined pharmacological activities, and in many instances Ca^{2+} channel activity has been demonstrated only indirectly.

It is now recognized that, in parallel to the several discrete structural classes of Ca^{2+} channel ligands, there exist discrete classes of voltage-dependent Ca^{2+} channels with significantly different kinetic and pharmacologic properties [Miller, 1985; Nilius et al., 1985; Nowycky et al., 1985; Cognard et al., 1986a]. These recent discoveries accommodate, at least in part, the many observations that the existing major structural categories of Ca^{2+} channel ligands are not equally effective in all tissues and, in particular, are comparatively ineffective in neuronal preparations [Rosenberger and Triggle, 1978; Triggle, 1984; Miller and Freedman, 1984; Miller, 1985].

These preliminary considerations indicate that the analysis of structure-function rela-

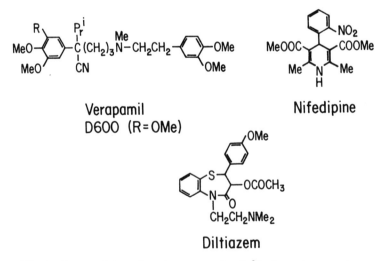

Fig. 2. *Structural formulae of representative Ca^{2+} channel antagonists.*

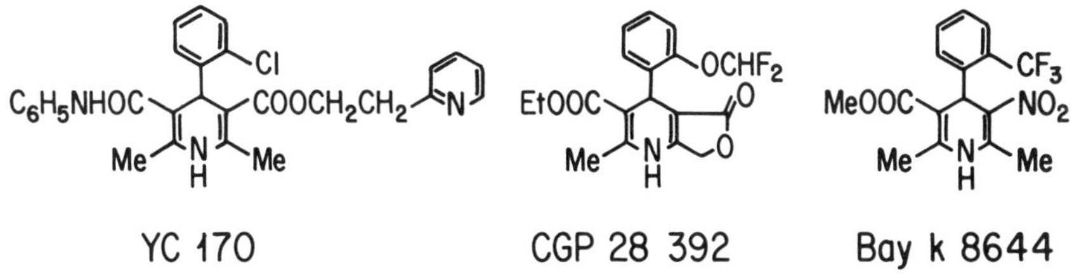

Fig. 3. *Structural formulae of 1,4-dihydropyridine* Ca^{2+} *channel activators.*

TABLE I. Summary of Available and Potentially Available Ca^{2+} Channel Antagonists

A) Phenylalkylamines
   Verapamil
   Gallopamil
   Tiapamil

B) Benzothiazepines
   Diltiazem

C) 1,4-Dihydropyridines

Nifedipine	Felodipine
Nitrendipine	Nicardipine
Nisoldipine	FR 34235
Nimodipine	PY 108-068
Niludipine	PN 200-110

D) Piperazines
   Cinnarizine
   Flurarizine
   Lidoflazine

tionships of Ca^{2+} channel ligands is a topic of some importance. The determination of structural requirements for antagonism and the delineation of the molecular features that discriminate activators and antagonists will be of the utmost significance to the optimization of current structures and to the activation of new structural leads. Structure-function relationships constitute a vital underpinning to biochemical efforts to isolate and reconstitute the Ca^{2+} channel. Structures currently available and those to be developed will play a vital role in the classification of channel types and will undoubtedly lead to the development of new clinical states for which Ca^{2+} channel ligands may be indicated. Finally, the existence of both activator and antagonist structures raises the question of endogenous control mechanisms and of possible endoge-

nous ligands that serve to regulate channel activity. The continued elucidation of structure-function relationships will be vital to all of these developments.

STRUCTURE-ACTIVITY RELATIONSHIPS: PHARMACOLOGIC STUDIES

Of the major structural classes of Ca^{2+} channel ligands, the most comprehensive structure-activity relationship studies to date are available for the 1,4-dihydropyridines. This is due unquestionably to the relative ease of synthesis of this structural category. Indeed, conservative estimates suggest that several thousand 1,4-dihydropyridines have been synthesized; however, only a very few have been subject to appropriately detailed and quantitative pharmacologic evaluation.

An early study measuring the *in vivo* hypotensive activities of a series of 1,4-dihydropyridines [Loev et al., 1974] defined the basic structural requirements for activity (Fig. 5; Table II):

1) Substitution in the 4-position of the 1,4-dihydropyridine ring increases the activity in the sequence, H < Me < alkyl < cycloalkyl < heterocyclic < phenyl < substituted phenyl.

2) Substitution into the 4-phenyl ring enhances activity in the sequence, ortho > meta >> para. Electron-withdrawing substituents enhance activity more than electron-releasing substituents.

3) The 1,4-dihydropyridine ring is essential: oxidized pyridines are dramatically less active and the presence of N_1-H is critical.

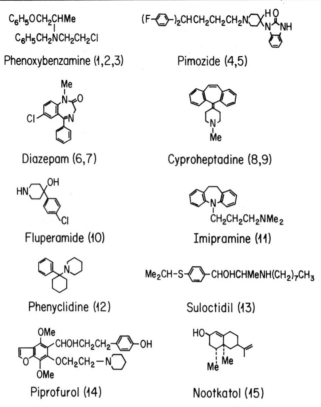

C6H5OCH2CHMe
|
C6H5CH2NCH2CH2Cl

Phenoxybenzamine (1,2,3)

Pimozide (4,5)

Diazepam (6,7)

Cyproheptadine (8,9)

Fluperamide (10)

Imipramine (11)

Phenyclidine (12)

Suloctidil (13)

Piprofurol (14)

Nootkatol (15)

Fig. 4. *Structural formulae of a miscellaneous series of Ca^{2+} channel antagonists (see text for further discussion). 1) Bevan et al., 1963; 2) Swamy and Triggle, 1972, 1973; 3) Gengo et al., 1984; 4) Gould et al., 1983; 5) Luchowski et al., 1984; 6) Cantor et al., 1984; 7) Mestre et al., 1985; 8) Lowe et al., 1981; 9) Bolger et al., 1983; 10) Reynolds et al., 1984; 11) Isenberg and Tamargo, 1985; 12) El-Fakahany et al., 1984; 13) Chatelain et al., 1984; 14) Pourrias et al., 1985; 15) Shoji et al., 1984.*

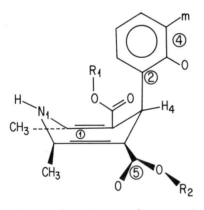

Fig. 5. *Structural requirements for antagonist action in 1,4-dihydropyridines (see text for further detail). Symbols ①, ②, ④, and ⑤ represent critical features:① 1,4-dehydropyridine ring;② 4-phenyl substituent;④ o-. and m- substituents in phenyl ring;⑤ ester groups in 3- and 5- positions.*

4) Ester groups at C-3 and C-5 of the 1,4-dihydropyridine ring confer optimum activity. The absence of a substituent or the presence of electron-withdrawing substituents, including -COMe, -CN, and lactone (2,3), reduces antagonist activity.

Although the study by Loev et al. [1974] was executed in an in vivo system with the customary attendant difficulties, the general conclusions drawn are paralleled by in vitro studies. The more comprehensive of such in vitro studies have focused on the ester substitution pattern at C-3 and C-5 and the substituents in the 4-phenyl ring.

The activities of a series of 2,6-dimethyl-3,5-dicarbomethoxy-4-substituted phenyl-1,4-

TABLE II. Hypotensive Action of Substituted 1,4-Dihydropyridines on Cat Blood Pressure*

Structure: 1,4-dihydropyridine with EtOOC and COOEt at positions 3 and 5, Me groups at positions 2 and 6, R_4 at position 4, N–H ring.

R_4	Dose (mg kg^{-1})	Hypotensive Activity[a] Degree[b]	Duration[c]
H	2.0	+	+
Me	0.5	+	+
Cyclohexyl	1.5	+ + +	+ +
2-Pyridyl	0.5	+ + +	+ + +
2-Thienyl	0.1	+	+
2-Furyl	0.5	+ +	+ + +
C_6H_5	0.1	+ + +	+ + +
$2\text{-}ClC_6H_4$	0.015	+ +	+ +
$2\text{-}O_2NC_6H_4$	0.01	+ + +	+ +
$2\text{-}F_3CC_6H_4$	0.05	+ + +	+ + +
$3\text{-}F_3CC_6H_4$	0.05	+ + +	+ +
$4\text{-}F_3CC_6H_4$	6.5	+ + +	+ +
$2,6\text{-}Cl_2C_6H_3$	0.05	+ + +	+ + +
C_6H_5[d]	0.5	+	+
$2\text{-}F_3CC_6H_4$[d]	1.5	+	+
C_6H_5[e]	6.0	+ + +	+
C_6H_5[f]	19.3	+	+ + +
C_6H_5[g]	0.5	+	+
$2\text{-}F_3CC_6H_4$[g]	0.5	+	+

*Data from Loev et al., 1974.
[a]Cardiovascular activity was measured in anesthetized cats following i.v. administration.
[b]+ + +, indicates b.p. fall > 50 mm; + +, indicates fall 40–50 mm; +, indicates fall 30–39 mm.
[c]+ + +, indicates duration > 5 min; + +, 3–5 min; +, < 3 min.
[d]R_1 = Me.
[e]R_2, R_6 = H.
[f]R_3, R_5 = CN.
[g]R_3, R_5 = COMe.

dihydropyridines in cardiac tissue have been analyzed [Rosenberger and Triggle, 1978; Rodenkirchen et al., 1979; Mannhold et al., 1982]. For a series of ortho-substituted derivates, activity was described by (Table III):

$$\log 1/ED_{50} = 5.06 + 0.8\,B_1, \qquad (1)$$

where B_1 is the substituent minimum width parameter [Verloop et al., 1976]. The effects of ester group variation were described [Table III] by a dependence on Rm (or π):

$$\log 1/EC_{50} = 6.67 - 0.66\,Rm, \qquad (2)$$

indicating that activity decreases with increasing lipophilicity. The latter conclusions contrast with those drawn by Loev et al. (1974) for in vivo hypotensive effects and by other workers [Towart et al., 1981; Bolger et al., 1983; Triggle, 1982] with in vitro vascular and nonvascular smooth muscle preparations, showing that activity is maintained or increased with increasing ester size. Conceivably, this reflects the assumption that the size and character of these ester substituents contribute to the tissue selectivity of 1,4-dihydropyridines. It should be noted, however, that the data set analyzed for Equations 1 and 2 covers a very restricted activity range.

TABLE III. Inhibitory Activities of 1,4-Dihydropyridines in Cat Papillary Muscle*

R; R^1	R''	EC_{50}, M
Me	H	1.2×10^{-6}
Me	2-NO$_2$	3.7×10^{-7}
Me	2-CN	4.3×10^{-7}
Me	2-OMe	1.1×10^{-6}
Me	2-SMe	3.5×10^{-7}
Me	2-Cl	4.5×10^{-7}
Me	2-CF$_3$	1.9×10^{-7}
Me	2-Me	3.8×10^{-7}
Me	3-Cl	1.2×10^{-6}
Me	3-OMe	1.6×10^{-6}
Me	3-NO$_2$	5.8×10^{-7}
Me	3-N$_3$	1.4×10^{-6}
Me	4-OMe	4.6×10^{-5}
Me	4-Me	2.5×10^{-5}
Me	4-Cl	3.7×10^{-5}
CH$_2$CH$_2$OC$_3$H$_7$	3-NO$_2$	2.0×10^{-6}
C$_2$H$_5$[b]	3-NO$_2$	1.4×10^{-6}
Me[c]	3-NO$_2$	7.5×10^{-7}
CHMe$_2$[d]	3-NO$_2$	1.3×10^{-6}

*Data from Rodenkirchen et al., 1979.
[b]R^1 = CHMe$_2$.
[c]R^1 = C$_2$H$_5$.
[d]R^1 = CH$_2$CH$_2$OMe.

The influence of the ester and phenyl substitution patterns are likely expressed independently. In a series of phenyl substituted 1,4-dihydropyridines carrying a 3-carbomethoxy substituent and carboethoxy, carbomethoxy, isobutyloxy, or 2-N-benzyl-N-methylamino carboethoxy substituents at C-5, the same rank order of activity is conferred by phenyl substituent independent of the nature of the ester group (Fig. 6). With nonidentical substituents at C-3 and C-5 of the 1,4-dihydropyridine ring, C-4 becomes chiral and stereoselectivity of pharmacologic activity is observed (Table IV).

The role of the substituent in 1,4-dihydropyridines bearing an ortho-substituted phenyl ring likely reflects both the ability of the substituent to bind to a complementary site on the 1,4-dihydropyridine receptor and to promote a noncoplanar arrangement of the phenyl and 1,4-dihydropyridine rings (Fig. 7). The adoption of this arrangement is shown in the solid state structures of a number of 1,4-dihydropyridines [Triggle et al., 1980; Fossheim et al., 1982; Langs and Triggle, 1985]. Its importance is shown in a series of rigid analogs bridged between the phenyl and 1,4-dihydropyridine rings (Fig. 8) [Seidel et al., 1984] where activity increases with increasing inter-ring angle. The phenyl substituent also influences the planarity of the 1,4-dihydropyridine ring, and a correlation exists between ring planarity and pharmacological activity (Fig. 9) [Fossheim et al., 1982]. However, these conformational features cannot be the sole determinants of activity; similar conformations are adopted by active and inactive compounds [Fossheim et al., 1982]. Furthermore, almost identical conformations are adopted by both activator and antagonist ligands, and some 1,4-dihydropyridines display opposing enantiomeric selectivity of action, whereby one enantiomer is an antagonist and the other is an activator (Fig. 10) [Hof et al., 1985; Franckowiak et al., 1985]. There is, currently, insufficient information to permit a quantitative comparison of the structural requirements for the expression of activator and antagonist properties in the 1,4-dihydropyridines.

The 1,4-dihydropyridine antagonists are recognized pharmacologically and therapeutically to be selective for smooth muscle, vascular and nonvascular, over cardiac muscle. A limited number of studies have attempted to compare structural requirements for activity in cardiac and smooth muscle and in different smooth muscle systems [Triggle, 1981; Triggle and Janis, 1984a,b; Langs and Triggle, 1984; Yousif and Triggle, 1986]. In a comparison of activities in papillary muscle and guinea pig intestine, the same rank order of activity is observed (Fig. 11) indicating that an identical (or very similar) structure-activity relationship is observed despite quantita-

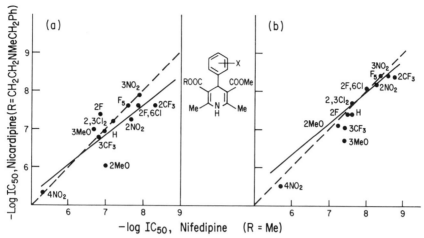

Fig. 6. *Comparison of pharmacologic activities of two series of aryl substituted 1,4-dihydropyridine (aryl substituents noted) bearing different ester substituents against methylfurmethide-induced contractile responses in guinea pig ileal longitudinal smooth muscle. a) phasic component; b) tonic component. (A. Joslyn and R. Klockowski, unpublished data).*

TABLE IV. Stereoselectivity of Pharmacological Action of 1,4-Dihydropyridine Antagonists

R	R^1	Ileum, K^+	Bladder, K^+	Rabbit aorta, K^+
Me	$CH_2CH_2NMeCH_2Ph$			
	(+)	3.1×10^{-10}	1.4×10^{-9}	3.0×10^{-9}
	(−)	1.3×10^{-9}	2.1×10^{-9}	1.5×10^{-8}
		(1)	(2)	(3)
Me	$CHMe_2$			
	(+)R	4.1×10^{-9}	4.0×10^{-9}	1.4×10^{-8}
	(−)S	4.2×10^{-10}	5.6×10^{-10}	1.5×10^{-9}
		(4)	(2)	(5)
Et	$CHMe_2$			
	(+)R	4.9×10^{-9}	—	—
	(−)S	1.9×10^{-9}		
		(5)		
$MeOCH_2CH_2$ (nimodipine)	$CHMe_2$			
	(+)R	—	—	1.6×10^{-8}
	(−)S			3.0×10^{-9}
				(6)
				(+) 1.5×10^{-9}
				(−) 2.0×10^{-10}
				(6; Rabbit basilar)
				(+) 2.6×10^{-9}
				(−) 6.0×10^{-10}
				(6; Rabbit saphenous)

Numbers in parentheses refer to: 1) D.J. Triggle, unpublished observations; 2) Yousif et al., 1985; 3) Takenaka et al., 1982; 4) Bolger et al., 1983; 5) Towart et al., 1981; and 6) Towart et al., 1982.

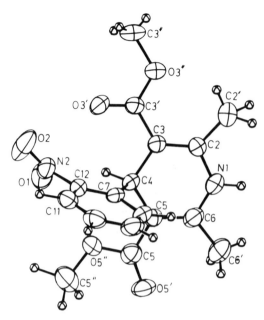

Fig. 7. *Solid state structure of nifedipine. Reproduced with permission of the American Chemical Society [Triggle and Sheflex, 1980].*

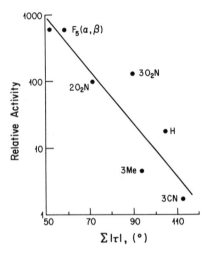

Fig. 9. *Correlation between pharmacological activity (inhibition of tension response of smooth muscle) and distortion of planarity of 1,4-dihydropyridine ring in a series of analogs of nifedipine (substituents indicated). Reproduced with permission of the American Chemical Society [Fossheim et al., 1982].*

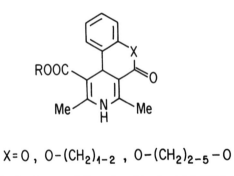

$$X = O, \ O-(CH_2)_{1-2}, \ O-(CH_2)_{2-5}-O$$

Fig. 8. *Structural formulae of bridged "rigid" 1,4-dihydropyridine analogs of nifedipine.*

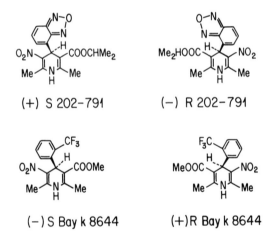

(+) S 202-791   (−) R 202-791

(−) S Bay k 8644   (+)R Bay k 8644

Fig. 10. *Enantiomeric pairs of 1,4-dihydropyridines. The S enantiomers are activators and the R enantiomers antagonists.*

tive differences in apparent potency. Similarly, when the sensitivities of a series of smooth muscles, subject to an identical K^+ depolarizing stimulus, to a common series of antagonists are compared, the same rank order of expression is observed despite the existence of comparative activity shifts (Fig. 12) [Yousif and Triggle, 1986].

In contrast to the amount of pharmacologic data available for 1,4-dihydropyridines, lim-

ited data only are available for verapamil and its analogs, and almost no comparative data for the diltiazem series. The negative inotropic activities of verapamil and some analogs have been measured by Mannhold and his colleagues [Mannhold et al., 1978, 1981, 1982] (Table V). For the series containing

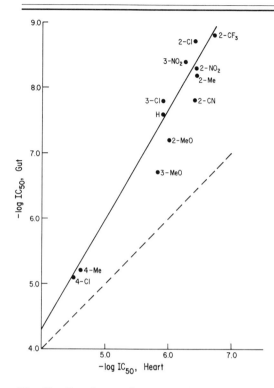

Fig. 11. *Correlation of activities of a series of analogs of nifedipine (substituent indicated) as antagonists of mechanical response in intestinal smooth muscle [Bolger et al., 1983] and cat papillary muscle [Rodenkirchen et al., 1979]. Solid line is regression and dashed line is 1:1 equivalency.*

substituents in the phenyl rings, activity is correlated with the substituent constant, F, and the molar refraction parameter, MR:

$$\log 1/ED_{50} = 0.93\ F - 0.59\ MR, \quad (3)$$

indicating that electron-withdrawing substituents enhance activity. However, only a small series of compounds was examined, and the range of activities is small.

Stereoselectivity of action is noted in a variety of smooth and cardiac muscle systems (Table VI). Quaternary ammonium derivatives of verapamil and D 600 are inactive in cellular preparations but function when injected intracellularly [Hescheler et al., 1982]. This suggests an intracellular locus of action for these compounds. A similar situation may

apply to the 1,4-dihydropyridines [Uehara and Hume, 1985].

Although the structure-activity studies reported for cellular preparations have been of substantial use, particularly in establishing the validity of the radioligand binding assay (see below), they are not without very serious quantitative limitations. Studies to date have used only restricted series of compounds and have not been cognizant of the state-dependence of activity of these agents whereby antagonist activity increases with increasing frequency of stimulation or membrane depolarization (see below).

STRUCTURE-ACTIVITY RELATIONSHIPS: RADIOLIGAND BINDING STUDIES

Structure-activity relationships derived from pharmacologic studies have been complemented in the past several years by data obtained in radioligand binding assays. Originally employed for nitrendipine, the binding assay has been extended to include other 1,4-dihydropyridines, verapamil and analogs, and diltiazem (Fig. 13). The general technique employed has been that of equilibrium binding to tissue homogenates or microsomal fractions usually in dilute suspension at 20–37°C in a Tris-based buffer with rapid filtration over glass fiber filters to separate bound and unbound material. Very few studies have measured binding to whole functional cells, and there are also few studies presenting a true comparison of ligand binding between tissues or within a single tissue. Several comprehensive reviews of Ca^{2+} channel ligand binding data are available [Janis and Triggle, 1984; Triggle and Janis, 1984c, 1987; Glossmann and Ferry, 1985].

There is general agreement that this binding assay does reflect events at ligand-sensitive Ca^{2+} channels and that the general binding behavior and pharmacologic specificity shown is that of ligand behavior at Ca^{2+} channels. Accordingly, the principal emphasis here will be on those experimental aspects that relate to structure-activity relationships.

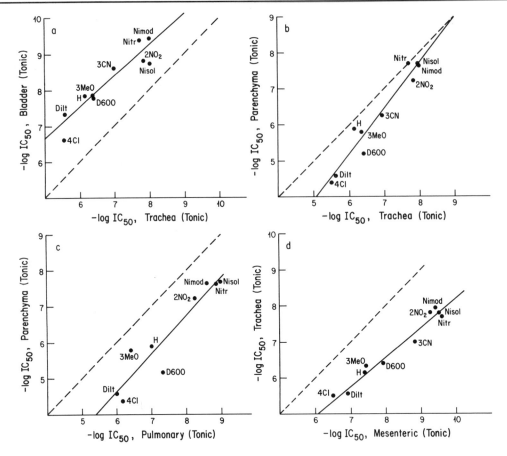

Fig. 12. *Comparison of activities of series of Ca^{2+} channel antagonists to inhibit tension responses to K^+ depolarization in the smooth muscles shown. The substituents indicated are for the nifedipine series.*

Nimod, nimodipine; nisol, nisoldipine; nitr, nitrendipine. Solid lines represent regression and dashed lines represent 1:1 equivalency. (Data from Yousif and Triggle, 1986.)

Equilibrium binding data, currently available for 1,4-dihydropyridines, are summarized in representative fashion in Table VII. Saturable high-affinity binding found with [^{3}H]1,4-dihydropyridines listed in smooth muscle, cardiac muscle, and neuronal preparations is of high affinity, 10^{-9}–10^{-11} M, and is generally described as representing one category of binding site. Binding to skeletal muscle is of lower affinity by one to two orders of magnitude, but binding site density is very much higher than in other preparations.

Although the general pharmacologic specificity of these binding sites represents that of ligand interaction with Ca^{2+} channels, comprehensive studies of the relationships between radioligand binding and pharmacologic activities are rare [Bolger et al., 1983; Bellemann et al., 1983; Janis et al., 1982, 1984; Janis and Triggle, 1984; Triggle and Janis, 1984c; Yousif et al., 1985; for review, see Janis et al., 1987]. There is an excellent and virtually 1:1 correlation between binding (inhibition of [^{3}H]nitrendipine-bound) and pharmacologic (inhibition of depolarization-

TABLE V. Negative Inotropic Activities of Verapamil Derivatives*

Name or No.	R_1	R_2	R_3	R_4	R_5	R_6	R_7	R_8	ED_{50}, M
Verapamil	OMe	OMe	H	Pr^i	Me	OMe	OMe	H	3.5×10^{-6}
D 600	OMe	OMe	OMe	Pr^i	Me	OMe	OMe	H	1.2×10^{-6}
D 557	H	OMe	H	Pr^i	Me	OMe	OMe	H	1.6×10^{-5}
PR 23	OMe	OH	H	Pr^i	Me	OMe	OMe	H	1.1×10^{-5}
D 595	Cl	Cl	H	Pr^i	Me	OMe	OMe	H	7.9×10^{-7}
T 13	CF_3	H	H	Pr^i	Me	OMe	OMe	H	2.6×10^{-6}
SZ 48	H	F	H	Pr^i	Me	OMe	OMe	H	6.6×10^{-6}
D 559	Me	Me	H	Pr^i	Me	OMe	OMe	H	8.1×10^{-6}
SZ 51	H	Bu^t	H	Pr^i	Me	OMe	OMe	H	3.0×10^{-5}
D 490	OMe	OMe	H	C_2H_5	Me	OMe	OMe	H	1.9×10^{-5}
D 586	OMe	OMe	H	$(CH_2)_7CH_3$	Me	OMe	OMe	H	1.3×10^{-4}
D 525	OMe	OMe	H	$CH_2C_6H_5$	Me	OMe	OMe	H	3.5×10^{-6}
SZ 45	H	H	H	Pr^i	Me	H	H	H	4.0×10^{-5}
D 784	OMe	H	OMe	Pr^i	Me	OMe	H	OMe	2.0×10^{-6}
D 894	OEt	H	OEt	Pr^i	Me	OEt	H	OEt	1.5×10^{-5}
F_3	OPr^n	H	OPr^n	Pr^i	Me	OPr^n	H	OPr^n	3.5×10^{-5}
F_8	OPr^i	H	OPr^i	Pr^i	Me	OPr^i	H	OPr^i	$>10^{-4}$
SZ 117	OBu^n	H	OBu^n	Pr^i	Me	OBu^n	H	OBu^n	$>10^{-4}$

*Data from Mannhold et al., 1978, 1981, 1982.

TABLE VI. Stereoselectivity of Action of Verapamil and D 600 in Pharmacologic Systems

System	D 600 (−):(+) ratio	Verapamil (−):(+) ratio
Smooth muscle		
Guinea pig ileum		
Ach	180[a]	—
Ca^{2+}/K^+	10[a]	—
Rat portal vein, NE	25[a]	—
Rat vas deferens,		
Ca^{2+}/K^+	40[a]	—
Rabbit aorta, Ca^{2+}/K^+	60[a]	10[b]
Cardiac muscle		
Canine heart		
AV block	—	10[c]
Negative chronotropic	—	3[c]
Cat heart, papillary	100	10[d,e,f]
Canine heart		
Negative inotropic	—	15[g]
Negative chronotropic	—	5[g]

[a]Jim et al., 1981.
[b]Raschach and Engelman, 1980.
[c]Kaumann and Serurs, 1975.
[d]Kaufmann et al., 1974.
[e]Ludwig and Nawrath, 1977.
[f]Nawrath et al., 1981.
[g]Satoh et al., 1980.

induced tension response) activities in guinea pig intestinal smooth muscle (Fig. 14a) [Bolger et al., 1983]. Analogous correlations, but of a more limited scope, are also available for other smooth muscles [Janis et al., 1982; Miller and Moore, 1984; Yousif et al., 1985]. Similar correlations exist for cardiac muscle, but the relationship is not 1:1 (Fig. 14b); this apparent dissociation reflects high-affinity binding and the low-affinity cardiac pharmacology that describes the smooth muscle selectivity expressed by the 1,4-dihydropyridines. It is noteworthy that the same high-affinity binding is expressed in both tissues (Fig. 14c). Apparently identical binding sites are found in brain preparations, the properties of which correlate very well with those derived from functional studies in smooth muscle (Fig. 14d). Similarly, despite the enormous concentrations of binding sites in skeletal muscle, there is little evidence of any pharmacologic function of Ca^{2+} channel blockers.

Binding studies have also permitted comparisons of the stereochemical requirements with those expressed in pharmacologic studies (Tables VIII, IX). In smooth and cardiac muscle there is agreement between the stereoselectivities observed in pharmacologic and binding studies.

STRUCTURE-ACTIVITY CORRELATIONS

Comparisons of structure-function relationships for pharmacologic and radioligand binding studies have been instructive in several important aspects in addition to their serving to establish the general validity of the radioligand binding assay. There is a generally permissible conclusion that the basic structure-activity patterns deduced either from pharmacologic or binding data are clearly complementary. There are, however, significant limitations to currently available data. The majority of the pharmacologic data have, thus far, necessarily been obtained from tension studies in intact tissues. It is very important that structure-activity studies also be carried out at the channel level with electrophysiologic techniques. Such data are likely to reveal differences that are not resolved using the blunt techniques thus far available [Rosenberg et al., 1986].

Nonetheless, despite these limitations, comparisons of pharmacologic and radioligand binding data have achieved some important objectives. In particular, they have focused attention on quantitative discrepancies between binding affinities, on the functional interrelationships between binding sites, and on the stoichiometry of the binding sites for the several ligand classes. From the structure-function perspective, analyses of the quantitative discrepancies between binding and pharmacologic data have been of particular value. In principle, a number of mechanisms may underlie the observed quantitative discrepancies between binding and behavior. These include: 1) differences in distribution, 2) differences in Ca^{2+} mobilization patterns, 3) differences in properties of ligand binding sites between tissues, 4) different affinity

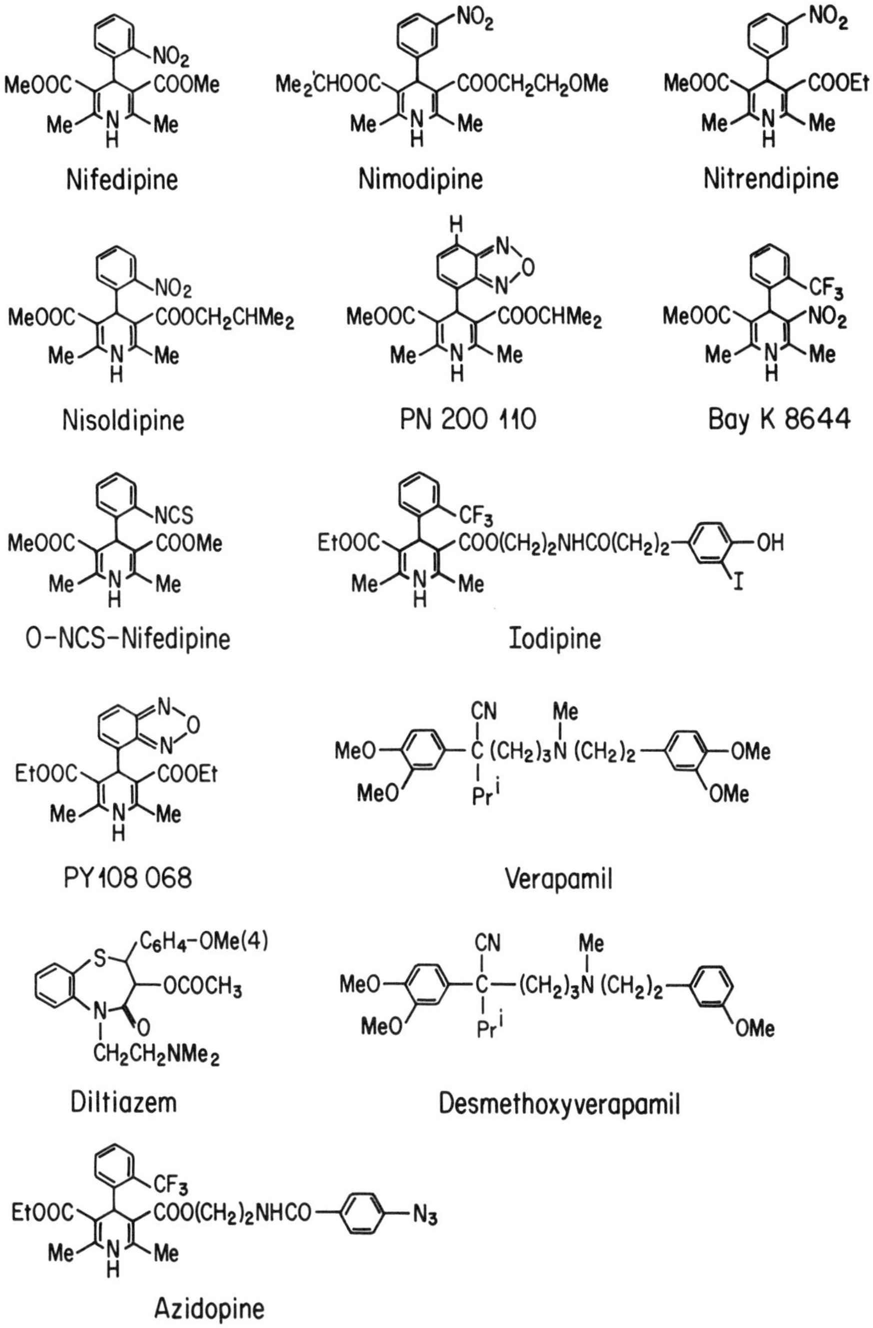

Fig. 13. *Ca^{2+} channel ligands used in binding assays.*

TABLE VII. Representative Radioligand Binding Data

System	Ligand	K_D ($\times 10^{-9}$ M)	B_{max} (fmol mg^{-1} protein)	Reference[a]
Heart (guinea pig)	Nitrendipine	0.29	122	1
Heart (rabbit)	Nitrendipine	0.14	335	2
Heart (rat)	Nimodipine	0.24	400	3
Ileum (guinea pig)	Nitrendipine	0.16	1,100	4
Ileum (guinea pig)	(+)PN 200 110	0.04	820	5
Skeletal muscle (rabbit)	Nitrendipine	1.7	56,000	6
Skeletal muscle (guinea pig)	Nimodipine	3.6	80,000	7
Brain (rat)	Nitrendipine	0.17	114	8
Brain (guinea pig)	Nimodipine	0.62	570	9
Heart (rabbit)	Bay K 8644	2.4	840	10
Brain (guinea pig)	Bay K 8644	3.0	808	10
Heart (pig)	Verapamil	50	1,250	11
Skeletal muscle (rabbit)	Verapamil	27	55,000	12
Skeletal muscle (rabbit)	Desmethoxyverapamil	1.5	70,000	12

[a]1. Schwartz and Vells, 1985; 2. Janis et al., 1984a; 3. Janis et al., 1982; 4. Bolger et al. 1983; 5. Rampe et al., 1986; 6. Fosset et al., 1983; 7. Ferry et al., 1983; 8. Yamamura et al., 1982; 9. Glossmann et al., 1983; 10. Janis et al., 1984b; 11. Garcia et al., 1984; 12. Galizzi et al., 1984a.

states of binding sites, 5) differences in properties of binding sites during cellular disruption, 6) different classes of channels with differing Ca^{2+} channel ligand sensitivities, 7) lack of or variable coupling of ligand binding sites to functional Ca^{2+} channels, and 8) presence of endogenous molecules regulating channel function.

These several mechanisms may operate at different levels ranging from whole animal to isolated channel, and they are not necessarily mutually exclusive. Clearly, inability of drugs to penetrate the CNS could explain the absence of pharmacologic effects. However, these agents do penetrate, and the same discrepancies occur in isolated preparations. Thus, considerations of access are probably unimportant. Similarly, when tension or Ca^{2+} mobilization experiments are employed to determine pharmacologic affinities, discrepancies between binding affinities may arise if the stimulus employed mobilizes Ca^{2+} through routes other than or additional to the ligand-sensitive Ca^{2+} channel. This is particularly important for smooth muscle preparations [Triggle and Swamy, 1983; Bolger et al., 1983; Yousif et al., 1985; Yousif and Triggle, 1986].

Two major lines of reasoning dominate most of the remaining mechanisms advanced to accommodate the discrepancies between binding and function. These phenomena of state-dependent binding interactions and channel classes with differing ligand sensitivities are also discussed elsewhere (see Kass and Krafte, this volume, and Miller, this volume).

The voltage-dependence of interaction of 1,4-dihydropyridines, the dominant ligand category for binding experiments, has been established by several groups [Sanguinetti and Kass, 1984a,b; Hess et al., 1984; Uehara and Hume, 1985; Williams et al., 1985; Cognard et al., 1986] and clearly demonstrates that 1,4-dihydropyridine affinity increases with increasing membrane depolarization. This reflects a preferential binding to a channel state favored by depolarization. This likely represents the inactivated state, either liganded by direct occupancy or via access through the open channel state. According to these observations (for further details, see Kass and Krafte, this volume, and Miller, this volume) experimental conditions that favor the dominance of one channel state over others will alter the apparent affinity of ligands. Thus, in

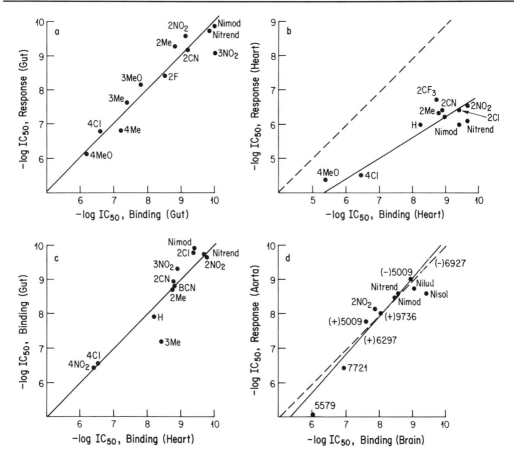

Fig. 14. *Correlations between pharmacologic and radioligand binding activities in 1,4-dihydropyridine series. a) Binding and pharmacology in intestinal smooth muscle [Bolger et al., 1983]. b) Binding and pharmacology in cardiac tissue [Rodenkirchen et al.,* *1979; Janis et al., 1984]. c) Binding in intestinal and cardiac muscle. d) Binding in brain and pharmacology in vascular smooth muscle [Bellemann et al., 1983]. The solid lines represent regression; the dashed lines represent 1:1 equivalency.*

the modulated receptor hypothesis [Hille, 1977; Hondeghem and Katzung, 1977, 1984], the apparent affinity of a ligand will be determined by the equilibrium among two or more conformational states and by the actual ligand affinity for each state. Thus, for a drug binding to the resting (R) and inactivated (I) states of the Ca^{2+} channel, we may write [Bean, 1984]:

$$Kapp = \frac{1}{(h/K_R) + (1-h)/K_I}, \quad (4)$$

where h is the fraction of channels in the R state in the absence of drug, and K_R and K_I are the affinity constants for each state. This is depicted for a specific situation in Figure 15 and depicts the dissociation constant of nitrendipine for the inactivated state to be $\sim 10^{-10}$ M and for the resting state to be $\sim 10^{-6}$ M. According to the experimental equilibrium between channel states, the apparent affinity of nitrendipine will lie somewhere between these two values which cover a range of approximately 10^4.

It will be noted that, according to this model, the high-affinity binding state corresponds to that commonly observed in radioligand binding experiments. This is reasonable since these experiments are performed on depolarized membrane fragments where channels may exist dominantly in the inactivated (high affinity) state. It would be predicted that ligand binding to whole functional cells or organelles should be sensitive to membrane potential. Several reports of voltage-dependent binding have appeared which suggest the

existence of a low-affinity dihydropyridine site converted upon depolarization to a high-affinity state [Green et al., 1985; Schilling and Drewe, 1986; Reuter et al., 1986].

The implications of such a state-dependent phenomenon to the definition and interpretation of structure-activity relationships are profound. Accordingly:

1) Different channel states exhibit different affinities. Thus, the apparent affinity of a drug or drug series will depend (and vary) according to experimental conditions.

2) The time- and voltage-dependent characteristics of interstate channel conversion likely vary according to cell type. This will also alter the expression of drug affinities.

3) Because drugs stabilize different states of a channel, they will also alter the kinetics and voltage-dependence of state interconversion.

These factors will exert a major impact on the interpretation of structure-activity relationships and to the expression of drug action according to cell type. These factors will affect the quantitative and qualitative expression of structure-activity relationships. The observation that quantitative shifts of activity occur in a series of compounds between tissues may well be a reflection of such state-dependent binding [Bolger et al., 1983; Yousif et al., 1985; Yousif and Triggle, 1986; Su et al., 1986]. Furthermore, the implications regarding the function of drugs that selectively stabilize one or another state, i.e., resting, open, and inactivated, are quite different.

TABLE VIII. Stereoselectivity of 1, 4-Dihydropyridines in Radioligand Systems

1,4-Dihydropyridine	IC$_{50}$ (K$_i$) $\times 10^{-9}$ M System	
	Rat brain	Pig brain
Nitrendipine		
(−)	0.43[a]	2.0[c]
(+)	8.8	30.0
Nimodipine		
(−)	1.04[a]	1.0[c]
(+)	2.4	30.0
PN 200 110		
(−)	14.9[b]	−
(+)	0.06	−
Nicardipine		
(−)	2.90[b]	−
(+)	0.37	−
Bay e 6927		
(−)	0.09[a]	0.1[c]
(+)	27.5	30.0

[a]Belleman et al., 1983.
[b]Lee et al., 1984.
[c]Holck et al., 1983.

TABLE IX. Stereoselectivity of Phenylalkylamines in Radioligand Systems

Systems	IC$_{50}$ $\times 10^{-9}$ M					
	Verapamil		D 600		Desmethoxyverapamil	
	(−)	(+)	(−)	(+)	(−)	(+)
Skeletal muscle[a]	77	30	15	67	−	−
Skeletal muscle[b]	40	10	20	60	−	−
Skeletal muscle[c]			12	55	3	7
Cardiac muscle[d]	21	550	21	560	10	280

[a]Goll et al., 1984.
[b]Gallizzi et al., 1984b.
[c]Goll et al., 1984.
[d]Ruth et al., 1985.

Thus, at the most simplistic level, drugs that stabilize open channel states will be activators, drugs that stabilize inactivated states will affect most profoundly those systems where channels are maintained in an activated state, and drugs that stabilize resting states may be pharmacologically silent but block the actions of drugs that interact preferentially with other channel states. Finally, there may be qualitative shifts in the expression of structure-activity relationships. A specific example is given by the recent discovery that activator and antagonist properties in 1,4-dihy-

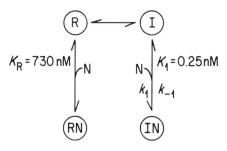

Fig. 15. *State dependence of nitrendipine block of cardiac Ca^{2+} channels with differing dissociation constants for resting (R) and inactivated (I) Ca^{2+} channels. It has been assumed that binding to open channels (not shown) is not important at the concentrations of nitrendipine employed. (Reproduced with permission from Bean, 1984.)*

dropyridines are enantiomer-specific [Hof et al., 1985; Franckowiak et al., 1985; Williams et al., 1985; Wei et al., 1986] where antagonist properties reside in one enantiomer and activator properties in the other. This likely indicates the opposing stereoselectivities of the open and inactivated states of the Ca^{2+} channel [Triggle, 1987].

It is now, also, quite clear that a second major contributor to observed discrepancies between binding and biologic expression is the existence of different classes of Ca^{2+} channels. This is not a surprising conclusion in light of the diversity of pharmacologic receptor subclasses and the recent demonstration that discrete mRNAs exist coding for brain Na^+ channels [Noda et al., 1986]. Two, and possibly three, electrophysiologically and pharmacologically distinct classes of voltage-dependent Ca^{2+} channels have been reported [Miller, 1985, this volume; Miller and Freedman, 1984; Nowycky et al., 1985; Nilius et al., 1985; Armstrong and Matteson, 1985; Bean, 1985; Cognard et al., 1986a]. It is very clear that these channels exhibit differential sensitivity to Ca^{2+} channel ligands (Table X), with the conventional, slowly inactivating channel being sensitive to currently defined agents including the 1,4-dihydropyridines.

TABLE X. Properties of Major Ca^{2+} Channel Types[1]

Property	Channel type	
	Persistent	Transient
Activation	-10 mV	-50 mV
Peak	$+20$ mV	-10 mV
Tails	Fast	Slow
Inactivation	Slow, incomplete	Fast, complete
Permeation	$Ba^{2+} > Sr^{2+} > Ca^{2+}$	$Ca^{2+} \sim Sr^{2+} \sim Ba^{2+}$
Stability	Labile	Stable
M^{2+}	Sensitive	Less sensitive
Organic antagonists	Sensitive[2]	Insensitive or much less sensitive

[1]This table was compiled using data from a variety of publications encompassing several tissue types. It is not intended to indicate that there are only two channel classes with precisely the above defined characteristics. Other classes and subclasses likely exist.
[2]Sensitivity of this channel type to 1, 4-hydropyridine is $\leqslant 10^{-9}$ M in smooth and cardiac muscle, but $\geqslant 10^{-6}$ M in many neuronal systems.

Because of the recent discovery of the multiple classes of Ca^{2+} channels, little can be said concerning ligand action. However, there are a number of recently discovered toxins including maitotoxin, a Ca^{2+} channel activator sensitive to known categories of antagonists [Takahashi et al., 1982; Ohizumi and Yasumoto, 1983; Login et al., 1985]; toxins from *Conus geographus* [Kerr and Yoshikami, 1984; Olivera et al., 1985]; leptinotarsin-h, an apparent activator of presynaptic neuronal channels [Crusland et al., 1984]; and atrotoxin from *Crotalus atrox*, an activator of cardiac Ca^{2+} channels [Hamilton et al., 1985]. These, and other toxins, may well serve as probes with which to further differentiate and identify Ca^{2+} channels and, of equal importance, to provoke the search for small molecule regulators of other categories of Ca^{2+} channels.

CONCLUSIONS

The determination of structure-activity relationships, first from pharmacologic and then from radioligand binding studies, has been of use in several important respects. It has permitted the definition of specific ligand binding sites associated with at least one category of voltage-dependent Ca^{2+} channels. This definition has, in turn, made possible the quantitation and localization of Ca^{2+} channels in both peripheral tissues and neuronal tissues of the central nervous system. The recognition of the specificity of action of the Ca^{2+} channel ligands has made them particularly valuable tools with which to dissect Ca^{2+} channels by both electrophysiologic [Beaty et al., this volume; Kass and Krafte, this volume; Miller, this volume] and biochemical techniques [Fosset and Lazdunski, this volume]. The molecular understanding of channel function that is thus being achieved with the aid of currently available ligands is proving to be of crucial significance to the definition of the basis of tissue selectivity and clinical indications. Finally, the observations of the inactivity or apparent inactivity of the commonly

available ligands in many neuronal Ca^{2+} channels have aided in the definition of new Ca^{2+} channel classes.

"If happiness is activity in accordance with excellence, it is reasonable that it should be in accordance with the highest excellence."
—Aristotle

REFERENCES

Armstrong CM, Matteson DR (1985): Two distinct populations of calcium channels in a clonal line of pituitary cells. Science 227:65–67.

Bean BP (1984): Nitrendipine block of cardiac calcium channels: high-affinity binding to the inactivated state. Proc Natl Acad Sci USA 81:6388–6392.

Bean BP (1985): Two kinds of calcium channels in canine atrial cells. J Gen Physiol 86:1–30.

Belleman P, Schade A, Towart R (1983): Dihydropyridine receptor in rat brain labeled with [³H] nimodipine. Proc Natl Acad Sci USA 80:2356–2360.

Bevan JA, Osher JV, Su C (1963): Response of vascular smooth muscle to potassium and its antagonism by phenoxybenzamine. J Pharmacol Exp Ther 139:216–221.

Bolger GT, Gengo P, Klockowski R, Luchowski E, Siegel H, Janis RA, Triggle AM, Triggle DJ (1983): Characterization of binding of the Ca^{2+} channel antagonist, [³H]nitrendipine, to guinea pig ileal smooth muscle. J Pharmacol Exp Ther 225:291–301.

Cantor EH, Kenessey A, Semenuk G, Spector S (1984): Interaction of calcium channel blockers with non-neuronal benzodiazepine binding sites. Proc Natl Acad Sci USA 81:1549–1552.

Chatelain P, Demol D, Roba J (1984): Inhibition by suloctidil of [³H]nitrendipine binding to cerebral cortex membranes. Biochem Pharmacol 33:1099–1103.

Cognard C, Lazdunski M, Romey G (1986a): Different types of Ca^{2+} channels exist in mammalian skeletal muscle cells in culture. Proc Natl Acad Sci USA 83:517–521.

Cognard C, Romey G, Galizzi J-P, Fosset M, Lazdunski M (1986b): Dihydropyridine-sensitive Ca^{2+} channels in mammalian skeletal muscle cells in culture: Electrophysiologic properties and interactions with Ca^{2+} channel activator (Bay k 8644) and inhibitor (PN 200-110). Proc Natl Acad Sci USA 83:1518–1522.

Crusland RD, Hsiao TH, McClure WO (1984): Purification and characterization of β-leptinotarsin-h, an activator of presynaptic calcium channels. Biochemistry 23:734–741.

El-Fakahany EE, Eldefrawi AT, Murphy DL, Aquayo LG, Triggle DJ, Alburquerque EX, Eldefrawi ME

(1984): Interactions of phencyclidine with crayfish muscle membranes. Sensitivity to calcium channel antagonists and other drugs. Mol Pharmacol 25:369–378.

Ferry DR, Goll A, Glossmann H (1983): Differential labelling of putative skeletal muscle channels by [³H]nifedipine, [³H]nitrendipine, [³H]nimodipine and [³H]PN 200-110. Naunyn-Schmied Arch Pharmacol 323:276–277.

Flaim S, Zelis R (eds) (1982): "Calcium Blockers. Mechanisms of Action and Clinical Applications." Baltimore, Maryland: Urban and Schwarzenberg.

Fleckenstein A (1977): Specific pharmacology of calcium in myocardium, cardiac pacemakers, and vascular smooth muscle. Ann Rev Pharmacol Toxicol 17:149–166.

Fleckenstein A (1983): "Calcium Antagonism in Heart and Smooth Muscle." New York: John Wiley and Sons.

Fleckenstein A, van Breemen C, Gross R, Hoffmeister F (eds) (1986): "Cardiovascular Effects of Dihydropyridine Type Calcium Antagonists and Agonists." Berlin: Springer Verlag.

Fosset M, Jaimovich E, Delpont E, Lazdunski M (1983): [³H]Nitrendipine labelling of the Ca^{2+} channel in skeletal muscle. Eur J Pharmacol 86:141–142.

Fossheim R, Svarteng K, Mostad A, Rømming C, Shefter E, Triggle DJ (1982): Crystal structures and pharmacological activity of calcium channel antagonists: 2,6-dimethyl-3,5-dicarbomethoxy-4-(unsubtituted, 3-methyl-, 4-methyl-, 3-nitro-, 4-nitro, and 2,4-dinitrophenyl)-1,4-dihydropyridine. J Med Chem 215:126–131.

Franckowiak G, Bechem M, Schramm M, Thomas G (1985): The optical isomers of the 1,4-dihydropyridine Bay k 8644 show opposite effects on Ca channels. Eur J Pharmacol 114:223–226.

Galizzi J-P, Fosset M, Lazdunski M (1984a): Characterization of the Ca^{2+} coordination site regulating binding of Ca^{2+} channel inhibitors d-dis-diltiazem, (±)bepridil and (−)desmethoxyverapamil to their receptor sites in skeletal muscle transverse tubule membranes. Biochem Biophys Res Commun 118:239–245.

Galizzi J-P, Fosset M, Lazdunski M (1984b): Properties of receptors from the Ca^{2+}-channel blocker verapamil in transverse-tubule membranes of skeletal muscle. Eur J Biochem 144:211–215.

Garcia ML, Trumble MJ, Reuben JP, Kaczorowski GJ (1984): Characterization of verapamil sites in cardiac membrane vesicles. J Biol Chem 259:15013–15016.

Gengo PJ, Yousif F, Janis RA, Triggle DJ (1984): Interaction of phenoxybenzamine with muscarinic receptors and calcium channels. Biochem Pharmacol 33:3445–3449.

Glossmann H, Ferry DR (1985): Assay for calcium channels. Meth Enzymol 109:513–551.

Glossmann H, Ferry DR, Lübbecke F, Mewes R, Hofmann F (1983): Identification of voltage operated calcium channels by binding: Differentiation of subclasses of calcium antagonists with [³H]-nimodipine radioligand binding. J Rec Res 3:177–190.

Godfraind T, Vanhoutte PM, Govoni S, Paoletti R (eds) (1985): "Calcium Entry Blockers and Tissue Protection." New York: Raven Press.

Goll A, Ferry DR, Glossmann H (1984): Target size analysis and molecular properties of Ca^{2+} channels labelled with [³H]verapamil. Eur J Biochem 141:177–186.

Goll A, Ferry DR, Striessnig J, Schober M, Glossmann H (1986): (−)[³H]Desmethoxyverapamil, a novel Ca^{2+} channel probe. FEBS Lett 176:371–373.

Gould RJ, Murphy KMM, Reynolds IJ, Snyder SH (1983): Antischizophrenic drugs of the diphenylbutylpiperidine type act as calcium channel antagonists. Proc Natl Acad Sci USA 80:5122–5125.

Green FJ, Farmer BB, Wiseman GL, Jose MJL, Watanabe AM (1985): Effect of membrane depolarization on binding of [³H]nitrendipine to rat cardiac myocytes. Circ Res 56:576–585.

Hamilton SL, Yatani A, Hawkes MJ, Redding K, Brown AM (1985): Atrotoxin: A specific agonist for calcium currents in heart. Science 229:182–184.

Hescheler J, Pelzer D, Trube G, Trautwein W (1982): Does the organic calcium channel blocker D 600 act from inside or outside on the cardiac cell membrane? Pflüg Arch 393:287–291.

Hess P, Lansman JB, Tsien RW (1984): Different modes of Ca channel gating behaviour favored by dihydropyridine Ca agonists and antagonists. Nature 311:538–544.

Hille B (1977): Local anesthetics: Hydrophilic and hydrophobic pathways for the drug-receptor reaction. J Gen Physiol 69:497–515.

Hof RP, Rüegg UT, Hof A, Vogel A (1985): Stereoselectivity at the calcium channel: Opposite action of the enantiomers of a 1,4-dihydropyridine. J Cardiovas Pharmacol 7:689–693.

Holck M, Thorens S, Haeusler G (1983): Does [³H]nifedipine label the calcium channel in rabbit myocardium. J Rec Res 3:191–198.

Hondeghem LM, Katzung BG (1977): Time- and voltage-dependent interactions of antiarrhythmic drugs with cardiac sodium channels. Biochim Biophys Acta 372:373–398.

Hondeghem LM, Katzung BG (1984): Antiarrhythmic agents: The modulated receptor mechanism of action of sodium and calcium channel-blocking drugs. Ann Rev Pharmacol Toxicol 24:387–423.

Isenberg G, Tamargo J (1985): Effects of imipramine on calcium and potassium currents in isolated bovine ventricular myocytes. Eur J Pharmacol 108:121–131.

Janis RA, Maurer SC, Sarmiento JG, Bolger GT, Triggle DJ (1982): Binding of [³H]nimodipine to cardiac and smooth muscle membranes. Eur J Pharmacol 82:191–194.

Janis RA, Rampe D, Sarmiento JG, Triggle DJ (1984a): Specific binding of a calcium channel activator, [^{3}H]Bay k 8644, to membranes from cardiac muscle and brain. Biochem Biophys Res Commun 121:317–323.

Janis RA, Sarmiento JG, Maurer SC, Bolger GT, Triggle DJ (1984b): Characteristics of the binding of [^{3}H]nitrendipine to rabbit ventricular membranes: Modification by other Ca^{2+} channel antagonists and by the Ca^{2+} channel agonist Bay k 8644. J Pharmacol Exp Ther 231:8–15.

Janis RA, Silver P, Triggle DJ (1987): Drug action and cellular calcium regulation. Adv Drug Res., in press.

Janis RA, Triggle DJ (1983): New developments in Ca^{2+} channel antagonists. J Med Chem 26:775–785.

Janis RA, Triggle DJ (1984): 1,4-Dihydropyridine Ca^{2+} channel antagonists and activators: A comparison of binding characteristics with pharmacology. Drug Dev Res 4:257–274.

Jim K, Harris A, Rosenberger LB, Triggle DJ (1981): Stereoselective and nonstereoselective effects of D 600 (methoxyverapamil) in smooth muscle preparations. Eur J Pharmacol 76:67–72.

Kaufmann R, Bayer R, Hennekes R, Kalusche D, Mannhold R (1974): Antidysrhythmic and Ca-antagonistic actions of verapamil with D 600. Naunyn-Schmied Arch Pharmacol 285:R39.

Kaumann AJ, Serurs JR (1975): Optical isomers of verapamil on canine heart. Naunyn-Schmied Arch Pharmacol 291:347–358.

Kerr LM, Yoshikami D (1984): A venom peptide with a novel presynaptic blocking action. Nature 308:282–284.

Langs DA, Triggle DJ (1984): Chemical structure and pharmacological activities of Ca^{2+} channel antagonists. In Paton W, Mitchell J, Turner P (eds): "IUPHAR 9th International Congress of Pharmacology: Proceedings," Vol 2. London and Basingstoke: Macmillan, pp 323–328.

Langs DA, Triggle DJ (1985): Conformational features of calcium channel agonists and antagonist analogs of nifedipine. Mol Pharmacol 27:544–548.

Lee HR, Roeske WR, Yamamura HI (1984): High affinity specific [^{3}H](+)PN 200-110 binding to dihydropyridine receptors associated with calcium channels in rat cerebral cortex and heart. Life Sci 35:721–732.

Loev B, Goodman MM, Snader KM, Tedesche R, Macko E (1974): "Hantzsch-type" dihydropyridine hypotensive agents. J Med Chem 17:956–965.

Login IS, Judd AM, Cronin MJ, Koiko K, Schettini G, Yasumoto T, MacLeod RM (1985): The effects of maitotoxin on $^{45}Ca^{2+}$ flux and hormone release in GH_3 rat pituitary cells. Endocrinology 116:622–627.

Lowe DA, Matthews EK, Richardson BP (1981): The calcium antagonistic effects of cyproteptadine on contraction, membrane electrical events and calcium influx in the guinea pig taenia coil. Br J Pharmacol 74:651–663.

Luchowski EM, Yousif F, Triggle DJ, Maurer SC, Sarmiento JG, Janis RA (1984): Effects of metal cations and calmodulin antagonists on [^{3}H] nitrendipine binding in smooth and cardiac muscle. J Pharmacol Exp Ther 230:607–613.

Ludwig C, Nawrath H (1977): Effects of D-600 and its optical isomers on force of contraction in cat papillary muscles and guinea pig auricles. Br J Pharmacol 59:411–417.

Mannhold R, Rodenkirchen R, Bayer R (1982): Qualitative and quantitative structure-activity relationships of specific Ca antagonists. Prog Pharmacol 5:25–52.

Mannhold R, Steiner R, Haas W, Kaufmann R (1978): Investigations on the structure-activity relationships of verapamil. Naunyn-Schmied Arch Pharmacol 302:217–226.

Mannhold R, Zierden P, Bayer R, Rodenkirchen R, Steiner R (1981): The influence of aromatic substitution on the negative inotropic action of verapamil in the isolated cat papillary muscle. Arzneim Forsch 31:773–780.

Mestre M, Carriot T, Belin C, Uzan A, Renault C, Dubroeucq MC, Guérémy C, Doble A, LeFur G (1985): Electrophysiological and pharmacological evidence that peripheral type benzodiazepine receptors are coupled to calcium channels in the heart. Life Sci 36:391–400.

Miller RJ (1985): How many types of calcium channels exist in neurones. Trends Neurosci 8:45–47.

Miller RJ, Freedman SB (1984): Are dihydropyridine binding sites voltage-sensitive calcium channels. Life Sci 34:1205–1221.

Miller WC, Moore JB (1984): High affinity binding sites for [^{3}]nitrendipine in rabbit uterine smooth muscle. Life Sci 34:1717–1724.

Nawrath H, Blei I, Gegner R, Ludwig C, Zang X-G (1981): No stereospecific effects of the optical isomers of verapamil and D-600 on the heart. In Zanchetti A, Krikler DM (eds): "Calcium Antagonists in Cardiovascular Therapy." Amsterdam: Excerpta Medica, pp 52–63.

Nilius B, Hess P, Lansman JB, Tsien RW (1985): A novel type of cardiac calcium channel in ventricular cells. Nature 316:443–446.

Noda M, Ikeda T, Kayano T, Suzuki H, Takeshima H, Kurasaki M, Takahashi H, Numa S (1986): Existence of distinct sodium channel messenger RNAs in rat brain. Nature 320:188–192.

Nowycky MC, Fox AP, Tsien RW (1985): Three types of neuronal calcium channel with different calcium agonist sensitivity. Nature 316:440–443.

Ohizumi Y, Yasumoto T (1983): Contractile response of the rabbit aorta to maitotoxin, the most potent marine toxin. J Physiol 337:711–721.

Olivera BM, Gray WR, Zeikus R, McIntosh JM, Varga J, Rivier J, de Santos V, Cruz LJ (1985): Peptide neurotoxins from fish-hunting cone snails. Science 230:1338–1343.

Opie LH (ed) (1984): "Calcium Antagonists and Cardiovascular Disease." New York: Raven Press.

Pourrias B, Huerta F, Santamaria R, Bowe C (1985): Calcium blocking properties of piprofurol. Arch Int Pharmacodyn 274:233–239.

Preuss KC, Gross GJ, Brooks HL, Warltier DC (1985): Slow channel activators, a new group of pharmacological agents. Life Sci 37:1271–1278.

Rahwan RG, Witiak DT (eds) (1982): "Calcium Antagonists." Washington, DC: American Chemical Society.

Rampe D, Luchowski E, Rutledge A, Janis RA, Triggle DJ (1986): Comparative aspects of [^{3}H]1,4-dihydropyridine Ca^{2+} channel antagonist and activator binding to neuronal and muscle membranes. Can J Physiol Pharmacol, in press.

Raschack M, Engelman K (1980): Calcium antagonistic activity and myocardial ischemia protection by both stereoisomers of verapamil. International Society for Heart Research 10th Intl. Congess, Moscow USSR (abs).

Reuter H, Porzig H, Kokobun S, Prod'hom B (1986): Voltage dependent binding and action of 1,4-dihydropyridine enantiomers in intact cardiac cells. In Hille B, Fambrough (eds): "Proteins In Excitable Membranes." New York: John Wiley and Sons, in press.

Reynolds IJ, Gould RJ, Snyder SH (1984): Loperamide: Blockade of calcium channels as a mechanism for antidiarrheal effects. J Pharmacol Exp Ther 231:628–632.

Rodenkirchen R, Bayer R, Steiner R, Bossert F, Meyer H, Möller E (1979): Structure-activity studies on nifedipine in isolated cardiac muscle. Naunyn-Schmied Arch Pharmacol 310:69–78.

Rosenberg RL, Hess P, Reeves JP, Smilowitz H, Tsien RW (1986): Calcium channels in plana lipid bilayers: Insights into mechanisms of ion permeation and gating. Science 231:1564–1566.

Rosenberger LB, Triggle DJ (1978): Calcium, calcium translocation, and specific calcium antagonists. In Weiss GB (ed): "Calcium in Drug Action." New York: Plenum Press, pp 3–31.

Ruth P, Flockerzi V, van Nettelbladt E, Oeken J, Hofmann F (1985): Characterization of the binding sites for nimodipine and (−)desmethoxyverapamil in bovine cardiac sarcolemma. Eur J Biochem 150:313–323.

Sanguinetti MC, Kass RS (1984a): Voltage-dependent block of calcium channel current in the calf cardiac

Purkinje fiber by dihydropyridine calcium channel antagonists. Circ Res 55:336–348.

Sanguinetti MC, Kass RS (1984b): Regulation of cardiac calcium current and contractile activity by the dihydropyridine Bay k 8644 is voltage-dependent. J Mol Cell Cardiol 16:667–670.

Sato K, Yanagisana T, Taira N (1980): Coronary vasodilator and cardiac effects of optical isomers of verapamil in the dog. J Cardiovasc Pharmacol 2:309–318.

Schilling WP, Drewe JA (1986): Voltage-sensitive nitrendipine binding in an isolated cardiac sarcolemma preparation. J Biol Chem 261:2750–2758.

Schramm M, Thomas G, Towart R, Franckowiak G (1983): Novel dihydropyridines with positive inotropic action through activation of Ca^{2+} channels. Nature 303:535–537.

Schwartz A, Taira N (eds) (1983): Calcium Channel Blocking Drugs: A Novel Intervention for the Treatment of Cardiovascular Disease. Circ Res 52(II):1–180.

Schwartz J, Velly J (1985): Interference of sodium with [^{3}H]nitrendipine binding to cardiac membranes. Br J Pharmacol 84:511–515.

Seidel W, Meyer H, Born L, Kazda S, Dompert W (1984): Rigid calcium antagonists of the nifedipine type: Geometrical requirements for the dihydropyridine receptor. Washington, D.C.: American Chemical Society, 187th National Meeting, St. Louis, MO, April 8–14, Abs. 14 (Medicinal Chemistry).

Shoji N, Umeyama A, Asakawa Y, Takemoto T, Nomoto K, Onizumi Y (1984): Structural determination of nootkatol, a new sesquiterpene isolated from Alpinia oxyphylla miguel possessing calcium-antagonistic activity. J Pharmacol Sci 73:843–844.

Su CM, Yousif FB, Triggle DJ, Janis RA (1986): Structure-function relationships of 1,4-dihydropyridines: Ligand and receptor perspectives. In Fleckenstein A, van Breemen C, Gross R, Hoffmeister F (eds): "Cardiovascular Effects of Dihydropyridine-type Calcium Antagonists and Agonists." Berlin: Springer Verlag, pp 104–110.

Swamy VC, Triggle DJ (1972): 2-Halogeneothylamines and the role of Ca^{2+} in adrenergic α-receptor activation. Eur J Pharmacol 19:67–78.

Takahashi M, Ohizumi Y, Yasumoto T (1982): Maitotoxin, a Ca^{2+} channel activator candidate. J Biol Chem 257:7287–7289.

Takenaka T, Maeno H (1982): A new vasoconstrictor 1,4-dihydropyridine derivative, YC-170. Jpn J Pharmacol 32:139P.

Takenaka T, Miyazaki I, Asano M, Higuchi S, Maeno S (1982): Vasodilator and hypotensive effects of the optical isomers of nicardipine (YC-93), a new Ca^{2+} antagonist. Jpn J Pharmacol 32:665–670.

Triggle AM, Shefter E, Triggle DJ (1980): Crystal structures of calcium channel antagonists. 2,6-Dimethyl-3,5-dicarbomethoxy-4-[2-nitro-, 3-cyano-, 4-(dimethylamino)-, and 2,3,4,5,6-pentafluorophenyl]-1,4-dihydropyridine. J Med Chem 23:1442–1448.

Triggle DJ (1981): Calcium antagonists: Basic chemical and pharmacological aspects. In Weiss GB (ed): "New Perspectives on Calcium Antagonists." Bethesda, MD: American Physiology Society, pp 1–18.

Triggle DJ (1982): Chemical pharmacology of calcium antagonists. In Rahwan RG, Witiak DT (eds): "Calcium Regulation by Calcium Antagonists." Washington, DC: American Chemical Society, pp 17–37.

Triggle DJ (1984): Ca^{2+} channels revisited: Problems and promises. Trends Pharmacol Sci 5:3–4.

Triggle DJ (1987): Ca^{2+} channels and 1,4-dihydropyridine receptors. J Cardiovasc Pharmacol, in press.

Triggle DJ, Janis RA (1984a): Nitrendipine binding sites and mechanism of action. In Scriabine A, Varov S, Deck K (eds): "Nitrendipine." Baltimore: Urban and Schwarzenberg, pp 33–52.

Triggle DJ, Janis RA (1984b): The 1,4-dihydropyridine receptor: A regulatory component of the Ca^{2+} channel. J Cardiovasc Pharmacol 6:S949–955.

Triggle DJ, Janis RA (1984c): Calcium channel antagonists: New perspectives from the radioligand binding assay. In Back N, Spector S (eds): "Modern Methods in Pharmacology," Vol 2. New York: Alan R. Liss, pp 1–28.

Triggle DJ, Janis RA (1987): Calcium channels and calcium channel ligands. In Williams M, Glennon RA, Timmermans PBMWM (eds): "Receptor Pharmacology and Function." New York: Marcel Dekker, in press.

Triggle DJ, Swamy VC (1983): Calcium antagonists—Some chemical-pharmacologic aspects. Circ Res 52(Suppl I):17–28.

Towart R, Wehinger E, Meyer H (1981): Effects of unsymmetrical ester substituted 1,4-dihydropyridine derivatives and their optical isomers on contraction of smooth muscle. Naunyn-Schmied Arch Pharmacol 317:183–185.

Towart R, Wehinger E, Meyer H, Kazda S (1982): The effects of nimodipine, its optical isomers and metabolites on isolated vascular smooth muscle. Arzneim-Forsch 32:338–346.

Uehara A, Hume JR (1985): Interactions of organic calcium, channel antagonists with calcium channels in single frog atrial cells. J Gen Physiol 85:621–647.

Verloop A, Hooganstraaten W, Tipker J (1976): Development and application of new steric substituent parameters in drug design. In Ariens EJ (ed): "Drug Design," Vol 7. London and New York: Academic Press, pp 165–207.

Wei XY, Luchowski EM, Rutledge A, Su CM, Triggle DJ (1986): A pharmacologic and radioligand binding analysis of the actions of 1,4-dihydropyridine activator-antagonist pairs in smooth muscle. J Pharmacol Exp Ther 239:144–153.

Weiss GB (ed) (1978): "Calcium in Drug Action." New York: Plenum Press.

Weiss GB (ed) (1981): "New Perspectives on Calcium Channel Antagonists." Bethesda, MD: American Physiology Society.

Williams JS, Grupp IL, Grupp G, Vaghy PL, Dumont L, Schwartz A (1985): Profile of the oppositely acting enantiomers of the dihydropyridine 202-791 in cardiac preparations: Receptor binding, electrophysiological, and pharmacological structures. Biochem Biophys Res Commun 131:13–21.

Yamamura HI, Schoemaker H, Boles RG, Roeske WR (1982): Diltiazem enhancement of [^{3}H]nitrendipine binding to calcium channel associated drug receptor sites in rat brain synaptosomes. Biochem Biophys Res Commun 108:640–646.

Yousif FB, Bolger GT, Ruzycky A, Triggle DJ (1985): Ca^{2+} channel antagonist actions in bladder smooth muscle: Comparative pharmacologic and [^{3}H]nitrendipine binding studies. Can J Physiol Pharmacol 63:453–462.

Yousif FB, Triggle DJ (1986): Inhibitory actions of a series of Ca^{2+} channel antagonists against agonist and K^+ depolarization induced responses in smooth muscle: An assessment of selectivity of action. Can J Physiol Pharmacol 64:273–283.

Structure and Physiology of the Slow Inward Calcium Channel, pages 51–70
© 1987 Alan R. Liss, Inc.

3

Ca²⁺ Channel Ligands: Comparative Pharmacology

A. Scriabine

*Miles Institute for Preclinical Pharmacology, P.O. Box 1956,
New Haven, Connecticut 06509*

INTRODUCTION

The term "Ca^{2+} antagonists" as introduced by Fleckenstein [1971, 1983] referred to drugs which interfere with the mediator function of Ca^{2+} in the excitation-contraction coupling. They were considered specific if the interference was so predominant that at pharmacologic doses other properties were more or less negligible. With the discovery of receptors for Ca^{2+} channel antagonists, the term "Ca^{2+} channel ligands" was introduced. It is being used in this chapter for drugs which bind to Ca^{2+} channels or to specific receptors associated with the channels. Ca^{2+} channel ligands modulate the function of channels either by inhibiting or enhancing the entry of Ca^{2+} ions. Ligands may also exist which bind to the same receptors as antagonists or agonists, but exert no direct pharmacologic effects, although they may displace other ligands and, therefore, interfere with the pharmacologic effects of either antagonists or agonists.

The inhibition or entry of calcium ions through sarcolemma of vascular smooth muscle or of myocardial cells is a common property of a chemically heterogenous group of drugs. The first drugs observed to inhibit slow inward Ca^{2+} current were prenylamine, verapamil, and gallopamil [Fleckenstein et al., 1967, 1969]. The discovery of nifedipine [Vater et al., 1972] and demonstration of its high Ca^{2+} antagonistic activity [Fleckenstein,

1971] established 1,4-dihydropyridines (DHPs) as a class of highly specific inhibitors of Ca^{2+} entry. Subsequently, many previously known vasodilators, e.g., diltiazem [Sato et al., 1971; Nakajima et al., 1975] or perhexiline [Hudak et al., 1970; Fleckenstein-Grün et al. 1978] were found to block or reduce slow inward Ca^{2+} currents.

The discovery of Ca^{2+} channel activators or agonists [Schramm et al., 1983; Takenaka and Maeno, 1982; Truog et al., 1984] led to the realization that slight differences in the chemical structure may determine the consequences of binding [Hof et al., 1985; Francowiak et al., 1985; Kongsamut et al., 1985; Gjörstrup et al., 1986] and even stereoisomers of the same compound may have opposite pharmacological effects.

The purpose of this chapter is to compare pharmacological effects of drugs with known Ca^{2+} channel ligand activity and to analyze differences in their pharmacological properties.

Ca²⁺ CHANNEL ANTAGONISTS

Comparison Between Groups

We can differentiate now at least three major groups of Ca^{2+} channel antagonists: phenylalkylamines, 1,4-dihydropyridines, and benzothiazepines. In addition, it has been

TABLE I. Comparison of Three Major Groups of Ca^{2+} Channel Antagonists

Properties	Phenylalkylamines (e.g., verapamil)	1,4-Dihydropyridines (e.g., nifedipine)	Benzothiazepines (e.g., diltiazem)
Specificity for Ca^{2+} channels	Are likely to interact with other ion channels and/or receptors	At therapeutic doses, are specific for Ca^{2+} channels	At therapeutic doses, are specific for Ca^{2+} channels
Tissue specificity	SA and AV node, myocardium, vascular smooth muscle	Vascular smooth muscle, myocardium, neurones	Vascular smooth muscle
Clinical indications	Supraventricular arrhythmias, hypertension, angina, cytoprotection	Angina, hypertension, stroke, cytoprotection	Angina, hypertension

claimed that many drugs of different chemical structures have Ca^{2+} channel antagonistic effects, often as a secondary pharmacological property. Table I compares the general properties of the three major groups of Ca^{2+} channel antagonists. Drugs from each group reduce a slow, inward Ca^{2+} current. The receptor sites for each of the three groups appear to be different, although they are apparently allosterically linked [Bolger et al., 1983; Glossmann et al.,1984]. A Ca^{2+} channel ligand of one group can either reduce or enhance binding of a ligand from another group.

The specificity of Ca^{2+} channel ligands for their receptor sites varies from one group to another. Verapamil is known to interact not only with the receptors associated with Ca^{2+} channels, but also with adrenergic and muscarinic receptors [Karliner et al., 1981]; verapamil (but not nitrendipine) was shown to antagonize presynaptic inhibitory effects of dopamine at the adrenergic nerve endings [Johnson et al., 1983].

There are significant and clinically important differences in tissue specificity between various groups of Ca^{2+} channel antagonists. Phenylalkylamines are very effective in slowing impulse conduction in SA and AV nodes. This negative dromotropic property is of considerable clinical significance: it determines the effectiveness of phenylalkylamines in the treatment of supraventricular arrhythmias. It can, however, also lead to A-V block particularly when sympathetic tone is reduced (e.g., after β-adrenoceptor blockade). Phenylalkylamines have also a more pronounced negative inotropic action than either 1,4-DHPs or benzothiazepines. Some 1,4-DHPs (e.g., nimodipine) and other Ca^{2+} antagonists were found to have neuronal effects. It is presently not clear, however, whether a relative absence of CNS effects with phenylalkylamines and benzothiazepines is due to their failure to act on neuronal tissue or to a relative inability to enter CNS. Clinical indications for Ca^{2+} channel antagonists (Table I) reflect not only

their known pharmacological properties but also clinical experience with these drugs. Some Ca^{2+} channel antagonists were tested clinically only as antianginal or antihypertensive drugs, although they appear to be useful in other indications as well.

Phenylalkylamines. The best known phenylalkylamine with Ca^{2+} channel antagonistic properties is verapamil. Its pharmacology was first described 24 years ago by Haas and Härtfelder [1962]. The drug was shown to dilate vascular smooth muscle and was recommended as a coronary vasodilator. Its Ca^{2+} channel antagonistic action was described by Fleckenstein [1968], who found that verapamil was more potent and more selective than prenylamine as an inhibitor of Ca^{2+} entry. Shortly thereafter, Fleckenstein et al. [1969] identified gallopamil (D600) as being even more potent than verapamil.

During the last 20 years, verapamil was widely used as an antiarrhythmic, antianginal, and, more recently, also as an antihypertensive agent [Baky, 1984]. Extensive clinical experience with the drug is probably the most important advantage of verapamil over other phenylalkylamines. Table II lists the major phenylalkylamines with Ca^{2+} channel antagonistic properties. They differ from each other in potency, specificity for Ca^{2+} channels, duration of action, and pharmacokinetic parameters. They all depress A-V nodal conduction and prolong P-R interval. In vitro, they depress myocardial contractile force, but in vivo their afterload-reducing activity and reflex sympathetic stimulation tend to counteract their myocardial depressant action.

Tiapamil resembles verapamil in having coronary vasodilator, antihypertensive, and antiarrhythmic properties [Eigenmann et al., 1981; Saini and Antonaccio, 1982; Opie et al., 1985]. As a negative inotropic agent, tiapamil is approximately 100 times less potent than verapamil. The specificity of tiapamil for Ca^{2+} channels is lower than for many other Ca^{2+} channel antagonists; it is also an effec-

TABLE II. Phenylalkylamines

Drugs	Chemical structure	Major pharmacological properties	References
Verapamil		Depresses A-V nodal conduction; prolongs P-R interval; antagonizes Ca^{2+}-induced vasoconstriction; antiarrhythmic; hypotensive; as a Ca^{2+} channel antagonist $(-)$isomer, is more potent than $(+)$isomer	Haas and Härtfelder, 1962; Fleckenstein, 1968; Baky, 1984
Prenylamine		Vasodilator, has low specificity for Ca^{2+} channels; inhibited excitation-contraction coupling in the heart muscle	Fleckenstein, 1964, 1983; Lindner, 1960
Gallopamil		More potent than verapamil as myocardial Ca^{2+} antagonist	Fleckenstein et al., 1969; Haas and Busch, 1967
Fendiline		Negative chronotropic; increases coronary blood flow to ischemic areas; inhibits Ca^{2+}-induced contractions of skinned smooth muscle completely displace $[^3H]$nitrendipine	Leszkowsky et al., 1966; Czik et al., 1983; Spedding, 1983
Terodiline		Blocks Ca^{2+} uptake into smooth muscle and also releases Ca^{2+} from intracellular stores; weak Ca^{2+} antagonist—IC_{50} from 2×10^{-5} to 5×10^{-6} M; no	Larsson-Backstrom et al., 1985

Name	Structure	Activity	Reference
Tiapamil	(chemical structure)	substantial difference between potencies on myocardium or vascular tissue	Eigenmann et al., 1981; Saini and Antonaccio, 1982
Anipamil	(chemical structure)	Blocks Na$^+$ channels at the same concentrations as Ca^{2+} channels; blocks ^{45}Ca entry into vascular smooth muscle; coronary vasodilator; as negative inotropic, 100 times less potent than verapamil; inhibits [^{3}H]nitrendipine binding to cardiac membranes; antiarrhythmic	Gries and Raschack, 1984
Ronipamil	(chemical structure)	Cardioprotective; hepatoprotective; has longer duration of action than verapamil	Hock et al, 1985
HOE 263	(chemical structure)	Cardioprotective; hepatoprotective	Lindner et al., 1984
SC-30552	(chemical structure)	Equally effective on the heart and vascular smooth muscle; cardiac depressant; as Ca^{2+} channel antagonist, equal in potency to verapamil; weak inhibitor of [^{3}H]nitrendipine binding, but unlike verapamil, can	Radzialowski et al., 1985

Long-acting antihypertensive; reduces peripheral vascular resistance without tachycardia; has negative inotropic activity in vivo

tive inhibitor of Na^+ channels. The last property may be partially responsible for its antiarrhythmic efficacy.

Hoe-263 was found to be equipotent with verapamil and much more potent than prenylamine in decreasing the upstroke velocity of the slow inward current of K^+-depolarized papillary muscles from guinea pigs. As an inhibitor of K^+-mediated contractions of guinea pig pulmonary artery, Hoe-263 was slightly more potent than verapamil. The site of Hoe-263-action was also thought to be similar to that of verapamil, although displacement of [^{3}H]nitrendipine from its binding sites on dog heart membrane preparation was more complete by Hoe-263 than by verapamil [Lindner et al., 1984].

Anipamil and ronipamil were described as having cardioprotective and hepatoprotective effects as well as prolonging survival of rats subjected to traumatic shock [Gries and Raschak, 1984; Hock et al., 1985; Lefer and Papanicolau, 1985]. It is not clear whether these effects are significantly different from those of verapamil. An unexpected effect of ronipamil was observed in perfused cat livers. The drug produced a marked increase in bile formation and secretion; this effect was not observed with anipamil.

1,4-Dihydropyridines (DHPs). The best-known DHP with Ca^{2+} channel antagonistic activity is nifedipine (Table III). Its pharmacology was first described by Vater et al. [1972] and its Ca^{2+} channel antagonistic activity by Fleckenstein [1971]. These investigators reported high potency of nifedipine as a coronary vasodilator and specificity of its Ca^{2+} channel antagonist activity. Subsequent studies confirmed the initial findings [for reviews see Kroneberg, 1975; Kazda and Scriabine, 1986]. Nifedipine found its major use in the treatment of angina pectoris, where Ca^{2+} channel antagonists relax coronary spasms and reduce oxygen demand. Nifedipine is also effective in lowering arterial pressure and in preventing development of hypertension in experimental animals [Kazda et al., 1983a]. In hypertensive animals or humans nifedipine reduces peripheral vascular resistance with little or no tachycardia or sodium and water retention.

Other first-generation DHPs include SKF 24260 [Fielden et al., 1974], ryosidine [Fleckenstein, 1983], and niludipine [Fleckenstein et al., 1979] (Table IIIa). None of these compounds was marketed, although their pharmacologic effects suggest their possible therapeutic usefulness in the treatment of coronary heart disease or hypertension.

Subsequent research in the field of DHPs led to the development of second-generation compounds which differed from nifedipine in their relative potency, duration of action, lipid solubility (and, therefore, tissue distribution), and a relatively greater potency in certain vascular beads (e.g., cerebral circulation). The quantitative differences in their negative inotropic/vasodilator ratios and the intracellular effects of some of them (e.g., calmodulin antagonism by felodipine) were also reported. These second-generation compounds include: nitrendipine [Stoepel et al., 1981; Scriabine et al., 1984a,b], nisoldipine [Kazda et al., 1980, 1983b], nimodipine [Kazda et al., 1982; Hoffmeister et al., 1982; Scriabine et al., 1985], nicardipine [Takenaka et al., 1976], felodipine [Boström et al., 1981], amlodipine [Dodd and Machin, 1985] and others. Tables III$_a$ and III$_b$ summarize pharmacological effects of many known DHPs and their possible clinical advantages.

Although on isolated smooth or heart muscle preparations various DHPs may exhibit only minor quantitative differences in potency, their in vivo pharmacology may differ considerably. The ability of Ca^{2+} channel antagonists to enter the central nervous system may determine not only their CNS effects, but also their in vivo cardiovascular actions. Higuchi et al. [1985] reported a central hypotensive effect of nifedipine when administered into the brain stem of rats. Nicardipine, however, was recently reported to elevate arterial pressure by intrathecal administration to dogs, while lowering it by intravenous route [Chelly et al., 1986]. Central Ca^{2+} channel antagonism may apparently lead to sympathetic stimulation and a consequent rise in arterial pressure in dogs. A lesser tendency of nimodipine to lower arterial pressure [Kazda et al., 1982], therefore, can be conceivably explained by greater ability of that drug to enter CNS [Van den Kerckhoff and Drewes, 1985], to increase sympathetic tone, and consequently to antagonize its own peripheral hypotensive effect.

In an attempt to develop new and more selective 1,4-dihydropyridines [Bossert et al., 1979; Meyer et al., 1981] structural changes in the nifedipine molecule included changes in the ester function and substitutions in the 2, 3, or 4 positions of the phenyl ring. The resulting compounds had higher lipophilicity and higher vasodilator potency than nifedipine (e.g., nisoldipine). Introduction of a nitrogen-containing side chain in position R_3 led to a water soluble compound, nicardipine [Takenaka et al., 1976], which was shown to have vasodilator activity in peripheral, coronary, and cerebral circulation [Baky, 1985].

Substitution of the methyl group in the R_5 position with aminoethoxymethyl group led to the synthesis of amlodipine [Dodd and Machin, 1985; Beresford et al., 1985], which offers a different pharmacokinetic profile: longer plasma half-life and 100% oral bioavailability. These pharmacokinetic properties apparently are responsible for longer duration of action and the maintenance of a sustained antihypertensive effect by once-a-day administration.

The 1,4-dihydropyridine differ from each other, also, in the ratios of their vasodilator: negative inotropic actions. The asymmetric esters: nitrendipine and nisoldipine have a lower ratio of their EC_{50} for vasodilator to myocardial depressant actions than nifedipine [Kazda et al., 1980; Stoepel et al., 1981; Scriabine et al., 1984a]. Also, PN 200-110 and PY 108-068 were reported to be more potent coronary vasodilators than negative inotropic agents [Wada et al., 1985; Hof et al., 1982, 1984; Hof, 1985]. The last two compounds differ from each other in their effects on SA nodal automaticity and AV nodal conduction. PY 108-068 suppresses SA nodal automaticity and AV nodal conduction to the same extent. PN 200-110 is more potent in suppressing SA nodal automaticity than in prolonging AV nodal conduction [Wada et al., 1985].

During the last few years, many new 1,4-hydropyridines were developed: most of them are listed in Tables IIIa and IIIb. Some of the new compounds have distinctly different pharmacological properties. BMY 20064, for example, has, in addition to its Ca^{2+} channel antagonistic effects, also an α_1-adrenoceptor blocking activity [Stanton et al., 1986].

Absence of in vivo negative dromotropic action represents one of the significant advantages of DHPs. Reflex sympathetic activation after administration of DHPs tends to counteract their direct negative dromotropic action. In vitro, however, on isolated, spontaneously contracting SA-node preparations, of rabbits, Molyvdas and Sperelakis [1986] found that mesudipine, nilvadipine, nifedipine, and verapamil can (at 1×10^{-7} M and higher concentrations) depress slow action potentials and automaticity of the SA-node. The prolongation of the A-H interval may also be dependent on the degree of hypoxia. Before hypoxia, verapamil and nifedipine prolonged the A-H interval in isolated perfused rabbit hearts. During hypoxia, however, the intensity of AH prolongation was significantly attenuated by the same Ca^{2+} channel antagonists [Arno et al., 1986].

Benzothiazepines. As with 1,4-dihydropyridines, diltiazem inhibits contractile activity of vascular smooth muscle and is more effective against K$^+$ - than against norepinephrine-induced contractions [Sato et al., 1971; Flaim, 1984; Chaffman and Brogden, 1985]. In normal or ischemic hearts, diltiazem dilates coronary arteries as well as collateral blood vessels. In isolated rabbit heart, diltiazem was shown to suppress SA nodal function, AV node conduction, and to prolong the AV node refractory period [Kawai et al., 1981]. In dogs, in vivo diltiazem prolonged the AV nodal refractory period and shortened sinus node recovery time. These effects were seen at doses which produced no substantial effect on arterial pressure [Fujimoto et al., 1981]. In man, diltiazem, unlike phenylalkylamines or 1,4-dihydropyridines, has a negative chronotropic action. Conceivably, this property is of clinical advantage, since it may lead to greater reduction in myocardial oxygen consumption [Bourassa, 1985]. It may also represent a disadvantage since diltiazem may enhance bradycardia or A-V block, particularly in

TABLE IIIa. 1,4-Dihydropyridines With Ca^{2+} Channel Antagonistic Activity

Name and/or code No.	R$_1$	R$_2$	R$_3$	R$_4$	R$_5$	Major pharmacological properties	References
Nifedipine	H	NO$_2$	−COOCH$_3$	−COOCH$_3$	CH$_3$	Coronary vasodilator; hypotensive; uterine relaxant; protects tissue from Ca^{2+} overload	Vater et al., 1972
SKF 24260	H	CF$_3$	−COOC$_2$H$_5$	−COOC$_2$H$_5$	CH$_3$	Hypotensive; vasodilator; no direct comparison with nifedipine available	Fieldenetal, 1974
Ryosidine	H	−OCHF$_2$	−COOCH$_3$	−COOCH$_3$	CH$_3$	Indistinguishable pharmacologically from nifedipine	Fleckenstein, 1983
Niludipine	NO$_2$	H	−COOCH$_2$CH$_2$OC$_3$H$_7$	−COOCH$_2$CH$_2$C$_3$H$_7$	CH$_3$	Hypotensive; vasodilator; cerebral vasodilator; as potent as nifedipine	Fleckenstein et al., 1979
Nitrendipine	NO$_2$	H	−COOCH$_3$	−COOC$_2$H$_5$	CH$_3$	More potent and longer acting than nifedipine; has more peripheral than cerebral vasodilator activities	Stoepel et al., 1981; Scriabine et al., 1984a,b
Nisoldipine	H	NO$_2$	−COOCH$_3$	−COOCH$_2$CH(CH$_3$)CH$_3$	CH$_3$	As a vasodilator, is 10 times more potent than nifedipine; vasoselective; has longer duration of action; has less negative inotropic activity than nifedipine	Kazda et al., 1980, 1983
Nimodipine	NO$_2$	H	−COOCH$_2$−CH$_2$−OCH$_3$	−COOCH(CH$_3$)CH$_3$	CH$_3$	Enters CNS better than nifedipine; relatively selective cerebral vasodilator; less hypotensive than nifedipine; protects	Kazda et al., 1982; Hoffmeister et al., 1982; Scriabine et al., 1985

Compound						Activity	References
					CH$_3$	brain from ischemia; anticonvulsant	
Ryodipine, PP-1466	H	OCHF$_2$	–COOCH$_3$	–COOCH$_3$	CH$_3$	Similar to nifedipine; more stable when exposed to light; has longer half-life in dogs than nifedipine or nicardipine	Inoue et al., 1985; Parinov et al., 1985
Nicardipine	NO$_2$	H	–CO$_2$(CH$_2$)$_2$–N(CH$_3$)CH$_2$C$_6$H$_5$	–COOCH$_3$	CH$_3$	Potent and long-lasting coronary and cerebral vasodilator; used clinically as antihypertensive and antianginal	Takenaka et al., 1976; Baky, 1985
Felodipine	CL	Cl	–COOCH$_2$CH$_3$	–COOCH$_3$	CH$_3$	Long-acting peripheral vasodilator; in addition to Ca^{2+} channel blockade, may have calmodulin antagonist properties	Bostrom et al., 1981
Nilvadipine FR 34235	NO$_2$	H	–COOCH$_3$	–COOCH(CH$_3$)$_2$	CN	Renal vasodilator; poor antihypertensive; diuretic	Jim and Matthews, 1985; Allison et al., 1985
Amlodipine	H	Cl	–COOC$_2$H$_5$	–COOCH$_3$	CH$_2$OCH$_2$CH$_2$NH$_2$	Antihypertensive with slow onset and long duration of action	Beresford et al., 1985; Dodd and Machin, 1985
FR 7534	NO$_2$	H	–COOC$_2$H$_5$	–COOC$_2$H$_5$	CH$_2$OH	Four times less potent than nifedipine as coronary vasodilator and hypotensive	Jolly et al., 1981
BM 20064	NO$_2$	H	–COO(CH$_2$)$_3$–[piperazinyl-N-(2-methoxyphenyl)]	–COOCH$_3$	CH$_3$	Has also α$_1$-adrenoceptor blocking activity; equivalent to nifedipine in potency as a Ca channel antagonist	Stanton et al., 1986
KW 3049	NO$_2$	H	–COO–[1-benzylpiperidin-4-yl]	–COOCH$_3$	CH$_3$	Has slow onset and long duration of action	Kubo et al., 1985

TABLE IIIb. 1,4-Dihydropyridines With Ca²⁺ Channel Antagonistic Activity

Name and/or code No.	Chemical structure	Major pharmacological properties	References
Flordipine		Prodrug, converted to active metabolites, which have Ca channel antagonistic activity; increases coronary, skeletal, and cerebral blood flow in rabbits	Shlevin et al., 1983; Mayhan and Heistad, 1985
PN 200-110		Relatively vasoselective; at 2×10^{-8}M protects isolated hearts from global ischemia	Hof et al., 1984; Cook and Hof, 1985
Darodipine, PY 108-068		Produces little or no reflex tachycardia in man; depresses sinus node more than nifedipine; a potent coronary vasodilator	Hof et al., 1982
Mesudipine		Equipotent with nifedipine on guinea pig papillary muscles; cardiac effects are frequency-dependent; at 10^{-8} M blocks slow APs	Molyvdas and Sperelakis, 1983, 1986
FR 7534		Coronary vasodilator has relatively selective action for subepicardial region; hypotensive	Meils et al., 1981; Warltier et al., 1983
8363-S		By oral route, more potent and longer acting than either nifedipine or nicardipine	Matsumara et al., 1985

Oxodipine

Similar to PY 108-068; not photolabile; reduces NE- and K$^+$-induced ^{45}Ca efflux in rat aortic strips

Marin et al., 1985

TABLE IV. Benzothiazepines and Related Compounds

Name and/or code No.	Chemical structure	Major pharmacological properties	References
Diltiazem		Weaker vasodilator than nifedipine; at coronary vasodilator concentrations (10^{-6} M) has no negative inotropic action; antagonizes ischemia-induced arrhythmias; negative chronotropic in man	Nagao et al., 1972; Flaim, 1984; Bourassa, 1985; Chaffman and Brogden, 1985
RT 362		May have intracellular site of action; in normal Ca^{2+} medium, inhibited NE-, methoxamine-, or 5-HT-, but not KCl- or histamine-induced contractions of smooth muscle; negative inotropic on rabbit atria	Wakabayashi et al., 1985
Fostedil, KB 944		Depresses A-V node in dogs; blocks slow Ca channels, but also displays hyperpolarizing action; vasodilator; hypotensive	Morita et al., 1982; Patterson et al., 1984; Gatlin et al., 1983

combination with digitalis or β-adrenoceptor antagonists [Crawford, 1985].

Remarkably few benzothiazepines or related drugs were developed in spite of extensive clinical use of diltiazem. Of structural interest are RT 362 [Wakabayashi et al., 1985] and fostedil [Morita et al., 1982]; they are listed in Table IV. The development of fostedil was discontinued because of toxicological problems.

Miscellaneous Ca^{2+} channel antagonists. Lidoflazine, cinnarizine, and flunarizine are piperazine derivatives which were reported to have Ca^{2+} antagonistic properties. This group of drugs appears to be less specific for Ca^{2+} channels than either 1,4-dihydropyridines, diltiazem, or even verapamil-like phenylalkylamines. According to Fleckenstein [1983], lidoflazine [Van Nueten and Wellens, 1979; Vanhoutte and Van Nueten, 1983] is "predominantly Na-antagonistic rather than Ca-antagonistic," while cinnarizine [Godfraind and Sturbois, 1975; Vanhoutte, 1982; Godfraind, 1982] and flunarizine [Van Nueten and Vanhoutte, 1984] appear to be more specific as calcium antagonists than lidoflazine. Flunarizine was shown to inhibit Ca^{2+} entry into the cells [Godfraind, 1981] and to reduce binding of [^{3}H]nitrendipine to cell membrane fractions [Bolger et al., 1983]. Its use was recommended in the treatment of peripheral vascular and cerebrovascular diseases, migraine, epilepsy, and various conditions associated with cell hypoxia. Piperazines appear to act at verapamil, and not at diltiazem or DHP binding sites [Snyder and Reynolds, 1984].

There are many other miscellaneous compounds, which were reported to have Ca channel antagonistic activity, although it is not always clear whether their effects are specific for Ca^{2+} channels. These drugs include bepridil [Cosnier et al., 1977; Marshall et al., 1984], brovincamine [Katsuragi et al., 1984], perhexiline [Hudak et al., 1970], caroverine [Fleckenstein and Späh, 1982], and many others. Bepridil is probably the best known of these compounds. Unlike most Ca^{2+} channel antagonists, bepridil inhibits not only Ca^{2+} but also fast Na$^+$ channels and is in this

TABLE V. Inhibition of [^{3}H]Nitrendipine Binding to Membranes From Cerebral Cortex of Rats*

Drug	IC$_{50}$ (nM)
Pimozide	13
Clopimozide	17
Fluspirilene	21
Penfluridol	30
Lidoflazine	650
Spiperone	2,500

*Adapted from Gould, RJ et al., 1983.

respect similar to lidocaine. There is also evidence that bepridil interferes with the release of intercellular Ca^{2+} in the vascular smooth muscle [Mras and Sperelakis, 1981]. Clinically, bepridil is effective in the therapy of supraventricular, as well as ventricular, arrhythmias and in angina pectoris. Of concern are *torsades de pointes*, observed occasionally in patients receiving bepridil [Leclercq et al., 1983].

Ca^{2+} channel antagonistic activity is a likely secondary property of many well established or experimental drugs, which are either in clinical use or under development for a variety of therapeutic indications. An antidiarrheal drug, loperamide, was described to have a Ca^{2+} channel antagonistic property on intestinal smooth muscle and to modulate the activity of Ca^{2+} channels by an apparently verapamil-like action [Reynolds et al., 1984; Snyder and Reynolds, 1984]. An antiarrhythmic agent, asocainol [Späh, 1986], and a β-adrenoceptor antagonist, CGS 10078B [Gallo et al., 1985], were described to have Ca^{2+} channel antagonistic activity as a secondary pharmacologic property.

Neuroleptics were described to inhibit [^{3}H]-nitrendipine binding to membranes from cerebral cortex of rats (Table V) [Gould et al., 1983]. Diphenylbutylpiperidines were found to be much more potent Ca^{2+} channel antagonists than either butyrophenones or phenothiazines. It was suggested that the ability of diphenylbutylpiperidines to improve personal interaction and reduce emotional withdrawal may be attributed to Ca^{2+} channel antagonistic properties of these drugs [Snyder and Reynolds, 1984]. [^{3}H]Nitrendipine binding can

TABLE VI. Inhibition of [^{3}H]Nitrendipine Binding by Calmodulin Antagonists to Membranes From Guinea Pig Ileum*

Drug	IC$_{50}$ (μM)
Calmidazolium	0.07
Pimozide	0.1
Trifluoperazine	4.1
Chlorpromazine	25
Promethazine	90

*Adapted from Luchowski, EM et al., 1984.

be antagonized by some calmodulin antagonists, with or without neuroleptic activity (Table VI) [Luchowski et al., 1984]. No clear relationship was established, however, between therapeutic and calcium channel antagonistic properties of these drugs.

Ca^{2+} CHANNEL AGONISTS

From the five 1,4-dihydropyridines with Ca^{2+} channel agonist properties listed in Table VII, BAY K 8644 is the most potent and the most extensively studied compound. It was discovered by Schramm et al. [1983] and shown to have cardiotonic, as well as vasoconstrictor, properties. Its activity was attributed to its (−)−(4S)-isomer, while (+)−(4R)-isomer had Ca^{2+} channel antagonistic properties [Franckowiak et al., 1985]. As an antagonist, (+)-(4R)-isomer is much less potent than (−)−(4S)-isomer as an agonist.

The pharmacology of 1,4-dihydropyridines with Ca^{2+} channel agonist properties was reviewed by Schramm and Towart [1985] and Preuss et al. [1985]. The Bay K 8644-induced pressor and positive inotropic effects appear to be primarily due to the increase in Ca^{2+} entry into vascular smooth muscle or myocardial cells, respectively. The possibility of an additional enhancement of catecholamine release from the nerve endings or from adrenal medulla was not, however, excluded [Garcia et al., 1984]. BAY K 8644 was also used to study the role of Ca^{2+} in the excitation-secretion coupling. Recently, this drug was found to stimulate calcitonin and to suppress parathyroid hormone release from isolated parathyroid glands of rat pups [Cooper et al., 1986].

BAY K 8644 proved to be an extremely useful tool for studying Ca^{2+} channels in single cells. This drug was found to enhance Ca^{2+} channel current by promoting the form of gating (mode 2) which favors long openings of Ca^{2+} channels [Hess et al., 1985]. The activity of BAY K 8644 was found to depend on membrane potential. Only when currents were measured from a negative holding potential did BAY K 8644 increase Ca^{2+} currents [Sanguinetti and Kass, 1984].

Of particular importance for potential use of Ca^{2+} channel agonists as cardiotonics was the observation of Thomas et al. [1985] that BAY K 8644 increases Ca^{2+} influx primarily during the initial 50 msec of systole, with little or no increase during the later parts of action potential. Such initial increase in Ca^{2+} influx can conceivably lead to a more efficient utilization of calcium and reduced tendency to produce side effects associated with Ca^{2+} overload.

All of the presently known 1,4-dihydropyridines with Ca^{2+} channel agonist activity (BAY K 8644, YC-170, CGP 28392, H 160/51, and 202-791) increase Ca^{2+} entry into the vascular smooth muscle to the same or even greater extent as into myocardial cells. The resulting peripheral and coronary vasoconstriction tends to increase left ventricular afterload and to decrease myocardial perfusion. Only a few studies involving comparison of pharmacological effects of CGP 28392 and BAY K 8644 under the same experimental conditions have been published. Preuss et al. [1984] reported that in conscious dogs in vivo, CGP 28392, unlike BAY K 8644, had only hypertensive, and no positive inotropic action. Hypertension was associated with reflex bradycardia. In a comparative study on isolated rat portal vein, Mikkelsen et al. [1985] found that both drugs enhance mechanical activity, but the preparation was more sensitive to BAY K 8644 than to CGP 28392. Of interest was their observation that ultraviolet radiation diminished the effect of BAY K 8644 but not of CGP 28392.

Ca^{2+} channel agonist properties were also reported for substances other than 1,4-dihydropyridines. The first animal toxin reported

TABLE VII. Ca²⁺ Channel Agonists

Name or code No.	Chemical structure	Major pharmacological properties	References
YC-170		Vasopressor in anesthetized rats and dogs; vasoconstrictor on rabbit aorta; considerably less potent than BAY K 8644	Takenaka and Maeno, 1982
BAY K 8644		Stimulates Ca^{2+} entry into vascular smooth muscle, myocardium, endocrine cells and neurones; vasopressor and cardiotonic, CNS stimulant and convulsant; more potent than either YC-170 or CGP 28392	Schramm et al., 1983; Towart et al., 1985; Preuss et al., 1984
CGP 28392		In vitro, has effects qualitatively similar to BAY K 8644 but is less potent; displaces [³H]nitrendipine from its binding sites	Truog et al., 1984; Freedman and Miller, 1984
H 160/51		(−) Enantiomer is agonist, but racemate has similar agonist activity; EC_{50} on papillary muscles 1.8×10^{-6} M; vasoconstrictor on rat portal vein	Gjörstrup et al., 1986
202-791 S(+)-isomer		Contracts pig coronary artery at 0.1 nM–3.5 μM; has endothelium-dependent relaxant effect at higher concentrations	Kongsamut et al., 1985

to activate Ca^{2+} channels, was maitotoxin [Takahashi et al., 1983]. It contracted guinea pig ileum and taenia caeci at concentrations ranging from 100 pg to 300 ng per ml. However, maitotoxin did not displace [^{3}H]nitrendipine from rat brain synaptosomes, although its effect on ^{45}Ca influx was antagonized by Ca^{2+} channel antagonists [Miller et al., 1984]. Of greater interest is a more recently described atrotoxin, a protein from *Crotalus atrox* venom [Hamilton et al., 1985]. The atrotoxininduced increase in Ca^{2+} current was blocked by cobalt or nitrendipine. Atrotoxin also inhibited [^{3}H]nitrendipine binding to guinea pig ventricular membrane preparation, apparently by an allosteric mechanism.

Of considerable theoretical interest was the discovery by Mestre et al. [1985] that PK 11195 (1-(2-chlorophenyl)-N-methyl-N-(1-methylpropyl)-3-isoquinoline carboxyamide), an antagonist of peripheral-type benzodiazepine receptors, antagonizes negative inotropic effects of nitrendipine, verapamil, or diltiazem and the positive inotropic effects of BAY K 8644. The authors interpreted their findings as evidence that peripheral-type benzodiazepine receptors are coupled to calcium channels. Their results also suggest that drugs may exist which could interact with Ca^{2+} channels without having either Ca^{2+} antagonist or agonist effects.

CONCLUSIONS

Ca^{2+} channel ligands are defined as drugs which bind to Ca^{2+} channels or specific sarcolemmal receptors associated with Ca^{2+} channels. They include Ca^{2+} channel antagonists, agonists and possibly other drugs which can interact with the same receptors.

Chemically, Ca^{2+} channel antagonists are a heterogeneous group of drugs, but three major groups were identified: phenylalkylamines, 1,4-dihydropyridines, and benzothiazepines. Their specificity for Ca^{2+} channels, duration of action, lipid solubility, ability to enter CNS and to activate the sympathetic

nervous system either directly or by a reflex mechanisms, ability to penetrate sarcolemma and to exert additional effects on intracellular Ca^{2+} translocation distinguish various Ca^{2+} antagonists from each other and determine their pharmacological profiles.

Some of the pharmacological differences between the various Ca^{2+} channel antagonists described in this chapter determine clinical indications for these drugs. They include angina pectoris, essential and pulmonary hypertension, peripheral vascular disease, cerebrovascular incidents, conditions associated with brain hypoxia, and premature labor. Many other indications are also being actively explored.

Many drugs, which are well established in the therapy of a variety of diseases were found to compete with Ca^{2+} channel ligands for their binding sites. The importance of this interaction is not yet fully appreciated.

Ca^{2+} channel agonists are, at present, largely experimental tools, but their use in the treatment of heart failure is conceivable, particularly if cardioselective drugs can be identified. Conceivably, they can also be useful in the treatment of shock.

REFERENCES

Allison N, Dubb J, Alexander S, Bodenheimer S, Familiar R, Blumberg A, Stote, R (1985): Effect of nilvadipine on renal function in normal man. Fed Proc 44:1638 (Abs. 7179).

Anno T, Kodama I, Shibata S, Toyama J, Yamada K (1986): Effects of calcium, calcium entry blockers and calmodulin inhibitors on atrioventricular conduction disturbance induced by hypoxia. Br J Pharmac 88: 277–284.

Baik YH, Dube GP, Vaghy P, Rapoport R, Schwartz A (1985): Modification of effects of enantiomers of a 1,4-dihydropyridine (202–791) by endothelium and light in pig coronary artery. Pharmacologist 27:267.

Baky S (1984): Verapamil. In Scriabine A (ed): "New Drugs Annual: Cardiovascular Drugs." New York: Raven Press, pp 71–102.

Baky S (1985): Nicardipine hydrochloride. In Scriabine A (ed): "New Cardiovascular Drugs 1985." New York: Raven Press, pp 153–172.

Beresford AP, Humphrey MJ, Stopher DA (1985) Amlodipine, a calcium channel blocker with pharmacokinetic properties novel to dihydropyridines. Br J Pharmacol 85:333P.

Bolger GT, Gengo P, Klockowski R, Luchowski E, Siegel H, Janis RA, Triggle AM, Triggle DJ (1983): Characterization of binding of the Ca^{2+} channel antagonist, nitrendipine to guinea pig ileal muscle. J Pharmacol Exp Ther 225:291–309.

Boström SL, Ljung B, Mardh S, Forsen S, Thulin E (1981): Interaction of the antihypertensive drug felodipine with calmodulin. Nature 292:777–778.

Bossert F, Horstmann H, Meyer H, Vater W (1979): Einfluss der Esterfunktion auf die vasodilatierenden Eigenschaften von 1,4-dihydro-2,6-dimethyl-4-nitrophenylpyridine-3,5-carbonsäureestern. Arzneim Forsch 29:226–229.

Bourassa MG (1985): Hemodynamic and electrophysiologic effects of diltiazem. Acta Pharmacol Toxicol (Copenh) 57(Suppl 2)21–30.

Chaffman M, Brogden RN (1985): Diltiazem: A review of its pharmacological properties and therapeutic efficacy. Drugs 29:387–454.

Chelly J, Montastruc J-L, Doursout M-F, Dang-Trang L, Hysing E, Montastruc P (1986): Blockade of central calcium channels induces hypertension in dogs. Hypertension 8:(4) Suppl part 2: I–66–I–69.

Cook NS, Hof RP (1985): Cardioprotection by the calcium antagonist PN 200–110 in the absence and presence of cardiodepression. Br J Pharmacol 86: 181–189.

Cooper CW, Borosky SA, Farrell PE, Steinsland OS (1986): Effects of the calcium channel activator BAY K 8644 on in vitro secretion of calcitonin and parathyroid hromone. Endocrinology 118:545–549.

Cosnier D, Duchene-Marullaz P, Rispat G, Streichberger G (1977): Cardiovascular pharmacology of bepridil(1[3–isobutoxy-2-(benzylphenyl) amino]propyl pyrrolidine hydrochloride) a new potential antianginal compound. Arch Int Pharmacodyn 225:133–151.

Crawford MW (1985): Effectiveness of diltiazem for chronic stable angina pectoris. Acta Pharmacol Toxicol (Copenh) 57(Suppl 2): 44–48.

Czik V, Szekeres L, Udvary E (1983): Comparison of two calcium antagonists, verapamil and fendiline, in an experimental model of myocardial ischemia mimicking classical angina of effort. Br J Pharmacol 79:37–43.

Dodd MG, Machin I (1985): Anti-hypertensive effect of amlodipine a novel dihydropyridine calcium channel blocker. Br J Pharmacol 85:335P.

Eigenmann R, Blaber L, Nakamura K, Thorens S, Haeusler G (1981): Tiapamil, a new antagonist. I. Demonstration of calcium antagonistic activity and related studies. Arzneim Forsch 31:1393–1401.

Fielden R, Owen DAA, Taylor EM (1974): Hypotensive and vasodilator actions of SKF 24260, a new

dihydropyridine derivative. Br J Pharmacol 52:323–322.

Flaim SF (1984): Diltiazem. In Scriabine A (ed): "New Drugs Annual: Cardiovascular Drugs," Vol 2. 123–156. New York: Raven Press.

Fleckenstein A (1968): Experimentelle Pathologie der akuten und chronischen Herzinsuffizienz. Verh Dtsch Ges Kreisl-Forsch 34:15–34.

Fleckenstein A (1964): Die Bedeutung der energiereichen Phosphate für Kontraktilität und Tonus des Myokards. Verh Dtsch Ges Inn Med 70:81–99.

Fleckenstein A (1971): Specific inhibitors and promoters of calcium action in the excitation-contraction coupling of heart muscle and their role in the production of myocardial lesions. In Harris P, Opie L. (eds): "Calcium and the Heart," London-New York: Academic Press, pp 135–188.

Fleckenstein A, Fleckenstein-Grün G, Byon YK, Haastert HP, Späh F (1979): Vergleichende Untersuchungen über di Ca^{2+} antagonistischen Grundwirkungen von Niludipin (Bay a 7168) und Nifedipin (BAY a 1040) auf Myokard, Myometrium und glatte Gefässmuskulatur. Arzneim Forsch 29:230–246.

Fleckenstein A, Kammermeier H, Döring HJ, Freund HJ (1967): Zum Wirkungs-Mechanismus neurartiger Koronardilatatoren mit gleichzeitig Sauerstoffeinsparenden Myokard-Effekten, Prenylamin und Iproveratril. Z Kreisl-Forsch 56:716–744, 839–853.

Fleckenstein A, Tritthart H, Fleckenstein B, Herbst A, Grün G (1969): A new group of competitive Ca-antagonists (Iproveratril, D600, Prenylamine) with highly potent inhibitory effects on excitation-contraction coupling in mammalian myocardium. Pflügers Arch Ges Physiol 307:R25.

Fleckenstein A, Späh F (1982): Excitation-contraction uncoupling in cardiac muscles. In: Adv. Pharmacol. Therap. II, Vol. 3. Cardio-Renal and Cell Pharmacol. Proc. 8th Internat. Pharmacol. Congr., Tokyo, July 1981. Eds. Yoshida H, Hagihara Y and Ebashi S pp. 97–110. Pergamon Press, Oxford-New York.

Fleckenstein A (1983): Calcium Antagonism in Heart and Smooth Muscle." New York: John Wiley and Sons.

Fleckenstein-Grün G, Fleckenstein A, Späh F, Assmann (1978): Mechanism of action of Ca^{2+} antagonists in the treatment of coronary disease with special reference to perhexiline maleate. In Proceedings of the Symposium on Perhexiline Maleate, September 18, 1976. Amsterdam; Excerpta Medica, pp 1–22.

Franckowiak G, Bechem M, Schramm M, Thomas G (1985): The optical isomers of the 1,4-dihydropyridine BAY K 8644 show opposite effects on Ca channels. Eur J Pharmacol 114:223–226.

Freedman SB, Miller RJ (1984): Calcium channel activation: A different type of drug action. Proc Natl Acad Sci 81:5580–5583.

Fujimoto T, Peter T, Mandel WJ (1981): Electrophysiologic and hemodynamic action of diltiazem: Disparate temporal effects shown by experimental dose-response studies. Am Heart J 101:403–407.

Gallo A, Kobrin I, Pegram BL, Frohlich ED (1985): Hemodynamic effects of a new α- and β-adrenergic receptor inhibitor with calcium entry blocking effects (CGS 10078B) in WKY and SHR rats. Am J Med Sci 290:47–51.

Garcia AG, Sala F, Reig JA, Viniegra S, Frias J, Fonteriz R, Gandia L (1984): Dihydropyridine BAY K 8644 activates chromaffin cell calcium channels. Nature 309:69–71.

Gatlin M, Robertson L, TenEick R (1983): New class of calcium channel inhibitors: Cardiac membrane effects of phosphonates. Circulation 68:(suppl III):220.

Gjörstrup P, Harding H, Isaksson R, Westerlund C (1986): The enantiomers of the dihydropyridine derivative H 160/51 show opposite effects of stimulation and inhibition. Eur J Pharmacol 122:357–361.

Glossmann H, Ferry DR, Goll A, Rombusch M (1984): Molecular pharmacology of the calcium channel: Evidence for subtypes, multiple drug receptor sites, channel subunits and the development of a radioiodinated 1,4-dihydropyridine calcium channel label, ^{125}I-iodipine. J Cardiovasc Pharmacol 6:S608–S621.

Godfraind, T (1982): Pharmacology of calcium entry blockade. In Godfraind T, Albertini T, Paoletti R (eds): "Calcium Modulators." Amsterdam: Elsevier Biomedical Press, pp 51–65.

Godfraind T, Sturbois X (1975): Inhibition by cinnarizine of heart ionic changes induced by isoprenaline. In: Fleckenstein A, Rona G (eds): "Recent Advances in Studies on Cardiac Structure and Metabolism," Vol 6. Baltimore University Park Press, pp 127–134.

Godfraind T (1981): Mechanisms of action of calcium entry blockers. Fed Proc 40:2866–2871.

Gould RJ, Murphy KMM, Reynolds IJ Snyder SH (1983): Antischizophrenic drugs of diphenylbutylpiperidine type act as calcium channel antagonists. Proc Natl Acad Sci (USA) 80:5122–5125.

Granger SE, Hollingsworth M, Weston AH (1985): A comparison of several calcium antagonists on uterine, vascular and cardiac muscles from the rat. Br J Pharmacol 85:255–262.

Gries J, Raschack M (1984): Cardiovascular protection by the new calcium antagonist anipamil in normotensive rats, SHRSP and cardiomyopathic hamsters. Proc. 9th intern. Congress of Pharmacology. Abs. #894P, London: McMillan.

Haas H, Busch E (1967): Vergleichende Untersuchungen der Wirkung von α-Isopropyl-α-(N-methyl-N-homoveratryl)-γ-aminopropyl-3,4-dimethoxy-pheny acetonitril seiner Derivate, sowie einiger anderen Coronardilatatoren und β-Receptor-affiner Substanzen. Arzneim Forsch 17:257–271.

Haas H, Härtfelder G (1962): α-Isopryl-α-(N-methyl-N-homoveratryl)-γ-amino-propyl)-3,4-dimethoxyphenyl-acetonitril, eine Substanz mit coronargefässerweiternden Eigenschaften. Arzneim Forsch 12:549–558.

Hamilton SL, Yatani A, Hawkes MJ, Redding K, Brown AM (1985): Atrotoxin: A specific agonist for calcium currents in heart. Science 229:182–184, 1985.

Hess, P., Lansmann, J.B. and Tsien, R.W. (1985): Mechanism of calcium channel modulation by dihydropyridine agonists and antagonists. In: Fleckenstein A, van Breemen C, Gross R, Hoffmeister F (eds): "Cardiovascular effects of dihydropyridine-type calcium antagonists and agonists," Bayer Symposium IX. Berlin: Springer Verlag, pp 34–55.

Higuchi S, Takeshita A, Ito N, Imaizumi T, Matsuguchi H Nakamura M (1985): Arterial pressure and heart rate responses to calcium channel blockers administered in the brain stem in rats. Circ Res 57:244–251.

Hock CE, Daitch JJ, Lefer A (1985): Salutary effects of two verapamil analogs in traumatic shock. Pharm Res 3:130–134.

Hof RP (1985): PY 108–068: A calcium antagonists with an unusual pattern of cardiovascular activity. Gen Pharmacol 16:1–6.

Hof RP, Hof A, Scholtysik G, and Menninger K (1984): Effects of the new calcium antagonist PN 200-110 on the myocardium and the regional peripheral circulation in anesthetized cats and dogs. J Cardiovasc Pharmacol 6:407–416.

Hof RP, Hof A, Neumann P (1982): Effects of PY 108–068, a new calcium antagonist, on general hemodynamics and regional blood flow in anesthetized rats: A comparison with nifedipine. J Cardiovasc Pharmacol 4:352–362.

Hof RP, Ruegg UT, Hof A, Vogel A (1985): Stereoselectivity at the calcium channel: Opposite action of the enantiomers of a 1,4-dihydropyridine. J Cardiovasc Pharmacol 7:689–693.

Hoffmeister F, Benz U, Heise A, Krause HP, Neuser V (1982): Behavioral effects of nimodipine in animals. Arzneim Forsch 32:347–360.

Hudak WJ, Lewis RE, Kuhn WL (1970): Cardiovascular pharmacology of perhexiline. J Pharmacol Exp Therap 173:371–382.

Inoue Y, Nakayama K, Wachi M, Jumakura K, Matsumoto T, Iwamoto M, Motoyoshi Y, Aikawa K (1985): Absorption, distribution, metabolism and excretion of 2,6-dimethyl-3,5-dimethoxycarbonyl-4-(o-difluoromethoxyphenyl)-1,4-dihydropyridine (PP-1466) in rats. Arzneim Forsch Drug Res 35:813–818.

Jim KF, Matthews WD (1985): Comparison of the calcium antagonistic activity of nifedipine and RF 34234 in the canine saphenous vein. J Cardiovasc Pharmacol 7:458–462.

Johnson CE, Steinsland OS, Scriabine A (1983): Dopamine antagonist effect of verapamil on isolated perfused rabbit ear artery. J Pharmacol Exp Ther 226:802–805.

Jolly SR, Hardman HF, Gross GJ (1981): Comparison of two dihydropyridine calcium antagonists on coronary collateral blood flow in acute myocardial ischemia. J Pharmacol Exp Ther 217:20–25.

Karliner JS, Motulski HJ, Dunlap J, Brown JH, Insel PA (1981): Verapamil: An antagonist of adrenergic and muscarinic receptors in rat myocardium. Circulation, 64:IV-208.

Katsuragi T, Ohba M, Mori R, Kushika K, Furukawa T (1984): Calcium antagonistic action involved in vasodilation by brovincamine. Gen Pharmacol 15:43–45.

Kawai C, Konishi T, Maysayama E, Okazaki H (1981): Comparative effects of three calcium antagonists, diltiazem, verapamil and nifedipine on the sinoatrial and atrioventricular nodes. Experimental and clinical studies. Circulation 63:1035–1042.

Kazda S, Garthoff B, Krause HP, Schlossmann K (1982): Cerebrovascular effects of the calcium antagonistic dihydropyridine derivative, nimodipine in animal experiments. Arneim Forsch 32:331–338.

Kazda S, Garthoff B, Luckhaus G (1983a): Calcium antagonism in hypertensive disease: Experimental evidence for a new therapeutic concept. Postgrad Med 59 (Suppl 2):78–83.

Kazda S, Garthoff B, Meyer H, Schlossman K, Stoepel K, Towart R, Vater W, Wehinger E (1980): Pharmacology of a new calcium antagonistic compound, isobutyl methyl 1,4-dihydro-2,6-dimethyl-4-(2-nitrophenyl)-3,5-pyridine-dicarboxylate (nisoldipine, BAY K 5552). Arzneim Forsch 30:2144–2162.

Kazda S, Garthoff B, Rämsch K-D, Schlüter G (1983b): In Scriabine A (ed): "New Drugs Annual: Cardiovascular Drugs," Vol 1. pp 243–258. New York: Raven Press.

Kazda S, Scriabine A (1986): In Krebs R (ed): 10 Years of Adalat®. In print.

Kongsamut S, Kamp TJ, Miller RJ, Sanguinetti MC (1985): Calcium channel agonist and antagonist effects of the stereoisomer of the dihydropyridine 202–791. Biochem Biophys Res Comm 130:141–148.

Kroneberg, G (1975) Pharmacology of nifedipine (Adalat®). In Hashimoto K, Kimira E, Kobayashi T (eds): "1st International Nifedipine (Adalat) Symposium." Tokyo: University of Tokyo Press, pp 3–10.

Kubo, K, Karasawa A, Shuto K, Nakamizo N (1985): Antihypertensive effects of a novel dihydropyridine-type Ca-antagonist, KW-3049. Jap J Pharmacol (Suppl);39 217P.

Larsson-Backstrom C, Arrhenius E, Sagge K (1985): Comparison of the calcium-antagonistic effects of terodiline, nifedipine and verapamil. Acta Pharmacol Toxicol 57(1):8–17.

Leclercq JF, Kural S, Valere PE (1983): Bepridil et torsades de poines. Arch Med Coeur 76(3):341–348.

Lefer AM, Papanicolau G (1985): Beneficial actions of two novel calcium entry blockers in the isolated perfused hypoxic cat liver. Meth Find Exptl Clin Pharmacol 7(2):59–63.

Leszkovszky G, Tardos L, Erdély I, Harsanyi K (1966): The pharmacology of diphenylalkyl derivatives. I. Comparative studies of coronary dilator diphenylalkylamine derivatives. Acta Physiol Acad Sci Hung 29:283–297.

Lindner E (1960): Phenyl-propyl-diphenyl-propyl-amin, eine neue Substanz mit coronargefässerweiternden Wirkung. Arzneim Forsch 10:569–588.

Lindner E, Ruppert D, Kaiser J (1984): HOE 263, a new substance with calcium channel antagonistic activity. Pharmacology 29:165–172.

Luchowski EM, Yousif F, Triggle DJ, Sarmiento JG, Janis RA (1984): Effects of metal cations and calmodulin antagonists on [^{3}H]-nitrendipine binding in smooth and cardiac muscle. J Pharmacol Exp Ther 230:607–613.

Marin J, Salaices M, Tamargo J, Tejerina T (1985): Effects of oxodipine on vascular smooth muscle fibers. Brit J Pharmacol 86 (Suppl): Abs 500P.

Marshall RJ, Winslow E, Laman, JC and Apoil E (1984): Bepridol "New Drugs Annual: Cardiovascular Drugs," Vol 2, pp 157–176. New York: Raven Press.

Matsumara S, Sato H, Morishige E, Kawakami M, Uno M, Hirose F, Doteuchi M, Ueda M (1985): Studies on pharmacological characteristic of a bicyclic dihydropyridine derivative (8363-S). Jpn J Pharmacol 39(Suppl): 216P.

Mayhan WG, Heistad DD (1985): Effect of flordipine on cerebral blood flow. J Pharmacol Exp Ther 235:92–97.

Meils CM, Gross GJ, Brooks HL, Warltier DC (1981): Reduction of myocardial infarct size by the calcium antagonist FR 7534. Cardiology 68:146–160.

Mestre M, Cariot T, Belin C, Uzan A, Renault C, Dubroeuca MC, Gueremy C, Doble A, Lefur G (1985): Electrophysiological and pharmacological evidence that peripheral type benzodiazepine receptors are coupled to calcium channels in the heart. Life Sciences 36:391–400.

Meyer H, Bossert F, Wehinger E, Stoepel K (1981): Synthese und vergleichende pharmakologische Untersuchungen von 1,4-Dihydro-2,6-dimethyl-4-(3-nitrophenyl)pyridin-3,5-dicarbonsäureestern mit nicht-identischen Esterfunktion. Arzneim Forsch 31:407–409.

Mikkelsen EO, Nyborg NCB, Jakobsen P (1985): A comparison of effects of BAY K 8644 and CGP 28392, dihydropyridines with Ca agonistic properties on spontaneous mechanical activity in rat portal vein: Modification of effect by ultraviolet radiation. Acta Pharmacol Toxicol 57:340–344.

Miller RJ, Freedman SB, Miller DM, Tindall, DR (1984): Maitotoxin activates voltage sensitive calcium channels in cultured neuronal cells. Proc 9th Internat. Congr. Pharmacol. Abs. 901P, London: McMillan.

Molyvdas PA, Sperelakis N (1986) Effects of calcium antagonistic drugs on the electrical activity of rabbit sino-atrial node. Br J Pharmacol 88:249–258.

Molyvdas PA, Sperelakis N (1983): Comparison of the effects of several calcium antagonistic drugs (slow channel blockers) on the electrical and mechanical activities of guinea pig papillary muscle. J Cardiovasc Pharmacol 5:162–169.

Morita T, Ito K, Nose T (1982): Cardiac actions of KB-944, a new calcium antagonist. Arzneim Forsch 32:1053–1056.

Mras S, Sperelakis N (1981): Bepridil (CERM 1978) and verapamil depression on contractions of rabbit aortic rings. Blood Vessels 18:196–205.

Nagao T, Sato M, Iwasawa Y, Takada T, Ishida R Nakajima H, Kiyomoto A (1972): Studies on a new 1-5-benzothiazepine derivative (CRD-401). III. Effects of optical isomers of CRD-401 on smooth muscle and other pharmacological properties. Jap J Pharmacol 22:467–478.

Nakajima H, Hoshiyama M, Yamashita K, Kiyomoto A (1975): Effect of diltiazem on electrical and mechanical activity of isolated cardiac ventricular muscle of guinea pig. Jpn J Pharmacol 25:383–392.

Opie LH, Muller CA, Thandroyen FT, Lloyd EA, Mabin T, Commerford PJ, Eichler HG: (1985): Tiapamil—a new calcium antagonist. S Afr Med J 67:881–883.

Parinov VJ, Odinec AG, Gilev AP, Dubur GJ, Muceniece DH, Ozol JJ, Shatz VD, Goars, MP, Vigante BA (1985): Pharmacokinetics and metabolism of ryodipine in rats. Arzneim Forsch/Drug Res 35:808–813.

Patterson E, Montgomery DG, Lynch JJ, Lucchesi BR (1984): Cardiac electrophysiologic actions of KB-944 (Fostedil): A new calcium antagonist, in the anesthetized dog. J Pharmacol Exp. Ther 230:632–640.

Preuss KC, Cheung NL, Brooks HL, Warltier DC (1984): Cardiovascular effects of the nifedipine analog CGP 28392, in the conscious dog. J. Cardiovasc Pharmacol 6:949–953.

Preuss KC, Gross GJ, Brooks HL, Warltier DC (1985): Slow channel calcium activators, a new group of pharmacological agents. Life Sciences 37:1271–1278.

Radzialowski FM, Bittner SE, Mooney AK, Lee JY, Campion J, Walsh GM (1985): Antihypertensive and cardiac effects of a benzhydrylpiperidine calcium antagonist, SC 30552. Fed Proc 44: abs 7183, 1639.

Reynolds, IJ, Gould RJ, Snyder SH (1984): Loperamide: Blockade of calcium channels as a mechanisms of antidiarrheal effects. J Pharmacol Exp Ther 231:628–632.

Saini RK, Antonaccio MJ (1982): Antiarrhythmic, antifibrillatory activities and reduction of infarct size after calcium antagonists RO 11-1781 (tiapamil) anesthetized dogs. J Pharmacol Exp Ther 221:29–36.

Sanguinetti MC, Kass RS (1984): Voltage dependent block of calcium channel current in the calf cardiac Purkinje fiber by dihydropyridine Ca channel antagonists. Circ Res 55:336–348.

Sato M, Nagao T, Yamaguchi I, Nakajima H; Kiyomoto A (1971): Pharmacological studies on a new 1,5-benzothiazepine derivative (CRD-401). I. Cardiovascular actions. Arzneim Forsch 21:1338–1343.

Schramm M, Towart R (1985): Modulation of calcium channel function by drugs. Life Sciences 37:1843–1860.

Schramm M, Thomas G, Towart R, Franckowiak G (1983): Novel dihydropyridines with positive inotropic action through activation of Ca^{2+} channels. Nature 303:535–537.

Scriabine A, Garthoff B, Kazda S, Rámsch K-D, Schlüter G, Stoepel K (1984a): Nitrendipine. In Scriabne A (ed): "New Drugs Annual; Cardiovascular Drugs," Vol 2. pp 37-49.

Scriabine A, Battye R, Hoffmeister F, Kazda S, Towart R, Garthoff B, Schlüter, G., Rämsch K-D, Scherling D (1985): Nimodipine. In Scriabine A (ed): "New Cardiovascular Drugs 1985." New York: Raven Press pp. 197–218.

Scriabine A, Vanov S, Deck K (eds) (1984b): "Nitrendipine." Baltimore: Urban and Schwarzenberg.

Shlevin HH, Barrett JA, Smith RD, Wolf PS, Pruss TP (1983): Flordipine: Effects on coronary blood flow in normotensive anesthetized canines. Fed Proc 42:1291.

Snyder SH, Reynolds IJ (1984): Calcium antagonist drugs: Receptor interactions clarify therapeutic effects. N Engl J Med 313:995–1002.

Späh F (1986): Asocainol. In Scriabine A (ed): "New Cardiovascular Drugs 1986." New York: Raven Press.

Spedding M (1983): Direct inhibitory effects of some "calcium-antagonists" and trifluoperazine on the contractile proteins in smooth muscle. Br J Pharmacol 79:225–231.

Stanton HC, Rosenberger LB, Hanson RC, Fleming JS, Poindexter G (1986): BMY 20064, a potent calcium channel blocker with α_1-adrenoceptor antagonist properties. Fed Proc 45:abs 5280, 1062.

Stoepel K, Heise A, Kazda S (1981): Pharmacological studies of the antihypertensive effect of nitrendipine. Arzneim Forsch 31:2056–2061.

Takahashi M, Tatsumi M, Ohizumi Y, Yasumoto T

(1983): Ca^{2+} channel activating function of maito-toxin, the most potent marine toxin known, in clonal rat pheochromocytoma cells. J Biol Chem 258: 10944–10949.

Takenaka T, Maeno H (1982): A vasoconstrictive compound, 1,4-dihydropyridine derivative. Jpn J Pharmacol 32:139P.

Takenaka T, Nomura T, Sado T, Usuda S, Maeno H (1976): Vasodilator profile of a new 1,4-dihydropyridine derivative, 2,6-dimethyl-4-(3-nitrophenyl) 1,4-dihydropyridine-3,4-dicarboxylic acid 3-[2-N-ben-zyl-N-methyl amino)] ethyl ester 5-methyl ester hydrochloride (YC-93). Arzneim Forsch 26:2172–2178.

Thomas G, Chung M, Cohen CJ (1985): A dihydropyridine (BAY K 8644) that enhances calcium currents in guinea pig and calf myocardial cells: A new type of positive inotropic agents. Circ Res 56:87–96.

Towart R, Kazda S, Lamp B, Thomas G, Schramm M (1985): Effect of dihydropyridine calcium channel modulators on isolated peripheral and cerebral vessles. In Fleckenstein A, van Breemen C, Gross R, Hoffmeister F (eds): "Cardiovascular Effects of Dihydropyridine- Type Calcium Antagonists and Agonists," Bayer Symposium IX. Berlin: Springer Verlag, pp 272–287.

Truog AG, Brauner H, Criscione T, Falbert M, Kuhnis H, Meier M, Rogg H (1984): CGP 28392, a dihydropyridine Ca-entry stimulator. In Rubin RP, Weiss GB, Putney JW (eds): "Calcium in Biological Systems." New York: Plenum Press, pp 441–449.

Van den Kerckhoff W, Drewes LR (1985): Transfer of the Ca-antagonists nifedipine and nimodipine across the blood-brain barrrier and their regional distribution in vivo. J. Cerebr. Blood Flow and Metabolism 5:(1):459–460.

Vanhoutte P, Van Nueten JM (1983): Lidoflazine. In Scriabine A (ed): "New Drugs Annual: Cardiovascular Drugs," Vol 1. New York: Raven Press, pp 203–206.

Vanhoutte PM (1982): Cinnarizine, flunarizine, lido-flazine. In Godfraind T, Albertini A, Paoletti R (eds): "Calcium Modulators." Amsterdam: Elsevier, pp 351–362.

Van Neuten JM, Wellens D (1979): Tissue specificity of calcium-antagonistic properties of lidoflazine. Arch Int Pharmacodyn 242:329–331.

Van Nueten JM, Vanhoutte PM (1984): Flunarizine. In Scriabine A (ed): "New Drugs Annual: Cardiovascular Drugs," Vol 2. New York: Raven Press, pp 245–266.

Vater W, Kroneberg G, Hoffmeister F, Kaller H, Meng K, Oberdorf A, Puls W, Schlossmann K, Stoepel K (1972): Zur Pharmakologie von 4-(2-Nitrophenyl)-2,6-dimethyl 1,4-dihydropyridine-3,5-dicarbonsaure dimethylester (Nifedipin, BAY a 1040). Arzneim Forsch 22:1–14.

Wada Y, Satoh K, Taira N (1985): Separation of the coronary vasodilator from the cardiac effects of PN 200–110, a new dihydropyridine calcium antagonist, in the dog heart. J Cardiovasc Pharmacol 7:190–196.

Wakabayashi S, Satake N, Ueda S, Shibata S (1985): KT 362 (5-(N-(2-(3,4-dimethoxyphenyl)ethyl)β-alanyl)2,3,4,5-tetrahydro-benzo-1,5-thiazepine bi-fumarate, a new vasorelaxing agent: A possible intracellular Ca^{2+} inhibitory action. Fed. Proc. 44:Abs 4102,1112.

Warltier DC, Hardman HF, Brooks HL, Gross GJ (1983): Transmural gradient of coronary blood flow following dihydropyridine calcium antagonists and other vasodilator drugs. Basic Res Cardiol 78:644–653.

Structure and Physiology of the Slow Inward Calcium Channel, pages 71–88
© 1987 Alan R. Liss, Inc.

4

Electrophysiology of Ca Channels in Excitable Cells: Channel Types, Permeation, Gating, and Modulation

Robert S. Kass and Douglas S. Krafte

University of Rochester, Department of Physiology, Rochester, New York 14642

INTRODUCTION

Ca channels are important to cellular function in a wide variety of cells. As is the case for other voltage-dependent channels in excitable tissues, changes in membrane potential cause these channels to open and allow Ca ions to flow into the cells. This inward movement of positive charge depolarizes the membrane and contributes to spike initiation and rhythmic firing in neurons, rhythmic activity in some smooth muscle cells, impulse conduction in cardiac nodal tissue, and maintenance of the plateau phase of the action potential of several cardiac tissues [Hagiwara and Byerly, 1981, 1983; Reuter, 1983; Tsien, 1983; Miller, 1985]. A distinct feature of Ca channels is that, in addition to their role in controlling membrane potential, the movement of Ca ions through them acts as a cellular messenger for such diverse actions as hormone secretion by gland cells and initiation of contractile activity in heart and smooth muscle cells. It is, thus, not surprising that there is intense interest in the properties of these channels.

The purpose of this review is to summarize the electrophysiology of Ca channels that have been studied in heart, smooth muscle, and neuronal tissue. The review will focus on recent data that have described different types of Ca channels, channel gating, channel permeation, and modulation of channel activity by neurohormones and drugs. Other properties of the channels are described in several previously published review articles [Hagiwara and Byerly, 1981, 1983; Reuter, 1979, 1983; Tsien, 1983].

METHODS OF MEASUREMENT

Ca channel currents have been measured in large cells and multicellular preparations using microelectrode voltage clamps described in Kass and Bennett [1985], and in small, isolated cells using patch clamps in single channel and whole cell arrangements [Hamill et al., 1981]. In all experiments, steps must be taken to eliminate or minimize other membrane currents [see Hagiwara and Byerly, 1981; Tsien, 1983]. This problem of dissection of individual ion channel current is minimized in single channel recordings, provided only one type of channel is trapped in the patch of membrane under investigation.

ELECTRICAL EVIDENCE FOR MULTIPLE TYPES OF Ca CHANNELS

Electrophysiological studies have now clearly demonstrated the existence of several types of Ca channels. Recent reports have shown that at least two kinds of Ca channels co-exist in egg cells, neuronal tissue, heart cells, and smooth muscle cells. The evidence for multiple channel types has been most convincingly provided by whole cell and single channel studies using the patch clamp technique, but many of the criteria for distinguishing these channels were established in earlier studies using less direct measurements.

Hagiwara et al. [1975] first reported the existence of two Ca channel currents in starfish eggs, preparations chosen because of their suitability for study using microelectrodes. This group found two inward currents that could be separated by several characteristics, which they listed. 1) The currents could be separated by their voltage-dependence. One type (I) activates at negative voltages (near −55 mV), whereas the second (II) activates at voltages near −6 mV. Both channel types inactivate, but type I has a half-maximal voltage for inactivation near −53 mV, and type II has a half-maximal voltage near −18 mV (note that these values were obtained in artificial sea water that contained a total divalent cation concentration of 75 mM). 2) The kinetics of the currents differ. The decay of type I channel current is much faster than type II at any given membrane potential. 3) The current of channel I is more sensitive to Na than channel II and is less sensitive to cations that block Ca channels. Fox and Krasne [1984] later reported two populations of Ca channels in eggs of the marine polychaete *Neanthes arenaceodentatus*, and Deitmer [1984] used a two-microelectrode voltage clamp to study two types of Ca channels in a fresh water hypotrich ciliate.

Llinas and Yarom [1981a,b] used current clamp techniques and provided evidence for the existence of two Ca channel types based on action potentials recorded from guinea pig inferior olivary neurons. Similar to criterion 1 above, was the observation that complex action potentials could be elicited from these cells and that two Ca-dependent spikes could be separated by changes in holding potential.

One spike, which was generated only from hyperpolarized membrane potentials (relative to average resting potentials of −65 mV), had a negative threshold and was refractory. The fact that the response was refractory implied that the current that generates it inactivates. The second spike required stronger depolarizations to reach threshold (thus it was termed a high-threshold spike) and showed little characteristics of inactivation. Both low- and high-threshold responses were blocked by Co^{2+}.

More direct evidence for multiple Ca channel types in cultured vertebrate neurons was provided by Carbone and Lux using the patch clamp technique in whole cell [1984a] (see Fig. 1) and single channel [1984b] arrangements. From these experiments, it was concluded that there are at least two distinct Ca conductances in cultured dorsal root ganglion cells from chick and rat embryos. Evidence has recently been presented that there may be a third type of Ca channel in this preparation (see below). As in the previous work one component was found to activate at voltages between −60 and −40 mV (low voltage-activated channel). This channel inactivates completely and quickly and deactivates with a characteristically slow time-course. The second type of channel is consistent with the high threshold response reported by Llinas and Yoram. It has weak inactivation (with time constants on the order of seconds at 12°C) and is activated at voltages between −20 and 0 mV. Current through this channel deactivates very quickly upon repolarization.

The time-course of Ca channel deactivation was also used to dissect two Ca channels in lines of cultured pituitary cells. Slow and fast deactivating channels were identified in GH3 cells [Armstrong and Matteson, 1985] and GH4C1 cells [Cohen and McCarthy, 1985]. In both cases, the slowly closing channels activated in a relatively negative voltage range and inactivated quickly. The fast closing channels activated at more positive potentials and inactivated slowly. In addition, Armstrong and Matteson report that the channels

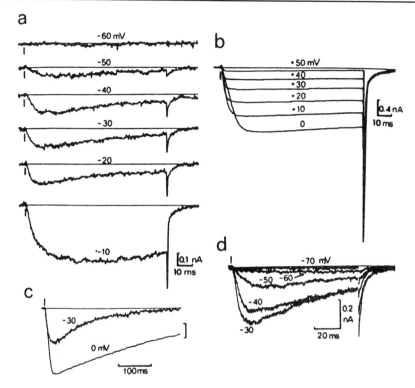

Fig. 1. *Two types of Ca channels in cultured chick dorsal root ganglion cells. Whole-cell clamp currents in 5 mM Ca (a and b). Time-course of inward Ca currents recorded from the same cell at the membrane potential indicated. Note the reduced amplification and the faster tail currents in b. c) Time-course of inward Ca currents during long-lasting depolarizations (400 ms). The conditions are the same as in a and b, but the cell is different. Note the nearly complete inactivation to a relatively low mem-* *brane potential (−30 mV) during the pulse and the slower inactivation time-course with stronger depolarization (to 0 mV). The holding potential is −80 mV. Vertical bar, 0.06 nA and 0.2 nA for the records at −30 mV and 0 mV, respectively. d) Inward currents in isotonic Ba recorded at low membrane potentials (−70 to −30 mV, potentials assigned to recordings). The holding and repolarization potential is −90 mV. (From Carbone and Lux, 1984a.)*

differ in the conduction of barium and calcium, whereas Cohen and McCarthy observed different sensitivities to dihydropyridine derivatives (see below).

Nowycky et al. [1985] have demonstrated that as many as three types of calcium channels may coexist in dorsal root ganglia obtained from cultured chick embryos. In this work, single channel and whole cell currents were measured using patch clamp arrangements, and single channel conductances were compared in addition to voltage-dependent and pharmacological properties. As in the previous studies, they identified a low-voltage

activated current that was termed "T" (for transient) because it inactivates quickly (30 ms at −30 mV). Current through these channels must be measured from negative holding potentials because steady-state inactivation is complete at voltages more positive than −40 mV. Activation is detectable positive to −50 mV, and the channel has a small slope conductance (about 8 pS measured in 110 mM Ba).

A second type of channel, termed "L" (for long-lasting) is consistent with previously identified "high threshold" responses. The single channel slope conductance is large (25 pS in 110 Ba), inactivation is weak and slow (hundreds of milliseconds), and activity is seen at voltages positive to -10 mV. A third type of channel was also identified with properties somewhat intermediate to "L" and "T" channels and were thus termed "N" (for neither L nor T) channels. These channels inactivate and thus require negative holding potentials (like T channels, they are completely inactivated at voltages more positive than -50 mV). In contrast to T channels, N channels require strong depolarizations (to voltages more positive than -20 mV) to cause channel openings. Finally, this channel type is characterized by a slope conductance on the order of 13 pS (in 110 Ba).

Identification of multiple types of Ca channels in heart and smooth muscle cells has recently gained intense interest because of improved procedures for cell isolation. Bean [1985] described two distinct kinds of Ca channels in cells isolated from dog atria (Fig. 2). In many respects, these currents appear very similar to L and T channel currents described above. A fast component is similar to T channel current in that it is present only if the membrane is held more negative than -50 mV, it inactivates quickly, and it peaks near -30 mV. This current is not affected by replacement of Ca by Ba. Another component of current, similar to L current, inactivates more slowly and only at voltages more positive than -30 mV. The single channel currents for the slow component are about twice as large as those for the fast component, and the slow component is enhanced when Ba replaces Ca as the charge carrier. Similar results have been reported for guinea pig ventricular cells [Mitra and Morad, 1985].

Single channel current records obtained from guinea pig ventricular cells have also provided evidence for two types of cardiac calcium channels [Nilius et al., 1985]. As in the atrial cells, a small conductance (8 pS), channel was detected with activation and approximately 90% complete steady-state inactivation at voltages near -50 mV, again

similar to T channels in neurons. The second channel resembles L neuronal channels, showing slower inactivation and activating at more positive potentials. The single channel conductance of the L-type channels is closer to 18–25 pS.

Two patterns of voltage-dependence of activation of Ca currents have also been reported in isolated smooth muscle cells [Isenberg and Klockner, 1984; Bean et al., 1985; Sturek and Hermsmeyer, 1985]. These channels, too, can be separated by the voltage-dependence of inactivation and activation. One activates at relatively negative potentials and inactivates quickly; the second activates at voltages positive to 0 mV and inactivates slowly (note that the voltage ranges reported will be greatly affected by the composition of the solutions in which the currents are measured).

In summary, at least two kinds of Ca channels have been identified by their electrophysiological properties in all cells for which they have been tested. The most common is the L-type channel which shows repeated openings at voltages more positive than -30 mV and inactivates with time constants that depend on membrane potential but range up to hundreds of milliseconds [Kass and Sanguinetti, 1984]. The second type is the T channel which activates at potentials more negative than -50 mV, inactivates with a fast time course, and is nearly completely inactivated in the steady-state at -50 mV. A third type of channel has been observed by Nowycky et al. [1985], but the generality of this channel has yet to be demonstrated.

These channels respond differently to neurohormones and drugs. Bean [1985] has shown that in dog atrial cells, L- but not T-type channels respond to isoproterenol, and several groups have reported that dihydropyridine agonists and antagonists modulate gating of L- but not T-type channels [Bean, 1985; Nowycky et al., 1985; Nilius et al., 1985; Sturek and Hermsmeyer, 1985; Mitra and Morad, 1985].

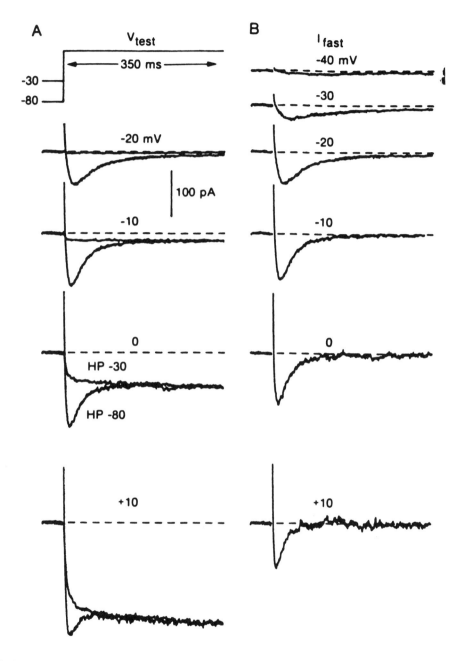

Fig. 2. *Two components of Ba current in dog atrial cells. 115 Ba, 10 μMTTX. A) Currents elicited by steps from −80 or −30 mV; for −30 traces, holding potential was changed to −30 mV for 2 sec before test pulse depolarization. Traces shown are averages of 3–6 sweeps, leak and capacity corrected. B) Difference currents from traces in A, along with current elicited by steps to −40 and −30 mV from −80 mV (leak and capacity corrected). 0.5 kHz filter. (From Bean, 1985.)*

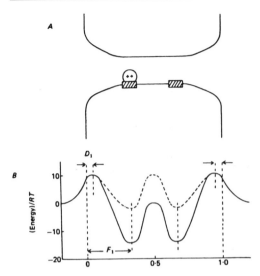

Fig. 3. *A) Schematic drawing of Ca channel with two binding sites (hatched), one of them complexed with a divalent cation. B) Energy profile of the Ca channel. The ordinate plots energy (in J/mol) divided by RT for an empty pore at zero membrane potential; the abscissa gives the fraction of the transmembrane potential experienced at any given point ("electric distance"). The energy profiles are symmetric about the midline (abscissa 0.5), with $D_1 = 0.05$ and $F_1 = 0.33$. Profiles shown are for Ca (continuous curve) and Na (dashed curve). (From Almers and McClesky, 1984.)*

PERMEATION

Under conditions where extracellular calcium levels are substantially lowered, preparations containing voltage-dependent calcium channels can conduct slow action potentials in the presence of certain monovalent cations [Takeda and Oomura, 1972; Rougier et al., 1969; Prosser et al., 1977; Yamamoto and Washio, 1979]. Kostyuk and Krishtal [1977] and Palade and Almers [1978] showed a large inward current in the presence of extracellular sodium under these same conditions. Based on kinetics and pharmacological characteristics [see Almers and McCleskey, 1984; Fukushima and Hagiwara, 1985], this current appears to be flowing through modified calcium channels as had been postulated in the earlier action potential studies. This interpre-

tation, at first, seemed somewhat confusing since it requires the calcium channel to be quite permeable to Na ions, a property the channel does not possess in the presence of mM Ca_0 [see Matsuda and Noma, 1984]. Recently, interest in this phenomenon has been renewed, with the hope that it may give some insight into the permeation mechanism of voltage-dependent calcium channels.

Hess and Tsien [1984] and Almers and McCleskey [1984] have explained the change in permeability of calcium channels when extracellular calcium is reduced in terms of a multi-ion single file pore model (i.e., there is more than one ion binding site within the channel pore) (see Fig. 3). The major piece of evidence leading to this conclusion is the presence of an anomalous mole fraction effect. If there is only one binding site within the channel for permeating ions, the total current in the presence of two permeant species cannot be less than the current in an equal concentration of either one of those ions alone. When this idea is tested experimentally, however, the result is that for certain mixtures of Ca and Ba, the total current is less than in an equal concentration of either ion, hence the name anomalous mole fraction effect. This result can be explained if the channel has two binding sites instead of one, allowing interaction between the ions at these sites. Hess and Tsien [1984] note in addition that the K_m for Ca binding is very different when estimated by saturation of Ca current through the channel, Ca block of Ba permeation, or Ca block of Na permeation. This is clearly inconsistent with a single binding site within the pore. The fact that there appear to be at least two ion binding sites within the calcium channel pore explains how the channel can show different permeabilities to monovalent cations under the conditions mentioned above. The presence of calcium at one of the sites can effectively reduce occupancy of other ions at the second site. In the absence of calcium, however, these other ions can occupy the binding sites within the channel and carry significant current.

The most interesting conclusion from this type of analysis is that calcium channels maintain selectivity by a different mechanism than other types of ion channels and that selectivity is derived as much from the calcium ion itself as from the molecular properties of the pore. Perhaps this is not surprising since Ca channels must overcome the fact that the calcium concentration is as much as two orders of magnitude lower than that of other ions in the medium (e.g., Na). This point is made by Hess and Tsien [1984] who state, "Ca is selected as much by deep-energy wells" (tight binding) "as by a relatively low-energy barrier ('selectivity filter')," the latter being the mechanism of selectivity proposed for other types of channels.

The above studies have centered on the L or slow type calcium channel. With the discovery of more than one channel type (see below), the question arises whether or not all calcium channels have a common permeation mechanism. Preliminary evidence [Bean, 1985] indicates that different types of channels show differing degrees of selectivity to divalent cations such as Ca and Ba, indicating permeation may not be the same. This is an area that merits further study.

GATING AND MACROSCOPIC CURRENTS

This section focuses on Ca channels that resemble those categorized as L-type channels (see above), because the properties of this kind of channel have been most thoroughly described to date.

Gating refers to the opening and closing of a channel which regulates ion flow through it. Channel gating is controlled, at least in part, by changes in cell membrane potential. When the voltage across a cell membrane containing L-type channels is changed to a value positive to the resting potential, the permeability of the membrane transiently increases to Ca^{2+}. The summation of currents through all individual channels that open and close in response to the change in potential is referred to as macroscopic, or whole cell cur-

rents. Macroscopic, or whole cell Ca currents rapidly increase and then decline if the depolarizing voltage pulse is maintained. The inward surge of current has been interpreted as activation of Ca channels, and the slower decline attributed to channel inactivation. This voltage-dependent change in cell permeability has suggested that Ca channels can exist in at least three different states: rested (closed, C), open (O), and inactivated (nonconducting, I). Transitions between these states are governed by rate constants, some or all of which may be voltage-dependent:

$$C \rightleftharpoons O \rightleftharpoons I. \qquad (1)$$

Single channel current measurements have provided data that suggest that activation, not inactivation, may be the rate limiting step in this sequence in some mammalian sodium channels [Aldrich et al., 1983]. Similar experimental tests are needed to determine whether this is also the case for Ca channel currents.

When the extracellular solution contains a total divalent cation concentration between 2 and 5 mM (see below for different solutions), inward Ca currents are measured in response to voltage steps to -30 mV or more positive voltages. Activation of the channels is seen as a very rapid inward surge of current that follows a sigmoidal time-course [Lee and Tsien, 1982; Adams and Gage, 1980; Brown et al., 1983; Lux and Brown, 1984]. The deactivation of this current, measured as the time course of inward tail currents after activating prepulses, has also been shown to consist of more than one exponential component [Byerly and Hagiwara, 1982; Fenwick et al., 1982; Brown et al., 1983]. These observations suggest that the change from rested (closed) to open states consists of a pathway via at least two closed (nonconducting states).

The steady-state voltage-dependence of the activation of these channels has been documented in several preparations [see Reuter, 1979]. Activation is determined from conductance changes during the first few milliseconds of depolarizing test voltage steps. Conductance is determined from peak inward currents normalized by driving force (test voltage minus reversal potential). Conductance becomes non-zero at voltages near -30 mV and reaches a saturating value at positive voltages (the absolute values of these voltages will depend on the composition of the solution in which the measurements are carried out, as discussed below). Deactivation is obtained from the time-course of current tails after prepulses to different test potentials [see Brown et al., 1983]. The probability of channel opening is obtained by normalizing these conductance/voltage curves to saturating value either at or after pulses to positive potentials. Thus, macroscopic measurements predict that at positive voltages there is unitary probability that Ca channels open upon depolarization of the cell membrane. Single channel studies, which reveal statistical properties of channel kinetics, differ with this prediction (see below).

The decline of ensemble, or macroscopic, currents measured during maintained depolarization is referred to as inactivation. Inactivation is also measured as the availability of Ca channels measured during depolarizing pulses applied from different conditioning potentials. In some cells, evidence has been provided that inactivation can be regulated by Ca_i [for complete review, see Eckert and Chad, 1984]. Recent reports of Ca channel inactivation in heart cells have indicated that inactivation of these channels is mediated by a combination of Ca_i and membrane potential [Kass and Sanguinetti, 1984; Lee et al., 1985]. These results resemble previous reports of dual regulation of Ca channel currents in some snail neurons [Brown et al., 1981]. In these experiments, it was shown that the time-course of inactivation was very sensitive to the divalent cation charge carrier, but that replacement of Ca_0 by barium did not eliminate inactivation at positive voltages. In fact, the time-course of inactivation at some potentials was very similar for Ca, Sr, or Ba currents (Fig. 4).

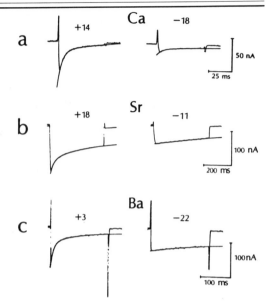

Fig. 4. *Time-course of Ca, Sr, and Ba current inactivation in the calf Purkinje fiber during depolarizing voltage pulses. The solutions contained 5.4 mM of the divalent cations indicated in a, b, and c. (From Kass and Sanguinetti, 1984.)*

One consequence of this finding is the importance of choice of membrane potential when testing for time-dependent inactivation. Furthermore, solutions containing high concentrations of divalent cations will shift the time constant vs. voltage relationship towards more positive potentials (see below) and cause time-dependent inactivation to occur at more positive potentials than it would in the presence of lower external divalent cation concentrations. This must be remembered in the categorization of types of Ca channels, because tests for inactivation are often carried out in solutions containing very high external divalent cation concentrations [see Bean, 1985].

SINGLE CHANNEL STUDIES

Activation

At the single channel level, depolarization of the cell membrane causes Ca channels to open and close in bursts [see Reuter et al.,

1982; Fenwick et al., 1982]. Analysis of the distributions of times during which the channel is open and times for which the channel is shut provides information about the number of states in which the channel can exist. In these experiments, open times and shut times can be measured directly from the records to determine either mean times or the time constants that describe these processes [methods described in Colquhoun and Hawkes, 1983] (Fig. 5). Analysis of the distribution of closed times has provided evidence for at least two closed states that precede the open state in Eq. 1 [Cavalie et al., 1983; Hess et al., 1984; Fenwick et al., 1982; Brown et al., 1984]. These results support the ensemble current measurements described above.

In single channel current experiments, the probability of channel opening can be determined directly by counting the appearances of unitary current events. The mean current can then be expressed as $I(t) = N * p(t) * i$, where N is the number of channels per membrane patch, $p(t)$ is the time-dependent probability that the channel is open at time t after a depolarizing voltage step, and i is the single channel current. The single channel current data resemble that for macroscopic current in that the probability of channel opening increases with depolarization [Reuter et al., 1982] and shows saturation at positive voltages [Cavalie et al., 1983]. In contrast to the macroscopic data, however, is the finding that the open state probability saturates at a value less than 1. This means that during pulses to positive potentials, there will be some sweeps in which there are no channel openings. Hess et al. [1984] report that this occurs roughly 30% of the time in their experience. Thus, at some times, the channel is unavailable for conduction out of the rested state.

There are at least two important interpretations of this finding. One is that there is a direct pathway that allows transitions from the rested to the inactivated state for a scheme such as that outlined in Eq. 1. Another, described below, is that this represents a change in the mode of gating of the channel.

Inactivation

Single channel measurements have confirmed whole cell measures of steady-state availability of Ca channels. In these experiments, Ca channel currents were measured either at fixed potentials [Reuter et al., 1982] or after conditioning pulses to different voltages [Cavalie et al., 1983]. The results showed channel openings occurring less frequently after positive conditioning pulses, but the amplitude of the single channel current was not affected.

Very little additional kinetic data about inactivation have been obtained from single channel current measurements because the inactivated state is a nonconducting state. Once channels inactivate, they remain unavailable for conduction until they leave this state, and thus, current recordings show no unitary currents through the channel.

DIFFERENT MODES OF GATING

The kinetic scheme illustrated by Eq. 1 allows for direct transitions between the open and inactivated states. In fact, in the scheme shown, the probability of channels entering the inactivated state is directly influenced by channels entering the open state. Thus conditions that alter the open state probability will influence the probability of channels reaching the inactivated state.

Hess et al. [1984] have suggested an alternate mechanism to account for different forms of Ca channel gating. This group has proposed that Ca channels can exist in one of three different "modes" of gating (Fig. 6). As shown in the figure, in two modes (1 and 2) the channel can make transitions between two closed and one open state, and in the other mode (0), the channel is unavailable for conduction (essentially inactivated). In modes 1 and 2, two distinct sets of rate constants are used to describe channel gating that is characterized by brief bursts of unitary currents (mode 1) or by periods of very long open times for the channel (mode 2). Transitions

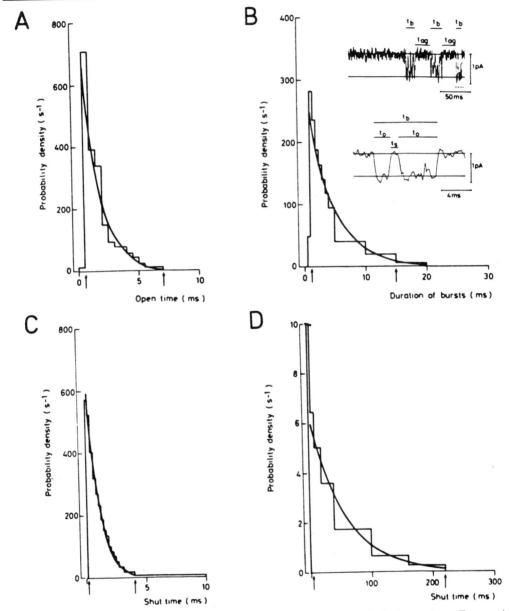

Fig. 5. *Single channel records and their analysis. L-type Ca channels recorded from single guinea pig ventricular cell. Distribution of open time (A) burst durations (B), and shut times (C,D) during 30 mV depolarizations (duration 300 ms). The pipette contained 50 mM Ba. Observations were grouped in bins of .5 ms in A and 0.2 ms in C throughout the histograms. In B, for burst durations up to 5 ms, .5-ms-long bins have been used, whereas longer bursts were grouped in 5-ms-long bins. Because of a lower total number of observations, shut intervals longer than 4 ms (D) were grouped in variable bins to avoid gaps between individual observations. Exponentials were fitted between the arrows by an exponential regression analysis routine. The inset (B) shows typical records at different time scales and bandwidths: the lower record is an expansion of the upper record as marked by the dotted line. Baseline and average elementary current amplitude levels are given by solid lines. t_b, burst length; t_{ag}, shut time between bursts; t_s, shut time within burst; t_o, open time. The top record was low-pass filtered at 1 kHz; the bottom record at 2.5 kHz. (From Cavalie et al., 1983.)*

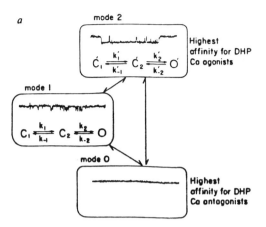

a

mode 2

$$\acute{C}_1 \underset{k_{-1}'}{\overset{k_1'}{\rightleftharpoons}} \acute{C}_2 \underset{k_{-2}'}{\overset{k_2'}{\rightleftharpoons}} \acute{O}$$

Highest affinity for DHP Ca agonists

mode 1

$$C_1 \underset{k_{-1}}{\overset{k_1}{\rightleftharpoons}} C_2 \underset{k_{-2}}{\overset{k_2}{\rightleftharpoons}} O$$

mode 0

Highest affinity for DHP Ca antagonists

Fig. 6. *Hypothetical modes of Ca channel gating. Transitions between modes are assumed to be much slower than gating transitions within modes; details of intermode connections are left unspecified and require further study. At the test potentials studied, mode 1 and mode 2 are distinguished by qualitatively different patterns of opening and closing. In these two modes, kinetic models for gating with two closed (C_1, C_2) and one open (O) state are indicated. No gating reactions are depicted for mode 0 because it represents condition(s) in which the channel is unavailable for conduction. (From Hess et al., 1984.)*

between the modes are allowed, but the voltage-dependence of the rate constants governing these transitions has not been specified. This scheme can account for recordings that show long open times, such as those in the presence of the dihydropyridine Bay K8644 (see below) and is consistent with the actions of the dihydropyridine antagonists such as nifedipine and nisoldipine (see below). In addition, it provides an explanation for slow transitions in which gating of the channel appears to occur via periods dominated by bursts of brief openings and periods of long-lasting channel openings in the absence of any drugs.

One drawback of this interpretation of single channel data is that a separate mode (0) is invoked to account for conditions in which the channel is unavailable for conduction. This condition is essentially the same as inactivation, described more often as a state of the channel (see Eq. 1). In some cases, inactivation may be coupled to voltage-dependent

channel opening [see Aldrich et al., 1983]. Such a connection is not obvious from the mode model in its present form. Future experiments are needed to clarify this important view of channel gating.

MODULATION OF Ca CHANNELS BY NEUROHORMONES AND DRUGS

Organic Compounds: Ca Channel Antagonists and Agonists

The material presented in the following section describes recent results reported for the modulation of Ca channels in a variety of cell types. All of the results relate to channels that resemble the L-type channels described earlier. The section is broken down into results obtained for whole cell or macroscopic currents and those obtained from single channel studies.

Ca channel antagonists. Ca channel antagonists form a major new class of drugs that has been investigated intensively by electrophysiological and biochemical techniques because of the wide and powerful range of applications of these compounds. Three different classes of these drugs have been identified based on electrophysiological and binding data. These are the papaverine derivatives (verapamil and D600), the benzothiazepine derivatives (diltiazem), and the dihydropyridine derivatives (such as nifedipine, nitrendipine, and nisoldipine). In each case, the drugs have been found to exhibit use- and frequency-dependent block [Ehara and Kaufmann, 1978; Kohlardt and Mnich, 1978; Pelzer et al., 1982; Tung and Morad, 1983; Lee and Tsien, 1983; Sanguinetti and Kass, 1984b; Bean, 1984; Uehara and Hume, 1985].

Results of studies of macroscopic currents have suggested that these compounds, particularly the dihydropyrines (DHP), interact with a particular state of the channel. Several findings suggest that the inhibitory actions of the DHP derivatives come about by interaction and promotion of the inactivated state. This conclusion is based on the observations that these drugs slow the recovery from inactiva-

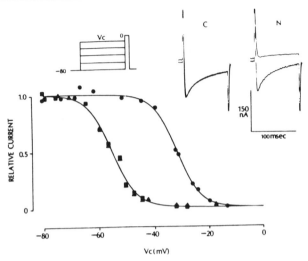

Fig. 7. *Nisoldipine (N) shifts the availability of Ca channels in the calf Purkinje fiber in the hyperpolarizing direction. Normalized plots of maximum inward current measured in response to test pulses (inset) to 0 mV after conditioning pulses (30 sec long) to the voltages indicated along the abscissa. Currents measured in the absence (●) and presence of nisoldipine (200 nM ▲, 400 nM ■). Inset shows current measured after conditioning pulses to −44 mV and −74 mV in the absence (C) and presence (N) of 200 nM nisoldipine. Curves: best fit of Boltzman functions to the data. $V_{1/2}$ shifted from −32 mV (control) to −53 mV (200 nM N) and −55 mV (400 nM N). (From Sanguinetti and Kass, 1984a.)*

tion after depolarizing voltage steps [Lee and Tsien, 1983; Sanguinetti and Kass, 1984; Uehara and Hume, 1985]; that the potency of the DHPs is increased dramatically with depolarizations that favor inactivated channels [Bean, 1984; Sanguinetti and Kass, 1984]; and that the relationship between Ca channel availability and membrane potential is shifted in the hyperpolarizing direction by the DHPs (Fig. 7).

These results were interpreted within the framework of the modulated receptor hypothesis [Hille, 1977; Hondeghem and Katzung, 1977] which proposes that drugs can bind to a site in or near a channel and that the affinity for this site varies depending upon the state of the channel, which in turn depends on membrane potential. An alternate interpretation has been proposed by Hess et al. [1984] based on the analysis of single channel data (see below).

Single channel data have shown that the predominant effect of the DHP antagonists, as well as D600, is to increase the number of sweeps in which no channel openings occur [Hess et al., 1984; Cavalie et al., 1984]. These observations are consistent with promotion of the inactivated state and with the alternative interpretation: stabilization of mode 0 gating. Hess et al. [1984] additionally reported that the DHP antagonist nitrendipine caused null sweeps to occur at a high frequency but also promoted the occurrence of sweeps with long channel openings (see below). Thus, this compound can have mixed activity. These results have also been confirmed for low concentration effects by Bean [1985] and Brown et al. [1985].

Ca channel agonists. Macroscopic current measurements have shown that Ca channel agonists such as Bay K8644 and CG 28392 promote large increases in Ca channel currents [Sanguinetti and Kass, 1984a; Hess et al., 1984; Thomas et al., 1984]. In addition to increasing current amplitude, Bay K8644 increases the apparent rate of inactivation of current, shifts the inactivation curve in the hyperpolarizing direction [Sanguinetti and Kass, 1985], and, depending on membrane

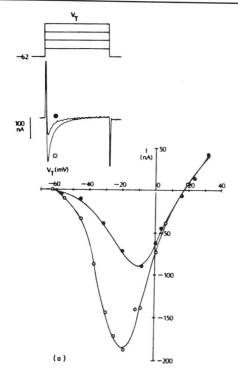
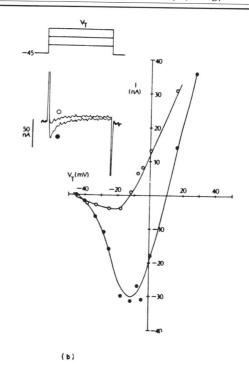

Fig. 8. *Influence of holding potential on the activity of Bay K8644 (0.5 μM) on membrane current in the calf Purkinje fiber. Membrane current was recorded in response to 100 ms test pulses (inset) applied to voltages from a holding potential of −62 mV (a) or −45 mV (b). The insets show currents in response to voltage pulses to −10 mV from each holding potential in control (●) and drug (○). The graphs show peak inward current plotted against test pulse voltage for control (●) and drug (○). (From Sanguinetti and Kass, 1984b.)*

potential, reduces or enhances peak currents (Fig. 8). These results show that the agonists, too, are voltage-dependent and have suggested an interpretation that links inactivation to the open state of the calcium channel [Sanguinetti and Kass, 1985].

The effects of these agonists on single channel currents have been reported by several groups [Hess et al., 1984; Ochi et al., 1984; Kokobun and Reuter, 1984; Brown et al., 1984]. The predominant effect of these drugs is to increase the mean open time of the channel during depolarizing voltage steps (Fig. 9). Single channel conductance is not affected, and activity of the channel is not induced in the absence of a change in potential. Ochi et al. [1984] have suggested that this change in channel kinetics is caused by a drug-induced

decrease in a rate constant for transition out of the open state. Such a change can account for increased channel openings, and, if inactivation is coupled to the open state, the same change accounts for the inhibitory actions of these drugs at more positive membrane potentials [Sanguinetti and Kass, 1985].

Hess et al. [1984] have interpreted their data in terms of changes in the modes of gating of the channels. In this view, the drugs do not alter a particular rate constant but bind to and favor channels that are gated in mode 2, a gating mode in which channel open times are long. Mode 2 gating can exist in the absence of drug, but it occurs with a much lower probability under these conditions.

The major difference between the interpretations based upon modes of gating and on

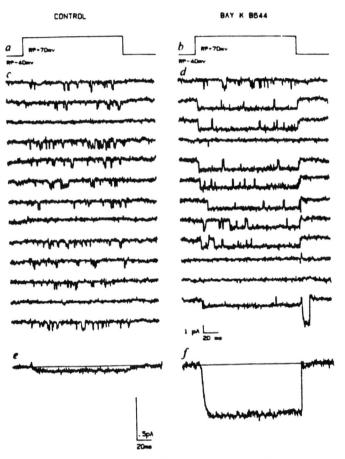

Fig. 9. *Influence of Bay K8644 on single channel currents in isolated rat ventricular cell. Single Ca channel activity in the absence (left) and presence of 5 μM Bay K8644 (right). Cell attached patch. a,b) Voltage protocol. RP, resting potential about −60 mV as determined by measurement of open channel current-voltage relations. Pulses applied once every 3 sec. c,d) Representative current signals (consecutive sweeps). Linear leak and capacity corrected. e,f) Averaged current signals from all sweeps in each run (vertical scale is different in c,d). (From Hess et al., 1984.)*

changes in single rate constants revolves around an understanding of the inactivated state. In terms of modes of gating, inactivation is represented by mode 0 gating, a mode in which no channel openings occur. Transitions into and out of this mode are not linked to channel openings per se, but to other modes of gating (see Fig. 6). The sequential picture of channel states (Eq. 1) allows for changes in population of the inactivated state that are directly influenced by occupancy of the open state. Resolution of experimental data and these two theoretical schemes will require additional single channel data obtained at potentials that promote inactivation of the channels.

Neurohormones: Beta Adrenergic Modulation

Macroscopic current measurements have shown that beta adrenergic stimulation has dramatic effects on heart Ca channels. In heart cells, norepinephrine causes at least a twofold increase in current amplitude at maximal concentrations [Reuter and Scholtz, 1977; Kass and Wiegers, 1982], but the mechanism responsible for this change has only recently begun to be understood.

Whole cell recordings from isolated heart cells have shown that injection of cAMP or of the catalytic subunit of the cAMP-dependent protein kinase exerts effects similar to bath application of catecholamines [Osterrieder et al., 1982; Brum et al., 1983]. Bean et al. [1984] used ensemble fluctuation analysis developed by Sigworth [1980] to define the mechanism behind these changes. This procedure relates the variance in whole cell currents to the mean current carried at a given membrane potential by the following equation: $var = iI - I^2/N_f$, where I is mean current, i is single channel current, and N_f is the number of functional, identical, independent functional channels having one non-zero conducting state. This analysis showed that isoprenaline, a pure beta agonist, increases the number of functional channels and slowed the time-course of both activation and inactivation. Also, in contrast to previous data from multicellular preparations, the enhancement of peak current by this catecholamine was influenced by membrane potential.

Single channel data have also shown that Ca channel kinetics are affected by catecholamines. Reuter et al. [1982] reported that isoprenaline does not change single channel current, but increases the mean open time and decreases interburst intervals of the channel, thus increasing the probability of channel opening. In another study, Cachelin et al. [1983] found that addition of 8-bromocyclic AMP to solutions bathing cultured cells from the hearts of neonatal rats also changed the probability of a channel opening. In this case, however, the largest effect seen was on the histogram of channel closed times. This suggested that the change in probability of opening was caused by a cAMP-dependent change in the forward rate constant leading to channel opening. This group also reported a reduction in the number of sweeps in which channels failed to open (see below) and that the number of functional channels in a given

patch did not appear to change. Brum et al. [1984] found similar effects of epinephrine and isoprenaline on single channel currents recorded from isolated bovine, cat, and guinea pig myocytes.

Fox et al. [1985] have proposed that, like the DHP derivatives, the effects of adrenergic stimulation can be explained, at least in part, by changes in modes of Ca channel gating. In this view, the reduction in null sweeps (sweeps with no channel openings) is caused by a catecholamine-induced swing towards mode 1 and away from mode 0 channel gating. Such a change in gating mode would account for the increased availability of channels for conduction during depolarization. Demonstration that this is in fact related to the cAMP-dependent phosphorylation is a very important area for future work.

In another system, chick dorsal root ganglion whole-cell recordings revealed that norepinephrine reversibly decreased Ca channel currents. Furthermore, this reduction of current did not appear to occur via a cAMP- or cGMP-mediated pathway. Further studies probing the basis for this action are needed [Forscher and Oxford, 1985].

Surface Potentials: Relationship to Channel Gating

The outer surface of cells is thought to have a negative surface charge layer that can be screened or reduced by monovalent and divalent cations in the extracellular solution [see Hille, 1984, for review]. This change in surface charge alters the transmembrane electric field, and thus affects voltage-dependent gating. According to this concept, elevation of extracellular divalent cation concentration should shift voltage-dependent gating to more positive potentials, and the magnitude of this shift should be related to divalent cation concentration in a predictable manner. Several groups have estimated the density of negative surface charges near Ca channels in a variety of cells using this approach and reported a fixed surface charge density near 1e/80 A^2 [Wilson et al., 1983; Ohmori and Yoshii,

1977; Krafte et al., 1985; for exception see Kostyuck et al., 1982].

It is very important to keep in mind changes in surface potential that occur in solutions of different divalent cations when comparing experimental data obtained in these solutions. For example, according to this theory, if the total divalent cation concentration in one solution is 5 mM, and that in another solution is 50 mM, voltage-dependent gating that occurs at 0 mV in the solution containing the lower divalent cation concentration will occur at +20 mV in the solution with the higher concentration. Since inactivation of Ca channels in whole cell and single channel experiments is often carried in the presence of very high concentrations of divalent charge carriers, comparison to multicellular data, obtained under more physiological conditions, must include compensations for changes in surface potential.

REFERENCES

Adams DJ, Gage PW (1980): Characteristics of sodium and calcium conductance changes produced by membrane depolarization in Aplysia neurone. J Physiol 291:467–481.

Aldrich RW, Corey DP, Stevens CF (1983): A reinterpretation of mammalian sodium channel gating based on single channel recording. Nature 306:436–441.

Almers W, McCleskey EW (1984): Non-selective conductance in calcium channels of frog muscle: Calcium selectivity in a single-file pore. J Physiol 353:585–608.

Armstrong CM, Matteson DR (1985): Two distinct populations of calcium channels in a clonal line of pituitary cells. Science 277:65–67.

Bean BP (1984): Nitrendipine block of cardiac calcium channels: High-affinity binding to the inactivated state. Proc Natl Acad Sci USA 81:6388–6392.

Bean BP (1985): Two kinds of calcium channels in canine atrial cells. Differences in kinetics, selectivity, and pharmacology. J Gen Physiol 86:1–30.

Bean BP, Nowycky MC, Tsien RW (1984): B-adrenergic modulation of calcium channels in frog ventricular heart cells. Nature 307:371–375.

Bean BP, Sturek M, Puga A, Hermsmeyer K (1985): Calcium channels in smooth muscle cells from mesenteric arteries. J Gen Physiol 86:23a.

Brown AM, Kunze DL, Yatani A (1985): Agonist effect of a dihydropyridine Ca channel blocker on guinea pig and rat ventricular myocytes. J Physiol 357:59P.

Brown AM, Lux HD, Wilson DL (1984): Activation and inactivation of single calcium channels in snail neurons. J Gen Physiol 83:751–769.

Brown AM, Morimoto K, Tsuda Y, Wilson DL (1981): Ca current-dependent and voltage-dependent inactivation in calcium channels in Helix aspersa. J Physiol (Lond) 320:193–218.

Brown AM, Tsuda Y, Wilson DL (1983): A description of activation and conduction in calcium channels based on tail and turn-on current measurements. J Physiol (Lond) 344:549–583.

Brum GV, Flockerzi F, Hofmann W, Osterrieder W, Trautwein W (1983): Injection of catalytic subunit of cAMP-dependent protein kinase into isolated cardiac myocytes. Pflugers Arch 398:147–157.

Brum GW, Osterrieder W, Trautwein W (1984): B-adrenergic increases in the calcium conductance of cardiac myocytes studied with the patch clamp. Pflugers Arch 401:111–118.

Byerly L, Hagiwara S (1982): Ca currents in internally perfused nerve cell bodies of Limnea stagnalis. J Physiol 322:503–528.

Cachelin AB, dePeyer JE, Kokubun S, Reuter H (1983): Calcium channel modulation by 8-bromo-cyclic AMP in cultured heart cells. Nature 304:462–464.

Carbone E, Lux HD (1984a): A low voltage-activated calcium conductance in embryonic chick sensory neurons. Biophys J 46:413–418.

Carbone E, Lux HD (1984b): A low voltage-activated, fully inactivating Ca channel in vertebrate sensory neurones. Nature (Lond) 310:502–510.

Cavalie A, Ochi R, Pelzer D, Trautwein W (1983): Elementary currents through Ca^{2+} channels in guinea pig myocytes. Pflugers Arch Eur J Physiol 398:284–297.

Cavalie A, Pelzer D, Trautwein W (1984): Modulation of the gating properties of single calcium channels by D600 in guinea pig ventricular myocytes. J Physiol 358:59P.

Cohen CJ, McCarthy RT (1985): Differential effects of dihydropyridines on two populations of Ca channels in anterior pituitary cells. Biophys J 47:513a.

Colquhoun D, Hawkes AG (1983): The principles of the stochastic interpretation of ion cell mechanisms. In Sackmann B, Neher E (eds): "Single Channel Recording" New York: Plenum Press, pp 135–176.

Deitmer JW (1984): Evidence for two voltage-dependent calcium currents in the membrane of the ciliate Stylonychia. J Physiol (Lond) 355:137–159.

Eckert R, Chad JE (1984): Inactivation of Ca channels. Prog Biophys Molec Biol 44:215–267.

Ehara T, Kaufmann R (1978): The voltage- and time-dependent effects of (−) verapamil on the slow inward current in isolated cat ventricular myocardium. J Pharmacol Exp Ther 207:49–55.

Fenwick EM, Marty A, Nehrer E (1982): Sodium and calcium channels in bovine chromaffin cells. J Physiol 331:599–635.

Forscher P, Oxford GS (1985): Modulation of calcium channels by norepinephrine in internally dialyzed avian sensory neurons. J Gen Physiol 85:743–763.

Fox AP, Hess P, Lansman JB, Nilius B, Nowycky MC, Tsien RW (1985): Shifts between modes of calcium channel gating as a basis for pharmacological modulation of calcium influx in cardiac, neuronal and smooth muscle-derived cells. In Poste G, Crooke ST (eds): "New Insights Into Cell and Membrane Transport Processes." Philadelphia: Smith Kline and French.

Fox AP, Krasne S (1984): Two calcium currents in Neanthes arenaceodentatus egg cell membranes. J Physiol (Lond) 356:491–505.

Fukushima Y, Hagiwara S (1985): Currents carried by monovalent cations through calcium channels in mouse neoplastic B lymphocytes. J Physiol 358:255–284.

Hagiwara S, Byerly L (1981): Calcium channel. Ann Rev Neurosci 4:69–125.

Hagiwara S, Byerly L (1983): The calcium channel. Trends Neurosci 6:189–193.

Hagiwara S, Ozawa S, Sand O (1975): Voltage clamp analysis of two inward current mechanisms in the egg cell membrane of a starfish. J Gen Physiol 65:617–644.

Hamill O, Marty A, Neher E, Sackmann B, Sigworth FJ (1981): Improved patch-clamp techniques for high resolution current recordings from cells and cell-free membrane patches. Pflugers Arch 391:85–100.

Hess P, Lansman JB, Tsien RW (1984): Different modes of Ca channel gating behaviour favoured by dihydropyridine agonists and antagonists. Nature 311:538–544.

Hess P, Tsien RW (1984): Mechanism of ion permeation through calcium channels. Nature 309:453–456.

Hille B (1977): Local anesthetics: Hydrophilic and hydrophobic pathways for the drug-receptor reaction. J Gen Physiol 69:497–515.

Hille B (1984): "Ionic Channels of Excitable Membranes." Sunderland, MA: Sinauer Associates, Inc., p 426.

Hodeghem LM, Katzung BG (1977): Time- and voltage-dependent interactions of antiarrhythmic drugs with cardiac sodium channels. Biochim Biophys Acta 472:373–398.

Isenberg G, Klockner U (1985): Calcium currents of smooth muscle cells isolated from the urinary bladder of the guinea-pig: Inactivation conductance and selectivity is controlled by micromolar amounts of [Ca]o. J Physiol 358:60-P.

Kass RS, Bennett PB (1985): Microelectrode voltage clamp: The cardiac Purkinje fibre. In Smith TG, Lecar H, Redman S, Gage P (eds): "Voltage and Patch Clamping with Microelectrodes." New York: Waverly Press, pp 178–191.

Kass RS, Sanguinetti MC (1984): Calcium channel inactivation in the cardiac Purkinje fibre: Evidence for voltage- and calcium-mediated mechanisms. J Gen Physiol 84:705–726.

Kass RS, Wiegers SE (1982): The ionic basis of concen-

tration-related effects of noradrenaline on the action potential of calf cardiac Purkinje fibres. J Physiol 322:541–558.

Kohlhardt M, Mnich Z (1978): Studies on the inhibitory effect of verapamil on the slow inward current in mammalian ventricular myocardium. J Mol Cell Cardiol 10:1037–1052.

Kokubun S, Reuter H (1984): Dihydropyridine derivatives prolong the open state of Ca channels in cultured cardiac cells. Proc Natl Acad Sci 81:4824–4827.

Kostyuk PG, Krishtal OA (1977): Effects of calcium and calcium-chelating agents on the inward and outward current in the membrane of mollusc neurones. J Physiol 270:569–580.

Kostyuk PG, Mironov SL, Doroshenko PA, Ponomarev VN (1982): Surface charges on the outer side of mollusc neuron membrane. J Mem Biol 70:171–179.

Krafte D, Coplin B, Bennett P, Kass RS (1985): Surface charge modification influences blocking activity of dihydropyridine Ca channel antagonists. Biophys J 47:512a.

Lee KS, Marban E, Tsien RW (1985): Inactivation of calcium channels in mammalian heart cells. Joint dependence on membrane potential and intracellular calcium. J Physiol 364:395–411.

Lee KS, Tsien RW (1982): Reversal of current through calcium channels in dialyzed single heart cells. Nature (Lond) 297:498–501.

Lee KS, Tsien RW (1983): Mechanism of calcium channel block by verapamil, D600, diltiazem, and nitrendipine in single dialyzed heart cells. Nature 302:790–794.

Llinas R, Yarom Y (1981a): Electrophysiology of mammalian inferior olivary neurones in vitro. Different types of voltage-dependent ionic conductances. J Physiol 315:549–567.

Llinas R, Yarom Y (1981b): Properties and distribution of ionic conductances generating electroresponsiveness of mammalian inferior olivary neurones in vitro. J Physiol 315:569–584.

Lux HD, Brown AM (1984): Patch clamp and whole cell calcium currents recorded simultaneously in snail neurons. J Gen Physiol 83:727–750.

Matsuda H, Noma A (1984): Isolation of calcium current and its sensitivity to monovalent cations in dyalised ventricular cells of guinea pig. J Physiol 357:553–573.

Miller RJ (1985): How many types of calcium channels exist in neurones? Trends Neurosci 8:45–47.

Mitra R, Morad M (1985): Evidence for two types of calcium channels in guinea pig ventricular myocytes. J Gen Physiol 86:22a.

Nilius BP, Hess P, Lansman JB, Tsien RW (1985): A novel type of cardiac calcium channel in ventricular cells. Nature 316:443–446.

Nowycky MC, Fox AP, Tsien RW (1985): Three types of neuronal calcium channels with different calcium agonist sensitivity. Nature 316:440–443.

Ochi R, Hino N, Niimi Y (1984): Prolongation of calcium channel open time by the dihydropyridine derivative Bay K8644 in cardiac myocytes. Proc Jpn Acad 60B:153–156.

Ohmori H, Yoshii M (1977): Surface potential reflected in both gating and permeation mechanisms of sodium and calcium channels of the tunicate egg cell membrane. J Physiol (Lond) 267:467–495.

Osterrieder W, Yan QF, Trautwein W (1982): Effects of Ba on the membrane currents in S-A node. Pflugers Arch 394:78–84.

Palade PT, Almers W (1978): Slow Na^+ and Ca^{++} currents across the membrane of frog skeletal muscle fibres. Biophys J 21:168a.

Pelzer DW, Trautwein W, McDonald TF (1982): Calcium channel block and recovery from block in mammalian ventricular muscle treated with organic channel inhibitors. Pflugers Arch 394:97–105.

Prosser CL, Kreulen DL, Weigel RJ, Yau W (1977): Prolonged action potentials in gastrointestinal muscles induced by calcium chelation. Am J Physiol 233:C19–C24.

Reuter H (1979): Properties of two inward membrane currents in the heart. Ann Rev Physiol 41:413–424.

Reuter H (1983): Calcium channel modulation by neurotransmitters and drugs. Nature 301:569–574.

Reuter H, Scholz A (1977): The regulation of Ca conductance of cardiac muscle by adrenaline. J Physiol 264:49–62.

Reuter H, Stevens CF, Tsien RW, Yellen G (1982): Properties of single calcium channels in cultured cardiac cells. Nature 297:501–504.

Rougier O, Vassort G, Garner D, Gargouil VM, Coraboeuf E (1969): Existence and role of a slow inward current during the frog atrial action potential. Pflugers Arch 308:91–110.

Sanguinetti MC, Kass RS (1984a): Regulation of cardiac calcium channel current and contractile activity by the dihydropyridine Bay K8644 is voltage-dependent. J Mole Cell Cardiol 16:667–670.

Sanguinetti MC, Kass RS (1984b): Voltage-dependent block of calcium channel current in the calf cardiac Purkinje fiber by dihydropyridine calcium channel antagonists. Circ Res 55:336–348.

Sanguinetti MC, Kass RS (1985): Voltage selects activity of the Ca channel modulator Bay K8644. Biophys J 47:513a.

Sigworth FJ (1980): The variance of sodium current fluctuations at the node of Ranvier. 307:97–129.

Sturek M, Hermsmeyer K (1985): Two different types of calcium channels in spontaneously contracting vascular smooth muscle cells. J Gen Physiol 86:23a.

Takeda K, Oomura Y (1972): Sarcotubular regenerative response induced by EDTA in proprionate solution. Proc Jpn Acad 48:753–757.

Tsien RW (1983): Calcium channels in excitable membranes. Ann Rev Physiol 45:341–358.

Tung L, Morad M (1983): Voltage- and frequency-dependent block of diltiazem on the slow inward current and generation of tension in frog ventricular muscle. Pflugers Arch 398:189–198.

Uehara A, Hume JR (1985): Interactions of organic calcium channel antagonists with calcium channels in single frog atrial cells. J Gen Physiol 85:621–647.

Wilson DL, Morimoto K, Tsuda Y, Brown AM (1983): Interaction between calcium ions and surface charge as it relates to calcium currents. J Mem Biol 72:117–130.

Yamamoto D, Washio H (1979): Permeation of sodium through calcium channels of an insect muscle membrane. Can J Physiol Pharmacol 57:220–223.

Structure and Physiology of the Slow Inward Calcium Channel, pages 89–108
© 1987 Alan R. Liss, Inc.

5

Molecular Model for the Binding of 1,4-Dihydropyridine Calcium Channel Antagonists to Their Receptors in the Heart: Drug "Imaging" in Membranes and Considerations for Drug Design

Leo G. Herbette and Arnold M. Katz

Biomolecular Structure Analysis Center (L.G.H.) and Cardiology Division (A.M.K.), University of Connecticut Health Center, Farmington, Connecticut 06032

OVERVIEW

Responses to Calcium Channel Antagonists in the Heart

The ability of calcium channel antagonists to inhibit the influx of Ca^{2+} across the plasma membrane (or sarcolemma) of the excitable cells of the heart reduces the amount of messenger Ca^{2+} that enters the interior of the cell. This, in turn, reduces the amount of Ca^{2+} that is available to bind to sites within the cell that initiate or regulate such key cellular processes as myocardial contraction and vasoconstriction in coronary and systemic arterial smooth muscle. These drugs also have electrophysiological effects because they can inhibit important depolarizing currents carried by Ca^{2+} influx. Thus, the ability of Ca^{2+} to serve as both a chemical signal that binds to proteins within the cell and as an electrical charge carrier across the sarcolemma may be partially controlled by antagonists (and agonists) which bind to specific receptors that are present in various membranes of these cells.

Calcium as a chemical messenger. The ability of Ca^{2+} to activate cardiac contraction arises from its ability to initiate interactions between the contractile proteins that lead to tension and shortening in the walls of the heart. This function reflects the presence of a family of high-affinity Ca^{2+}-binding proteins in the cytosol of these and other mammalian cell types [Kretsinger, 1979].

Calcium as the carrier of an electrical signal. In addition to serving as an intracellular chemical messenger, Ca^{2+}, because of its charge, carries an inward (depolarizing) current across the cardiac cell membrane [Reuter, 1979]. The inward current, generated by Ca^{2+} fluxes across the sarcolemma of the working cells of the atria and ventricles and the rapidly conducting cells of the His-Purkinje system, contributes to the plateau of the action potential. However, the initial depolarizing event in these cells arises from Na^+ entry through fast channels that are relatively insensitive to the calcium channel antagonists, so that these drugs do not affect impulse transmission in the atria, ventricles, and His-Purkinje system. In contrast, the pacemaker cells of the sino-atrial node and the slowly conducting cells of the atrioventricular node do not contain functionally active, fast Na^+ channels; instead, depolarization is initiated by an inward current carried by Ca^{2+}. As Ca^{2+} entry is responsible for normal pacemaker activity and atrioventricular conduction in the heart, these activities can be inhibited by the calcium channel antagonists.

Drug Interactions with Membranes

The effects of most drugs of cardiac function are initiated by the binding of the drug to a specific sarcolemmal "receptor," which recognizes and forms a tight complex with the molecular structure of the drug. The events that follow binding of the drug to the receptor have been the subject of considerable investigation, but little attention has been devoted to understanding mechanisms which explain the approach and subsequent binding of the drug with its sarcolemmal receptor. The drug may bind to a specific site in the aqueous (hydrophilic) region at or above the surface of the membrane, external to the membrane bilayer, or the drug may approach its binding site by diffusion through the aqueous medium outside the cell and bind to the interior of the receptor protein within the membrane bilayer via an aqueous channel within the protein. Some calcium channel antagonists have been suggested to block ion fluxes by insertion into the aqueous pore, or "mouth" of the channel. This mechanism can explain the phenomenon of "use dependence," where prior membrane depolarization, which opens both sodium and calcium channels, enhances the potency of drugs, like quinidine and verapamil, which block sodium and calcium channels, respectively. This potentiation of the inhibitory effects of these and other calcium channel antagonist drugs by prior use of the channels

can be explained if the drugs enter the channel when it is in the open state. There are, however, alternative explanations for the observation that the state of an ionic channel, or a receptor, influences its sensitivity to a specific drug.

Molecular Information, Drug-Membrane Receptor Mechanisms, and Drug Design

We have proposed a model for drug interaction with cardiac membranes which involves a partitioning of these lipophilic, and often amphiphilic, drug substances into the sarcolemmal bilayer matrix where the drug can become oriented, followed by lateral diffusion throughout this matrix to a specific protein receptor site (Fig. 1) [Rhodes et al., 1985; Herbette et al., 1986]. Models similar to this hydrophobic pathway have been previously suggested for other systems but not investigated [Hille, 1977; Schwarz et al., 1977; Courtney, 1980; Broughton et al., 1984]. The physical interaction of the drug with the sarcolemmal bilayer is precisely governed by inter- and intramolecular forces which together result in a specified location (depth within the bilayer), orientation (directional coordinates with respect to some reference axis within the lipid bilayer), and intramolecular conformation (internal drug structure) of the drug substances. The nature of this interaction, how it may influence the binding properties of cardiovascular agents, and how this may in turn alter cellular functions are the topics of this chapter.

Briefly, our approach to reviewing and critically evaluating this molecular model focuses on the review of the current molecular data that defines the nature of the binding site of calcium channel antagonists in a variety of tissues, as well as the nature of the specific protein complex and the properties of the sarcolemmal membrane that contains this protein complex. Subsequently, we summarize pertinent data which have led to a definition of this molecular model for drug binding, including structural work on the sarcolemmal membrane, physical chemistry of calcium

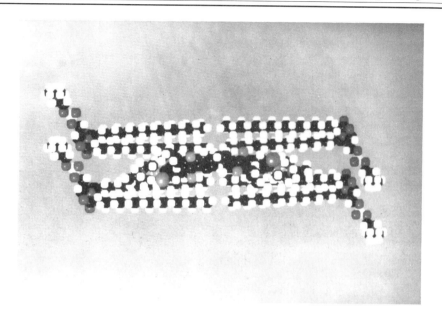

Fig. 1. *Electron density profile structure superimposed on a space-filling molecular model of a lipid molecule. The most prominent electron dense maxima corresponds with the phosphoryl moiety of the lipid headgroup; the lower flat electron-dense region corresponds to the methylene segments of the fatty acyl chains; the lowest electron-dense corresponds to the terminal methyl region of the lipid molecule.*

channel antagonists, drug membrane interactions, and the theoretical basis for evaluating the various schemes by which these drugs may interact with their protein receptors. We review other studies which either support or do not support this molecular model for drug binding to receptors in the heart and provide an overall evaluation based on these studies as to the validity of such a model. We provide specific details as to the precise molecular events that may be involved in the interaction of these calcium channel antagonists with cardiac membranes. These include location, orientation, and conformation of these drug substances in cardiac membranes and how these physical parameters may define drug activity, selectivity, and clinical effectiveness. We describe a novel drug design modality as suggested by the molecular approach discussed. We speculate about future advances in drug "imaging" and drug interactions at the membrane, cellular, and organ levels and their impact on clinical medicine.

STRUCTURE OF THE CALCIUM CHANNEL

Our current knowledge of the structure of the calcium channels and the proteins to which the calcium channel antagonists bind is discussed in detail (see Lazdunski, and Venter, this volume). There are few data now available from these studies that help to define the mechanism by which these drugs interact with the receptors that are related to these channels. Several features of this mechanism are, however, now coming into focus. Notably, the channel is an oligomeric structure containing at least one integral membrane glycoprotein that binds several lectins which can be displaced from it by specific sugars [Glossman and Ferry, 1983; Curtis and Catterall, 1984; Borsotto et al., 1985; Rengasamy et al., 1985]. The finding that the dihydropyridine receptor can be extracted by detergents provides evidence that this receptor is contained on an integral membrane protein.

Radiation inactivation and sucrose velocity gradient centrifugation suggest that the native dihydropyridine receptor is a large macro-molecular structure having a molecular weight of 150–300,000 [Venter et al., 1983; Ferry et al., 1983a,b]. As reviewed by Lazdunski and Venter, this volume, the dihydropyridine receptor is an oligomer. Most reports suggest that the dihydropyridine calcium channel antagonists bind to a 32–45,000 dalton peptide of the dihydropyridine receptor [Campbell et al., 1984; Horne et al., 1984; Kirley and Schwartz, 1984; Venter et al., 1983].

SUMMARY OF OUR PERTINENT DATA FOR DEFINITION OF A MOLECULAR MODEL FOR DRUG BINDING
Structure and Function of the Sarcolemma

The sarcolemmal membrane is a complex structure with a unique composition. When the glycocalyx is removed, the membrane contains several different proteins, most of which are present in low concentrations [see Table I]. The dominant protein on a weight/weight basis (and density) is the Na/K ATPase; the Na/Ca exchanger, Ca^{2+} ATPase, and related enzymes are present in much lower concentrations. Other proteins that probably function in the earlier phases of regulation of ion fluxes across the sarcolemma are specific receptors or receptor/channel complexes that exist in extremely low concentrations (see Table I) consistent with their functional roles [Colvin et al., 1985]. Overall, the composition of the sarcolemma is much different than other membranes in the myocardial cell, especially more highly specialized membranes such as the sarcoplasmic reticulum which is involved in fewer regulatory processes.

The lipid content of the sarcolemma is also quite high; on a weight/weight basis, it is approximately 3 mg lipid/mg protein. This high lipid content is similar to that in myelin. This is in contrast to membranes, such as the sarcoplasmic reticulum (~ 0.7 mg lipid/mg protein), which contain a high concentration of the Ca^{2+} pump ATPase protein. Whereas

TABLE I. Estimation of Receptor Density in the Purified Sarcolemmal Membrane*

Receptor ligand	Mol lipid per mol site	Sites/m²	
		Lipid surface	Protein-corrected
Ouabain	8.5 10³	400	330
Quinuclidinyl-benzilate	5.3 10⁵	6	5
Dihydroalprenolol	1.4 10⁶	2	1.6
Nitrendipine	4.2 10⁶	0.8	0.6

*Receptor densities were estimated by comparison of B_{max} values obtained from Scatchard analysis of binding isotherms and lipid content of purified sarcolemmal vesicles, as described in Colvin et al., 1985.

the lipid bilayer is composed of a heterogeneous mixture of lipids and lipid-like substances, this heterogeneity is typical of other membranes in the myocardial cell, notably the sarcoplasmic reticulum, with differences occurring in the amounts of specific lipid species.

X-ray diffraction studies have shown that the width of the sarcolemmal membrane is similar to that for lipids extracted from either the sarcolemmal or the sarcoplasmic reticulum [Herbette et al., 1985]. In fact, the structure of the membrane, expressed as a plot of electron density against distance along the bilayer axis* is similar to that of the pure lipid extracts. Although protein is present in the sarcolemmal membrane, because the lipid content is high, x-ray diffraction has been able to only marginally detect the presence of this protein. However, these studies have shown that the lipid bilayer structure in sarcolemma stripped of its glycocalyx is similar to that in other membranes, with a phospholipid headgroup separation of 45° (see Fig. 1)

*This plot of electron density is made against a reference axis in the membrane. For these studies, this reference axis is parallel to the fatty acyl chains of the membrane bilayer (perpendicular to the membrane plane defined by the phospholipid headgroups). For this specific case, this plot is referred to as the electron density *profile* structure and may be interpreted as shown in Figure 1—relatively high electron density referable to phospholipid headgroups and lower electron density for the fatty acyl chains.

compared to both the sarcoplasmic reticulum and lipid extracts from the sarcoplasmic reticulum of around 40 Å. This 5 Å difference can be identified with the greater thickness of the hydrocarbon core in the sarcolemma and is consistent with the lipid composition of the sarcolemma compared to the sarcoplasmic reticulum.

The functional properties of the sarcolemma have been studied by several investigators. Of primary relevance to this review are studies which have demonstrated that ion transport or exchange reactions in the sarcolemma can be influenced by the presence of certain drug substances. Along these lines, extensive background work has been obtained to better define the biochemical reactions that are mediated by the sarcolemma. Na/Ca exchange has been one area of intense study. The characterization of the Na/Ca exchange protein along with other ion transport proteins, such as the Na/K ATPase, the Ca^{2+} ATPase and the Mg^{2+} ATPase, to mention a few, all apparently work in a harmonious fashion to balance ionic currents and establish different globally functional states for the sarcolemma. When taken into context with the membrane potential, the electrophysiological results are most significant. It is no surprise, then, that the various actions of drug substances with such a multifunctional and multiregulatory membrane are so widespread (see below).

Physical Chemistry of the Calcium Channel Antagonists

The class of 1,4-dihydropyridine calcium channel antagonists do not, in general, possess a formal charge at physiological pH. However, an inspection of their chemical structure would support the notion that these drug substances are amphiphilic and probably highly lypophilic. Table II is a summary of partition coefficients for several drug substances including some dihydropyridine calcium channel antagonists measured both in biological membranes against buffer and in octanol/buffer. First, there would appear to

TABLE II. Partition Coefficients

Drug	Biological membranes	Octanol/buffer
Amiodarone	921,000	350
Bay P 8857	125,000	40
Beta X-61	12,500	120
Nisoldipine	6,000	40
Nimodipine	5,000	260
Beta X-67	3,200	250
Beta X-57	350	3
Cimetidine	300	1
Propranolol	200	18
Acetylcholine	32	0.003
Timolol	16	0.7
Ethanol	3	0.6

be little correlation between these two sets of values. Apparently, a two-phase isotropic bulk solvent system such as octanol/buffer apparently cannot serve as a model for the highly anistropic chemical nature of a lipid bilayer. Thus, the proper measure of the lipophilicity of these drug substances must be made directly in biological membranes. Second, the partition coefficients in membranes are seen to be quite high, especially for the dihydropyridine calcium channel antagonists. Thus, these substances are very soluble in lipid bilayer structures. In fact, an interesting comparison between the concentration of drug in aqueous buffer can be made with its corresponding concentration in the membrane. Using nimodipine as our example, if we take the most conservative approach for calculating the concentration of nimodipine in the lipid bilayer, then the entire lipid bilayer can be used as the volume in which the nimodipine is "dissolved." The volume per lipid would equal the product of the length (30 Å) and average cross-sectional area (60 Å) which are taken directly from x-ray diffraction measurements [Levine, 1973]. Based on the partition coefficient measurements, at the k_d for nimodipine binding to its high affinity receptor which is 4.1×10^{-10} M, there is approximately one nimodipine molecule in 10^6 lipids. A simple calculation demonstrates that this is equivalent to a "membrane" concentration for nimodipine equal to approximately 1×10^{-6}

M, a factor of 10^4 higher than the aqueous nimodipine concentration. Even this is a lower limit estimate since neutron diffraction studies (see below) show that nimodipine occupies discrete positions in the lipid bilayer, not its entire volume. Thus, because of their high lipophilicity, these drugs assume high membrane concentrations at relatively low aqueous buffer concentrations. This may be important in the analytical treatment of kinetic data for specific drug binding to receptors in the sarcolemma. Table III summarizes other examples for membrane and aqueous buffer drug concentrations.

Drug-Sarcolemma and Drug-Drug Interactions in Sarcolemma

Recent studies have shown that the highly lipophilic calcium channel antagonists bind very rapidly to lipid bilayers. In fact, a lower limit estimate for the rate of binding of these drugs with lipid bilayers is at least 10^3 times faster than overall binding of these substances to their receptors in the sarcolemma. In addition, utilizing fluorescence redistribution after photobleaching (FRAP) techniques with fluorescent-labelled nisoldipine and labeled phospholipids, it was shown that these drug substances are diffusing at a rate similar to that of the lipids that comprise the sarcolemmal membrane bilayer. Thus, prior to actual binding of the calcium channel antagonists to their receptors, an equilibrium dissolution of the drug in the membrane bilayer is established. On-rates, off-rates, k_d and B_{max} values, displacement parameters, etc., for these antagonists have been the subject of numerous studies. In light of the above findings, the rate limiting step for the interaction of the calcium channel antagonists with their receptors must involve molecular interactions other than the binding of these antagonists to and diffusion within the lipid bilayer. Thus, these drugs may first interact with the lipid bilayer, and this may be a necessary prerequisite to their binding to protein receptors. However, other events, most probably related to conformational perturbations at the receptor site, must dominate the binding reaction.

TABLE III. Drug Concentrations in Membranes

Drug	Partition coefficient in a biological membrane	"Membrane" concentration (μmol) at 1 nmol aqueous concentration
Amiodarone	921,000	740
Bay P 8857*	125,000	100
Nimodipine*	5,000	4
Propranolol	200	0.16
Timolol	16	0.016

*1, 4 dihydropyridine calcium channel antagonists

Some of the calcium channel antagonists, notably verapamil, displace other classes of drugs from their specific receptors. This effect is seen at high drug concentrations, but can exhibit stereospecificity, similar to their effects in blocking calcium channels [Gerry et al., 1985]. Thus, while these effects are often attributed to nonspecific "detergent" actions, it is possible that, once dissolved in the bilayer, the individual drug molecules have targeted effects on proteins other than the calcium channel [Gruner, 1985].

Theoretical Considerations for Drug Binding Models

The rate at which a calcium channel antagonist, such as nimodipine, approaches its receptor in the sarcolemma can be calculated for different molecular schemes based on diffusion-limited processes. As shown in Figure 2, two distinctly different pathways would be 1) diffusion of the drug through the aqueous buffer to a receptor site that is external to the lipid bilayer, and 2) diffusion of the drug through the aqueous buffer to some point of contact with the lipid bilayer and lateral diffusion through the bilayer to a protein receptor site within the lipid bilayer. For an isotropic drug structure (which nimodipine is not), calculations of these diffusion-limited rates for the two pathways have been made as a function of the size of the drug molecule [Rhodes et al., 1985]. The rates of drug binding via the membrane pathway are 10^3–10^4 times faster than the rates via the aqueous pathway. If a physically reasonable degree of anisotropy is introduced (now more applica-

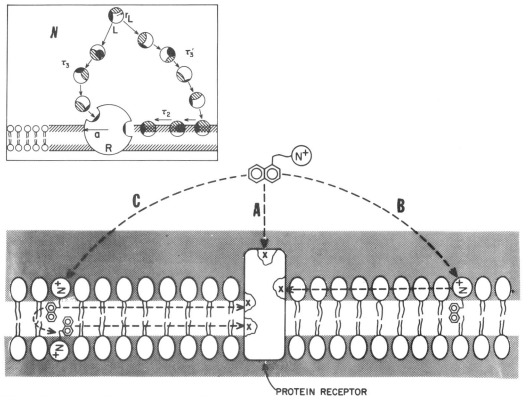

Fig. 2. *Theoretical (insert) and pictorial representation of the membrane vs. aqueous pathway models for drug binding to a protein receptor site. A, B, C represent different pathways for drug binding to a protein receptor. These may be characterized by different parameters such as time constants (τ_3, τ_3', τ_2), radius of the ligand r_L, and radius of the receptor a_R in a kinetic simulation as shown in the insert.*

ble to nimodipine), the rates for both pathways decrease, still preserving the 10^3 difference. Thus, independent of the degree of anisotropy, the rates for approach by the membrane bilayer pathway are at least three orders of magnitude faster than the rate of approach by the aqueous pathway. Thus, a rate enhancement has been achieved by reducing the dimensionality of the process from a drug diffusing in a three dimensional volume of fluid to a drug diffusing in a two dimensional plane. This may be significant for cases where the concentration of both the drug and the receptor are very low, such as in the heart.

The overall experimental on-rates for these calcium channel antagonists are less than either the isotropic maximum calculated rates for either pathway. However, these upper limit calculations are physically unreasonable since the drugs are highly anisotropic, as can be gleaned by inspection of their chemical and crystal structures. For the case of Bay P8857, another calcium channel antagonist, the measured on-rate is near to the maximum diffusion limited rate for the aqueous pathway (and greater than the physicially reasonable anisotropic rate). Thus, on a theoretical basis, Bay P8857 may reach its protein receptor by the membrane pathway.

LITERATURE REVIEW—MOLECULAR MODEL

The calcium channel blockers exhibit a property generally referred to as "use-dependence," in that their ability to block calcium channel function is potentiated at rapid heart rates, that is, when the channels are being used. Use-dependence is seen with the dihydropyridines and is especially marked in the case of verapamil and diltiazem [Bayer and Ehara, 1978; Ehara and Kaufman, 1978; Kohlhardt and Mnich, 1978; Hachisu and Pappano, 1983; Lee and Tsien, 1983; Trautwein and Cavalie, 1985]. While use-dependence is generally explained by assuming that the drug inserts into the mouth of the open channel [Schramm and Towart, 1985], this phenomenon can also be explained if the drugs bind preferentially to a specific conformation assumed by the channel during its open or refractory state. Reports that the inhibitory effects of calcium channel blockers are potentiated by partial membrane depolarization [Sanguinetti and Kass, 1984; Bean, 1984] are in accord with the hypothesis that the state of the channel determines its sensitivity to this class of drug [see Hondeghem and Katzung, 1984, for a review of this general area].

Other Studies Supporting the Membrane Pathway Model

The membrane pathway model for ligand receptor interaction has a firm basis in the biochemical literature. Although the application of this concept to calcium channels is relatively recent, similar models were suggested as early as 1977 by research on other membrane systems [Hille, 1977]. The development of this model was preceded by observations of numerous investigators of correlations of local anesthetic activity with oil/water partition coefficients or ability to penetrate membrane bilayers [McLaughlin, 1975]. Until recent data became available regarding the position, structure, and orientation of drugs in membrane bilayers [Herbette et al., 1983], the idea of a directed approach of an oriented drug to a binding site on a membrane-associated receptor protein was not considered [Rhodes et al., 1985]. Even today, there remains only circumstantial (albeit extensive) evidence that the membrane pathway model is operative in the case of 1,4-dihydropyridine calcium channel antagonists and agonists.

The work of Hille and colleagues with Na channels of the node of Ranvier was the first to suggest a membrane pathway (referred to as a "hydrophobic pathway") in order to explain the effects of charged and uncharged local anesthetics and their analogs [Hille, 1977]. These investigators used anesthetics which were permanently charged ("quaternary"), which carried titratable charge ("amine"), and which were uncharged ("neutral"). Table IV (adapted from this work) summarizes their results.

From these and other data, Hille proposed that the anesthetic receptor is in the channel near the inactivation gating subunit. With the inactivation gate open, binding is weak, but when the channel conformation changes to close the gate, affinity increases, stabilizing the closed state. The interactions must include not only a hydrophobic component, but also a polar component. However, since both permanently charged and uncharged molecules shift the inactivation curve, neither the drug-receptor reaction nor the use-dependent inactivation has a significant charge-charge component. Hille's model, then, allowed 1) neutral drugs to be in the inner or outer aqueous solution, within the membrane, or bound to receptor; 2) permanently charged drugs to be in the inner or outer aqueous solution or bound to the receptor (with access limited by the receptor ligand itself); and 3) amines to be in ionic equilibrium in the aqueous solvent within the membrane in the neutral state, or bound to the receptor site in an uncharged or charged state. In this manner, drugs could bind by either a hydrophobic pathway, in which a charged drug could reach the binding site directly from within the channel, or an uncharged drug could diffuse within the hydrophobic core of a membrane bilayer to reach the site. As Hille mentions, the behavior of this system is very similar to that of certain antiarrhythmic drugs applied to myocardial membranes, according to results published by Gettes and Reuter [1974].

Reuter's group later published some of the most convincing data to date, which indicate that binding of dihydropyridine calcium channel agonists and antagonists to calcium channels occurs via the membrane pathway [Ko-

TABLE IV. Summary of local anesthetic interactions with the sodium channel

Na-channel characteristic	Quaternary	Anesthetic type amine	Neutral
Modulated by holding potential	−	+	−
Modulated by [Ca^{2+}]	−	+	
h Shift by first pulse	−	+ −	+
Further h shift by many pulses	+	+	−
Large depolarization enhances block	+	+	−
Persistence time (sec)	>20	0.4–12	<0.2

kubun and Reuter, 1984]. Using cultured rat myocardial cells for patch-clamp studies, these investigators found that if a single calcium channel were included in a patch on a sealed, right-side-out cell, the dihydropyridine calcium channel antagonists added to the external solution, the drug would still exert its effects. This result, confirmed by Brown et al. [1984], strongly suggests that the membrane pathway is operative for this system, although alternative pathways could exist. For example, despite the very high membrane partition coefficients observed for 1,4-dihydropyridine calcium channel antagonists (Table II), it is possible that the drug diffused across the bilayer, desorbed into the cytosolic side of the membrane, and bound to the receptor from that medium.

There is further evidence regarding the sidedness of the binding sites on calcium channels from the work of Affolter and Coronado [1986] with charged and uncharged verapamil derivatives. These investigators demonstrated that when ionized, and therefore unable to traverse a bilayer, these drugs could only inactivate calcium channels when added to the cytosolic side of the membrane. Similar work with 1,4-dihydropyridine compounds did not indicate sidedness of binding. While this result does not conclusively demonstrate applicability of the membrane pathway, neither does it preclude it. Although the verapamil analogues bound only from the cytosolic side of the membrane, there is no indication that they did not first partition into that side of the bilayer; in fact, the structure of this compound suggests that it is highly lipophilic. At

least some of the dihydropyridines, which bear no formal charge, have been shown to diffuse across bilayers [Herbette et al., unpublished observation]. Therefore, added to the cytoplasmic side, these drugs could be partitioning into the bilayer, diffusing across to the cytosolic side, and then diffusing laterally.

In the case of phenylalkylamines, the drugs appear to bind preferentially at the inner, or cytosolic, opening of the calcium channel [Hescheler et al., 1982]. These data, along with evidence cited above, are consistent with the view that these drugs inhibit channel opening by an effect on the hydrophobic portion of the calcium channel itself. The ability of phospholipase A_2 to inhibit nitrendipine binding to brain, heart, and smooth muscle membranes [Goldman and Pisano, 1985] also indicates that membrane phospholipids play a role in the interaction between the calcium channel blockers and the calcium channels.

Overall Evaluation of the Molecular Model in View of Existing Literature

Based on the results discussed above, the approach most likely to be in effect (for these calcium channel antagonists added to the cytoplasmic side of the membrane) is the membrane pathway shown in Figure 2. In addition, because a formally charged drug added to the cytosolic side of the membrane is effective, the active site may be near the hydrocarbon core/water interface on that side of the membrane. If this is true, the position of nonspecific partitioning (relative to the bilayer normal) would be very close to the position of specific binding, which would be compliant with the restrictions necessary to make the membrane bilayer approach more "favorable." Even if the verapamil and dihydropyridine sites are not in close proximity, the fact that the dihydropyridines were able to reach a patch-included receptor and did not display sidedness indicates, at least, some involvement by the lipid bilayer. Although more work must be done before this model is conclusively demonstrated, there is clearly an increasing base of circumstantial evidence in support of the membrane bilayer pathway.

SIGNIFICANCE OF DRUG-MEMBRANE INTERACTIONS AT THE MOLECULAR LEVEL

Location, Orientation, and Conformation of Drugs in Cardiac Membranes

X-ray and neutron diffraction have been used to define the locations of several drug substances in both synthetic and native biological membranes. Previous studies focused on cardiovascular drugs with a formal charge at physiological pH, such as propranolol and timolol [Herbette et al., 1983]. More recent studies have turned to the calcium channel antagonists which do not possess a formal charge at physiological pH [Herbette et al., 1985]. These findings are summarized in Figure 3, where these drug substances have been shown to assume discrete positions near the hydrocarbon core/water interface of the membrane bilayer. Most recently, the position of amiodarone has been determined in the membrane bilayer, using x-ray diffraction. Amiodarone is apparently buried deep within the bilayer near the terminal methyl region (Fig. 4).

The x-ray and neutron diffraction results described above clearly indicate that cardiac drugs assume discrete locations within the lipid bilayer structure of both native and synthetic model membranes. The significance of this finding is not yet appreciated but may have to do with the interaction of specific classes of cardiac drugs with specific classes

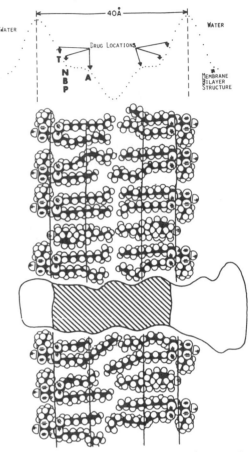

Fig. 3. *The locations of several drug substances in both model (dipalmitoyl and dimyristoyl lecithin, sarcolemmal lipid extracts) and native (sarcoplasmic reticulum) biological membranes have been determined. Dueteration and neutron diffraction were used to locate propranolol (P) and nimodipine (N) in a membrane bilayer; iodination and x-ray diffraction were used to locate Bay P 8857 (B) and amiodarone (A). The location of other substances such as timolol (T) and Bay Q 1280 (not shown) would be established by inference from these and other data. The general finding is that these lipid soluble drug substances prefer discrete regions of the membrane bilayer (e.g., near the hydrocarbon core/water interface).*

of protein receptors. Therefore, location of the drug molecule within the lipid bilayer matrix along the direction of the fatty acyl chains may prove to be an essential criterion for the binding of these agents to specific protein receptor sites also contained at the same depth within the lipid bilayer. Not only

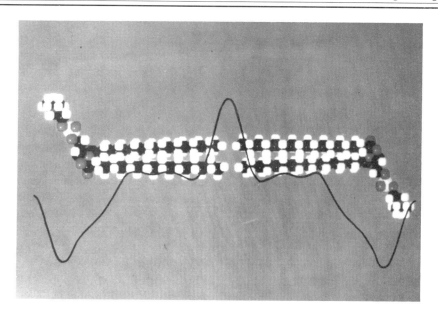

Fig. 4. *The determination of the position of amio-darone in a membrane bilayer by x-ray diffraction. Amiodarone was shown to penetrate 25 Å into the* hydrocarbon core near to the terminal methyl ($-CH_3$) region of the bilayer.

do these molecules assume a precise location in the membrane bilayer, but, at least for two of them studied to date, their orientation within the bilayer may be as well defined as their location. This orientation, which is referable to specific directional coordinates of the drug structure with respect to some reference axis within the lipid bilayer structure, may play an important role in the binding of these substances to protein receptor sites (Fig. 5). Finally, although we have not yet mapped out in detail the precise conformation of a drug molecule in a lipid bilayer, it is likely that because the orientation and location of these molecules in the membrane bilayer is very well defined, the conformation of the drug will also be well defined. We are developing two independent approaches, one using x-ray scattering and polymerizable lipids, and the other using neutron scattering in native membranes, for mapping out the precise conformation of a drug structure in a lipid bilayer matrix. We expect to find that the 1,4-dihydropyridine calcium channel antagonists have specific conformations within the lipid bilayer

matrix, so that for a given drug at a particular location and orientation in the membrane, the conformation will be unique to that drug structure. All three of these molecular parameters, namely location, orientation, and conformation, may play a crucial role in the actual binding of these molecules to high affinity sites on proteins, as schematically portrayed in Figure 5.

In addition to these basic molecular criteria, it is likely that there are several other structural determinants which will govern the binding reaction of the drug to its protein receptor. If the membrane bilayer mechanism is not operative for the binding of the 1,4-dihydropyridine calcium channel antagonists to their receptors in the heart, then the location of these molecules in membrane bilayers is not important. In addition, their orientation and conformation within the lipid bilayer will probably be of no consequence to the binding of the drug to the protein receptor. Their orientation and confirmation, however, will still be important factors which will determine their successful binding to a protein receptor

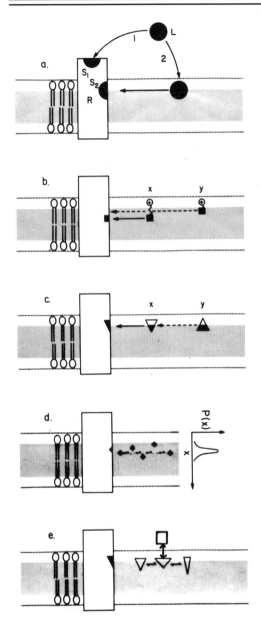

site, but these factors will only play a role specifically at the high affinity protein receptor site. At the high affinity binding site, the drug substance, which diffused through the aqueous layer to this site via isotropic tumbling of the drug molecule, will then assume a specific orientation with regard to some reference axis within the protein structure in order for it to successfully bind. With this orientation and a specific conformation, drug substances will either match the conformation of the protein site or not. However, in this regard the ultimate molecular criteria for drug binding will be the conformation of the drug molecule at the protein receptor site. Therefore, a detailed structural analysis of the conformation of the drug free in solution versus bound to a protein receptor site would be crucial for understanding drug activity and selectivity (see below). To date, there are no detailed structural tools, other than nuclear magnetic resonance, which can provide the structure of drug molecules free in solution. If the receptor protein can be isolated, purified, or produced in sufficiently high quantities, then a detailed x-ray and/or neutron diffraction study could provide the structure of the drug at the receptor site. In fact, there would be an advantage to having a deuterated drug bound to a fully protonated receptor, since a detailed structural analysis such as this would provide information that has not yet been obtained for any ligand receptor system.

Fig. 5. *Molecular parameters that may define the basis for the design of membrane active drugs. a) A drug L may reach a binding site S_1 or S_2 on a membrane-associated receptor protein (R) by 1) direct diffusion through the aqueous solvent or by 2) partitioning into the lipid bilayer and then diffusing laterally to the active site. b) The highly ordered structure of the lipid bilayer may restrict membrane-soluble drugs to a particular depth of penetration into the bilayer (drug x would be a reactive molecule since it is positioned at the proper depth of penetration for optimal reaction with a protein receptor site;*

drug y would be inactive). c) Bilayer constraints on the orientation of drug molecules relative to the active site might also affect their activity (drug x would be active, drug y would be inactive). d) Diffusion about the equilibrium position in the direction of the bilayer normal may be considered as a probability, P(x), that the drug will be found at a particular depth in the bilayer, x. e) Due to conformational equilibria not necessarily similar to those in bulk phases, a conformation suitable for binding to a receptor site may exist only as a metastable state. More than likely, the drug enters the bilayer, changing its conformation, and then binds with a well defined, stable, long-lived conformation to a site on a protein with a metastable conformation.

In summary, if the membrane bilayer model is the mechanism by which drugs bind to their protein receptor sites, then the above criteria, namely location, orientation, and conformation, will play key roles in understanding drug activity, selectivity, and pharmacokinetic properites.

Applications of Molecular Models for Defining Drug Activity and Selectivity

The location of a drug substance in a membrane bilayer, in addition to establishing one specific molecular criterion for drug binding, will also play a crucial role in the pharmacokinetic activity of drug substances. As some of the above data have shown, a molecule such as amiodarone, which is situated very deep within the membrane bilayer, also has associated with it a very long half-life or reactivity. It is probably fair to predict certain pharmacokinetic properties of a drug substance based on its location in the membrane bilayer. This may prove crucial in prescribing certain clinical agents for alleviating particular abnormalities, especially if short half-lifes for drug activity are preferred versus long half-lifes.

In summary, the precise molecular constraints for drug molecules in lipid bilayers, namely their location and possible orientation, may prove most useful in predicting, or at least rationalizing, pharmacokinetic behavior of drug substances.

The degree of activity of a drug substance (namely, inactive, partially reactive, fully active) and the selectivity of drug substances for protein receptor sites may also occur by a combination of the above three molecular criteria. For example, referring to Figure 5, a drug substance which does not penetrate to the precisely correct depth in the bilayer may still exhibit some partial reactivity due to thermal motion within the bilayer which would allow the drug substance to "bob" about an equilibrium position within the membrane bilayer. Even if the drug substance were a few angstroms from the optimal location in the bilayer, there could be some probability for

reactivity due to this bobbing effect. This could explain some of the partial reactivity of drug substances compared to others in which there is no activity (too far removed from the optimal location in the bilayer) to full activity (exactly at the right location within the membrane bilayer).

Drug molecules may partition to the right depth of penetration, but analogs of the same parent structure may not have the correct orientation at this particular depth of penetration. As shown in Figure 5, this may be one discriminating means by which the selectivity of drug substances for a particular receptor site is mediated. The conformation of a drug substance at a particular location and with a particular orientation is yet another discriminating factor for its activity and selectivity for a particular protein receptor site. This may also explain differences in the activity of antagonists versus agonists which appear to have very similar structures yet result in profound differences in the functioning of the receptor channel. Referring to Figure 5, two possible alternatives exist for this mechanism, based on the membrane bilayer model. In mechanism one, the drug may undergo conformational fluctuations in which only one of these conformations is the correct one for binding to a fixed (or "frozen") protein receptor site conformation. Alternatively, mechanism two would fix the conformation of the drug substance in the membrane bilayer which could then bind to only one conformation of a particular receptor channel, depending on the state of the receptor channel. Since the chemical environment within a lipid bilayer is highly constrained, it is likely that the conformation of the drug substance, once it incorporates into the membrane bilayer, remains constant. Based on the present consensus, it is highly likely that the receptor channel may have different conformations depending upon the state of the channel, i.e., mainly open, densensitized, or closed. For a given drug substance, only one of these states for the receptor channel may have the high-affinity site in the correct conformation for the binding of the drug to that site. Then, according to this latter mechanism, even though the antagonist and agonist structures are chemically similar, there may exist subtle conformational differences between the agonist and the antagonist such that either one binds to a particular state of the receptor channel. In this way, the membrane bilayer model provides a precisely controlled and subtle mechanism for the selectivity of an agonist or antagonist for a particular state of the receptor channel. This model is also particularly pleasing because it requires minimal free energies for converting one state to the other for the binding of an agonist versus an antagonist, an energetically favorable situation for the sarcolemmal membrane.

With these few examples, and the many others that exist, the membrane bilayer mechanism provides an exquisite theoretical basis for rationalizing how the interaction of specific drug structures with specific states of the receptor can lead to a number of different outcomes and alternatives. A few clinical and physiological observations that have been made will illustrate the utility of this model, as described below.

Clinical and Physiological Data in Perspective

Observations of drug activity at the molecular level, that is, interactions with different components of the membranes comprising the myocardial cell, can be related to both clinical and physiological observations. For example, the clinical half-lives for cardiovascular agents may be related to their locations in biomembranes. Two examples given above are nimodipine and amiodarone, which have much different locations, that is, depth of penetration in the membrane bilayer, and dramatically different clinical half-lives. Correlations such as these need to be made cautiously. However, they should be made in order to enhance our understanding of what we observe as the expression of these drugs on a more global scale. Many other examples which relate molecular data to clinical data provide interesting correlations.

A NOVEL DRUG DESIGN MODALITY SUGGESTED BY "IMAGING" DRUGS IN MEMBRANES

X-ray and Neutron Diffraction Approach (Crystal vs. Membrane Structures)

Because of the major role that membrane-associated receptor proteins play in regulating physiological function, many drugs, like the calcium channel antagonists, exert their effects through interaction with these proteins. The calcium channel antagonists clearly have hydrophobic or lipophilic properties which may be responsible for their side effects and/or specific activity, and it is feasible that the receptors to which they bind have amphiphilic helices in transmembrane regions. Whether one is interested in nonspecific drug membrane interactions or specific interactions of drugs with membrane-associated proteins, it is very important to understand the interaction of these small, lipophilic molecules with lipid bilayers and the constraints placed on the structure of membrane-associated proteins by bilayers. The various chemically distinct regions of the bilayer may impose a unique position, orientation, and conformation of a ligand, which may be significant to the binding process. Similarly, the secondary structure of membrane proteins may be significantly different from that of the water-soluble proteins. Dynamic fluctuations from the equilibrium positions, and conformations of both ligands and proteins, or transitions to various metastable conformations or transition states will affect binding rates. Even moderate substitutions may alter the position, orientation, and conformation of the ligand, thus perturbing the functional behavior of the molecule in the membrane. Similarly, perturbations of membrane protein structure, whether induced by ligand binding, solvent effects, or changes in the membrane bilayer itself, may profoundly affect the ligant-protein interaction.

In order to assess the importance of these interactions in the chemistry of ligand binding to membranes and membrane associated components, a detailed structural analysis must include: 1) a determination of the overall structure of synthetic and biological membranes; 2) identification of the equilibrium positions, orientations, and conformations of a series of drug substances (e.g., the calcium channel antagonists) partitioned into model membrane systems; 3) a determination of the structure of membrane-associated receptor proteins and the location of their active site within the membrane; and 4) a compilation of all this information (incorporating molecular modeling calculations) in order to a) better understand the chemistry of drug-membrane and drug-receptor interactions and b) enable informed, directed design of novel calcium channel antagonists which interact with different membrane systems.

Our ability to obtain structure data from membrane systems has been restricted by the limited resolution attainable, due, in large measure, to disorder of the lipid samples. Because of the flexibility of membranes and their fluidity in the lateral direction, one is not able to obtain ordered samples analogous to those used in crystallography. Some chemical features of lipid systems do allow structural data to be obtained. The intermolecular interactions that result in bilayer formation assert a degree of order; these molecules are aligned such that corresponding parts of adjacent molecules are at approximately the same depth in the membrane. For conventional lipids, however, there is no further orientation of these aligned molecules, and because the lipid-lipid interaction is nonspecific, these associated structures are quite flexible, and, thus, yield low resolution diffraction data. Better resolution might be obtained from polymerized lipids, which offer an additional restriction to the movement of the constituent molecules.

Polymerizable lipid systems have been the object of extensive investigation in recent years. A variety of cross-linking chemistries have been "borrowed" from polymer science, most involving initiation of polymerization with ultraviolet light, following which the vesicles are much more stable. Two effects of the polymerization will improve the resolution of the diffraction data. First, be-

cause adjacent lipids are covalently bound, they exhibit order in the lateral direction. Depending upon the position of the cross-link, this may not be a rigid constraint due to the many rotational degrees of freedom normally present in the aliphatic chain of the lipid molecules. Second, the membrane becomes more rigid, and movements of individual lipids in the direction of the bilayer normal become very small, greatly increasing order in the direction of the bilayer normal. To date, research on polymerizable lipids has focused on the polymerization chemistry, on spectroscopic studies of the polymerized structure, and on morphological studies. Emphasis is now being placed on the molecular, high resolution structure, since the improved order of these systems will allow high resolution structure data to be obtained for drug substances, such as the calcium channel antagonists, in these membranes.

Calcium channel antagonists incorporated into lipid bilayers before polymerization, followed by polymerization of the lipid, create a highly ordered "liquid crystal" of the monomolecularly dispersed drug in a lipid bilayer. For calcium channel antagonists with electron-dense atoms as part of their structure (e.g., Bay P8857), x-ray diffraction can provide higher resolution structures of the drug-lipid complex. A more powerful approach requires selective deuteration of the calcium channel antagonist to be used in a neutron diffraction experiment. This latter approach is more useful since 1) any drug substance that contains hydrogen can be selected so long as the specific hydrogen can be synthetically replaced with deuterium, and 2) the amount of structure information is vastly increased. For example, utilizing a limited series of specifically deuterated active analogs of the same calcium channel antagonist, the individual molecular moieties of the drug structure can be mapped out in a membrane bilayer in three dimensions utilizing the polymerized lipid matrix. This neutron diffraction approach could be extended to mapping out the structure (orientation and conformation) of the calcium channel antagonist bound to its receptor protein site, if the receptor could be reconstituted into a membrane at sufficient ($>1,000$ receptors/μm^2) concentrations.

Molecular mechanics could then be employed to calculate molecular energies (as a sum of constituent energies), bond stretch, steric interaction, electrostatic interaction, etc.), each represented as a potential function with parameters derived from experimental data. Using a particular minimization strategy and constraints appropriate to a specific system, one may calculate a minimum energy molecular configuration, a priori. These calculations are very powerful tools, in that they supplement experimental data, and allow one to make reasonable inferences and projections regarding data which are difficult or impossible to obtain.

A Molecular Scheme for Optimizing Drug Structures

The above tools can be coupled in order to provide a powerful means for understanding both the molecular basis for the interaction of calcium channel antagonists with membranes and the design parameters for new antagonists with improved properties. Referring to Figure 6, a biological substance, e.g., a membrane with bound calcium channel antagonist normally not possessing sufficient structural order, could be subjected to one of a number of orientation procedures [Herbette and Blasie, 1986] which would introduce some degree of order (crystalline, liquid crystalline, fiber, etc.). X-ray and/or neutron scattering approaches would provide an experimental structure that could be input to various molecular modeling schemes, along with relevant measurable physical properties of the drug-membrane complex, to calculate structural parameters (bond energies, total free energies, etc.) or predict new related structures. For the prediction of structural parameters, conditions used in the experiment could be altered (e.g., temperature, degree of hydration, pH, ionic strength, and composition, etc.) for this particular composition of drug and membrane structure, and properties could

be re-examined. Following prediction of new drug analogs in membranes, synthetic chemistry and/or molecular biology approaches could be employed to prepare new biological substances that could re-enter this scheme. This cyclic experimental-theoretical-experimental structure approach should allow the structure-based identification of important properties of the calcium channel antagonists, prediction of new analogs and their structures, and prediction of specific properties of these new analogs.

CONCLUSIONS AND SUMMARY
Future Advancements of Drug Imaging in the Membrane

The complexities and subtleties that exist in the interactions of drug substances with biological membranes have only recently been examined at the molecular level. A drug substance that is administered to a patient will be distributed throughout organs, cells, and membranes by several processes. Using the myocardial cell as an example, the process eventually involves partitioning of the drug substance between the fluids hydrating the myocardial cell membrane and the sarcolemma. Since it has been demonstrated that several classes of cardiovascular agents are highly lipid-soluble, these drug substances prefer to partition or dissolve in the membrane bilayer phase. The majority of the drug molecules that incorporate into the sarcolemmal lipid bilayer probably never interact with a specific protein receptor since the amount of receptor protein relative to the amount of lipid matrix and incorporated drug is very small.

We do not yet know the "history" of a drug substance that has gone from the interstitial cellular fluids to the high affinity binding sites on proteins; that is, we do not know if the particular drug that binds to a protein receptor ever actually enters the membrane bilayer prior to binding to a receptor. However, given the high lipid solubility of these cardiovascular agents resulting in partitioning of the drug

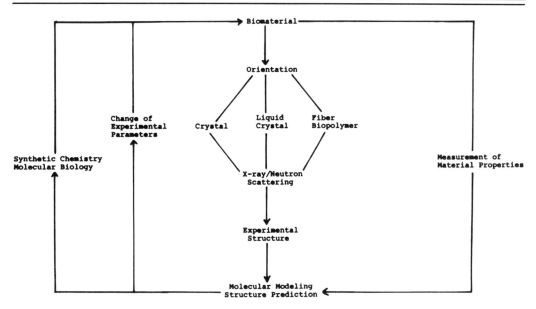

Fig. 6. *Drug design scheme. Experimental drugs can be studied by both x-ray and neutron diffraction. Biological samples can be oriented/ordered by a number of techniques. Crystal structures could be compared and contrasted to membrane-bound drug structures obtained by both x-ray and neutron diffraction methods, and these experimental structures could then be used in molecular model calculations. Calculated drug structures could allow the selection of a limited number of new drug compounds to then be synthesized and re-entered into the scheme. Measurements of physical properties, drug activity, etc., can also be imputed into the data base. It is anticipated that within a few cycles, optimal drug structures within a class of drugs could be determined.*

into the membrane bilayer, the low concentration of receptor proteins in the sarcolemma and the large amount of available lipid matrix, it is highly probably that a cardiovascular drug which does eventually bind to its protein receptor, probably first interacted with the sarcolemmal membrane bilayer. Since the ratio of interstitial fluid volume to membrane bilayer volume is not appreciably different, and the partition coefficients of the drugs favor this lipid bilayer component, the driving force for these drugs is to interact and remain incorporated in the membrane bilayer. Eventually, one of these drug molecules could bind to a protein receptor within the bilayer. If this is indeed the molecular pathway these drugs take to "locate" protein receptor sites, then an evaluation of the structure of the drug in the membrane bilayer is a necessary first step in understanding the molecular basis for drug-receptor interactions.

The x-ray and neutron diffraction approach described above will now provide some molecular information as to the interaction of drugs with the membrane bilayer; however, these techniques are limited to still relatively high drug concentrations (aqueous concentrations of 10^{-6} to 10^{-3} M). Presently, this information will most benefit a better definition of the pharmacokinetic properties of these drug substances. Future developments will seek to look at even lower drug concentrations. In addition, future studies must also focus on drug receptor structures, i.e., what is the structure of both the protein receptor site and the drug at the receptor site. With the advent of molecular biology techniques, it should be possible to obtain more highly concentrated receptor protein preparations which are more suitable to the diffraction techniques. In addition, advances in technology (greater x-ray and neutron fluxes, more efficient detection systems and (bio)material science applications in the area of liquid crystal technology) will allow more detailed drug-membrane structure studies.

Future Applications of Drug "Imaging" at the Cellular and Organ Levels

The interaction of site-selective antibodies to calcium channel receptors in the heart may allow new imaging techniques to be exploited. Two such imaging techniques are 1) magnetic resonance imaging (MRI), a newly developed approach currently being extensively tested and 2) x-ray holography, currently a laboratory curiosity which will require future technical developments based on appropriate coherent x-ray sources. Utilizing either antibodies with paramagnetic ions or possibly perdeuterated antibodies, MRI may be used to determine a voxel by voxel quantitation of the amount of antibody and, hence, concentration of specific protein receptors in the heart. Such data may then be correlated with detailed structure studies at the molecular level to aid our understanding of drug-receptor interactions and distributions within the heart. The likelihood of applications to the calcium channel antagonists is not unreasonable. The second technique, x-ray holography, if successful, would allow direct "images" of receptor-channel and antibody-receptor complexes on cellular surfaces to be made. These images, probably with 10–100 Å resolution, would provide new structural information related to the architecture of receptor-channel complexes at the cellular level as well as to local receptor distribution on cellular surfaces.

Clinical Applications of These Approaches

The practical implications of success in these analyses of the molecular basis of drug-receptor interactions arise from the "side effects" commonly seen with clinically useful drugs. The advantage of drugs with low toxic therapeutic characterization of specific receptor sites on membrane proteins would facilitate the design of drug molecules targeted to one or another membrane activity. Thus, it might be possible to obtain drugs that only inhibit calcium channels in a specific organ or tissue. It might also be possible to develop drugs that act only on a specific state of an ion channel, and even to design drug molecules that block only abnormal channels, such as those involved in coronary vasospasm.

ACKNOWLEDGMENTS

We would like to thank Dr. B.P. Schoenborn, Dr. A. Saxena, and associated staff at the High Flux Beam Reactor, Brookhaven National Laboratory, Upton, New York for their assistance, making it possible to carry out neutron diffraction studies. We extend our gratitude to Dr. A. Pappano for continual discussions regarding drug-membrane interactions, which further allow us to correlate these structural results with electrophysiological and pharmacological observations. This work was supported by research grants HL-33026 and HL-21812 from the National Institutes of Health, by a grant-in-aid from the American Heart Association and the Connecticut affiliate, a grant from the Whitaker Foundation, and gifts from The Patterson Trust Foundation and RJR Nabisco, Inc. We would like to thank Drs. Chester and Rhodes, who were supported by National Institutes of Health Research Training Grant HL-07420, for their valuable research contributions. Our sincere thanks to Ms. C. Cronin and Ms. T. Wojtusik for their dedication in preparing this manuscript for submission. L. Herbette acknowledges his affiliation as an Established Investigator of the American Heart Association.

REFERENCES

Affolter H, Coronado R (1985): Agonists Bay-K8644 and CGP28392 open calcium channels reconstituted from skeletal muscle transverse tubules. Biophys J 48:341–347.

Affolter H, Coronado R (1986): The sidedness of reconstituted calcium channels from muscle transverse tubules as determined by D600 and D890 blockade. Biophys J 49:197a.

Bayer R, Ehara T (1978): Comparative studies on calcium antagonists. Prog Pharmacol 2:31–37.

Bean BP (1984): Nitrendipine block of cardiac calcium channels: High affinity binding to the inactivated state. Proc. Natl. Acad. Sci. 81:6388-6392.

Borsotto M, Barhanin J, Fosset M, Lazdunski M (1985): The 1,4-dihydropyridine receptor associated with the skeletal muscle voltage-dependent Ca^{2+} channel. Purification and subunit composition. J Biol Chem 260:14255-14263.

Brown AM, Kunze DL, Yatani A (1984): The agonist effect of dihydropyridine on Ca channels. Nature 311:570-572.

Broughton A, Grant AO, Starmer FC, Klinger JK, Stambler BS, Strauss HC (1984): Lipid solubility modulates pH potentiation of local anesthetic block of Vmax reactivation in guinea pig myocardium. Circ Res 55:513-523.

Campbell KP, Lipshutz GM, Denney, G.H. (1984): Direct photoaffinity labelling of the high affinity nitrendipine binding site in subcellular membrane fractions isolated from canine myocardium. J Biol Chem 259:5384-5387.

Colvin RA, Ashavaid TF, Herbette LG (1985): Structure-function studies of canine cardiac sarcolemmal membranes. I. Estimation of receptor site densities. Biochim Biophys Acta 812:601-608.

Courtney KR (1980): Structure-activity relations for frequency-dependent sodium channel block in nerve by local anesthetics. J Pharmacol Exp Ther 213:114-119.

Curtis BM, Catterall WA (1984): Purification of the calcium antagonist receptor of the voltage-sensitive calcium channel from skeletal muscle transverse tubules. Biochemistry 23:2113-2118.

Ehara T, Kaufman R (1978): The voltage and time-dependent effects of (−) verapamil on the slow inward current in isolated cat ventricular myocardium. J Pharmacol Exp Ther 207:49-55.

Ferry DR, Goll A, Glossman H (1983a): Putative calcium channel molecular weight determination by target size analysis. Naunyn-Schmiedeberg's Arch Pharmacol 323:292-297.

Ferry DR, Goll A, Glossman H (1983b): Calcium channels: Evidence for oligomeric nature by target size analysis. EMBO J 2:1729-1732.

Gerry RH, Rauch B, Colvin RA, Katz AM, Messineo FC (1985): Verapamil interaction with the muscarinic receptor demonstrates stereoselectivity at two sites (Abstract). Circulation 72(suppl III):III-330.

Gettes LS, Reuter H (1974): Slow recovery from inactivation of inward currents in mammalian myocardial fibers. J Physiol 240:703-724.

Glossman H, Ferry DR (1983): Solubilization and partial purification of putative calcium channels labelled with ^{3}H-nimodipine. Naunyn-Schmiedeberg's Arch Pharmacol 323:279-291.

Goldman ME, Pisano JJ (1985): Inhibition of [^{3}H]nitrendipine binding by phospholipase A_2. Life Sci 37:1301-1308.

Gruner SM (1985): Intrinsic curvature hypothesis for biomembrane lipid composition: A role for non-bilayer lipids. Proc Natl Acad Sci 82:3665-3669.

Hachisu M, Pappano AJ (1983): A comparative study of the blockade of calcium-dependent action potentials by verapamil, nifedipine and nimodipine in ventricular muscle. J Pharmacol Exp Ther 225:112-120.

Herbette LG, Blasie JK (1986): Procedures for orienting synthetic and native biological membranes for time-averaged and time-resolved structure determinations. Submitted.

Herbette LG, Chester DW, Rhodes DG (1986): Structural analysis of drug molecules in biological membranes. Biophys J 49:91-94.

Herbette LG, Blasie JK (1986): Procedures for orienting synthetic and native biological membranes for time-averaged and time-resolved structure determinations. Methods in Enzymology, in press.

Herbette LG, MacAlister T, Ashavaid TF, Colvin RA (1985): Structure-function studies of canine cardiac sarcolemmal membranes. II. Structural organization of the sarcolemmal membrane as determined by electron microscopy and lamellar x-ray diffraction. Biochim Biophys Acta 812:609-623.

Hescheler J, Pelzer D, Trube G, Trautwein W (1982): Does the organic calcium channel blocker D600 act from inside or outside on the cardiac cell membrane? Pfleugers Arch 393:287-291.

Hille B (1977): Local anesthetics: Hydrophilic and hydrophobic pathways for the drug-receptor reaction. J Gen Physiol 69:497-515.

Hondeghem LM, Katzung BG (1984): Antiarrhythmic agents: the modulated receptor mechanism of action of sodium and calcium channel-blocking drugs. Ann Rev Pharmacol Toxicol 24:387-423.

Horne P, Triggle DJ, Venter JC (1984): Nitrendipine and isoproterenol induce phosphorylation of a 42,000 dalton protein that co-migrates with the affinity labeled calcium channel regulatory subunit. Biochem Biophys Res Commun 121:890-898.

Kirley TL, Schwartz A (1984): Solubilization and affinity labelling of a dihydropyridine binding site from skeletal muscle: Effects of temperature and diltiazem on ^{3}H dihydropyridine binding to transverse tubules. Biochem Biophys Res Commun 123:41-49.

Kohlhardt M, Mnich Z (1978): Studies on the inhibitory effect of verapamil on the slow inward current in mammalian ventricular myocardium. J Mol Cell Cardiol 10:1037-1052.

Kokubun S, Reuter H (1984): Dihydropyridine derivatives prolong the open state of Ca channels in cultured cardiac cells. Proc Natl Acad Sci USA 81:4824-4827.

Kretsinger RH (1979): The informational role of calcium in the cytosol. Adv Cyclic Nucleotide Res. 11:1-26.

Lee KS, Tsien RW (1983): Mechanism of calcium channel blockade by verapamil, D-600, diltiazem and nitrendipine in single dialyzed heart cells. Nature 278:269-271.

Levine YK (1973): X-ray diffraction studies of membranes. In Davison SG (ed): "Progress in Surface Science," Vol 3, Part 4. Elmsford, NY: Pergamon Press.

McDonald TF, Pelzer D, Trautwein W (1984): Cat ventricular muscle treated with D600: Characteristics of calcium channel block and unblock. J Physiol (Lond) 352:217-241.

McLaughlin S (1975): Local anesthetic and the electrical properties of phospholipid bilayer membranes in molecular mechanism of anesthesia. In Fink BR (ed): Vol I. New York: Raven Press, pp 193–221.

Rengasamy A, Ptasienki J, Hosey M (1985): Purification of the cardiac 1,4-dihydropyridine receptor/calcium channel complex. Biochem Biophys Res Commun 126:1-7.

Reuter H (1979): Properties of two inward membrane currents in the heart. Ann Rev Physiol 41:413-425.

Rhodes DG, Sarmiento JG, Herbette LG (1985): Kinetics of binding of membrane-active drugs to receptor sites: Diffusion-limited rates for a membrane bilayer approach of 1,4-dihydropyridine calcium channel antagonists to their active site. Mol Pharmacol 27:612-623.

Sanguinetti MC, Kass R.S. (1984): Voltage-dependent block of calcium channel current in the calf cardiac Purkinje fiber of dihydropyridine calcium channel antagonists. Circ Res 55:336-348.

Sanguinetti MC, Kass RS (1984): Regulation of cardiac calcium channel current and contractile activity by the dihydropyridine Bay K8644 is voltage-dependent. J Mol Cell Cardiol 16:667-670.

Schwarz W, Palade PT, Hille B (1977): Local anesthetics. Effect of pH on use-dependent block of sodium channels in frog muscle. Biophys J 20:343-368.

Schramm M, Towart R (1985): Modulation of calcium channel function by drugs. Life Sci 37:1843-1860.

Trautwein W, Cavalie A (1985): Cardiac calcium channels and their control by neurotransmitters. J Am Coll Cardiol 6:1409-1416.

Venter JC, Fraser CM, Schaber JS, Jung CY, Bolger G, and Triggle DJ (1983): Molecular properties of the slow inward calcium channel. J Biol Chem 258:9344-9348.

Structure and Physiology of the Slow Inward Calcium Channel, pages 109–121
© 1987 Alan R. Liss, Inc.

6

Molecular Properties of the Voltage-Dependent Calcium Channel

S. Martin Shreeve and J. Craig Venter

*Department of Pharmacology, College of Medicine,
University of Vermont, Burlington, Vermont 05405 (S.M.S.), and
Section of Receptor Biochemistry, LNP, NINCDS, National Institutes of Health,
Bethesda; Maryland 20892 (J.C.V.)*

INTRODUCTION

In an unstimulated cell, the concentration of free calcium in the cytoplasm is approximately 0.05–0.5 μM. Electrical or chemical stimulation can increase the cytoplasmic calcium ion concentration by one or two orders of magnitude and thereby trigger a variety of calcium-dependent processes including neurotransmitter release [Katz and Miledi, 1964; Katz, 1969] and muscle contraction [Ebashi and Endo, 1968]. Cytoplasmic-free calcium can be increased either as a result of the release of calcium from intracellular stores, or by the influx of calcium through the cell membrane, or both. Electrophysiological studies have demonstrated that calcium influx across cell membranes in response to electrical stimulation occurs through protein channels, or pores, which are embedded in and transverse the lipid bilayer of the membrane [Hagiwara and Byerly, 1981; McCleskey and Almers, 1985]. Since the extracellular medium contains a higher concentration of free calcium (1–10 mM) than the cytoplasm, the opening of the calcium channels enables calcium ions to move passively across the membrane down their electrochemical gradient into the cell.

Calcium channels have been classified into four basic types: 1) leak channnels, 2) stretch sensitive channels, 3) receptor operated channels, and 4) voltage-dependent channels [for review see Schramm and Towart, 1985]. Much work has yet to be done to characterize fully these channels and determine their relationship to membrane receptors. Voltage-dependent calcium channels are present in a variety of cells and are "opened and closed" as a result of changes in the membrane potential. Recently, electrophysiological studies have revealed that there is a variety of voltage-dependent calcium channels in different tissues, and even in the same cell membrane (e.g., neuronal and cardiac membranes), which can be distinguished by functional properties such as gating, conductance, and pharmacological sensitivity [Hagiwara and Byerly, 1981; Bean, 1985; Nowycky et al., 1985; Nilius et al., 1985].

Of the four basic classes of calcium channels, the voltage-dependent channels are the better characterized, particularly in cardiac muscle, where the pioneering work of Fleckenstein [1971, 1977] first demonstrated the importance of a class of drugs known as the "calcium channel antagonists." These drugs are currently the focus of much pharmacological and therapeutic attention. They are divided into three main groups: 1) the 1,4-dihydropyridines, which include such drugs as nitrendipine and nifedipine; 2) verapamil and D-600; and (3) diltiazem. Although drugs from all three groups antagonize the influx of calcium ions through calcium channels into certain cells (muscle cells, for example), they do not bind to a common site. Yousif and Triggle [1985] have suggested that the three groups of calcium antagonists should be regarded as allosteric effectors of calcium channel gating, interacting at allosterically linked binding sites. It appears as though the three binding sites are anatomically close to each other, as originally proposed by Murphy et al. [1983].

Pharmacological studies using calcium channel antagonists provide evidence in support of a variety of voltage-dependent calcium channels which are tissue-specific [Triggle and Swamy, 1983; Bean, 1985]. For example, from radioligand binding studies, the dissociation constants of the antagonists are different in skeletal muscle compared to other tissues [Gould et al., 1984]. However, based on Scatchard analysis, the 1,4-dihydropyridines appear to bind to only one class of sites in each tissue. This suggests that the various types of calcium channels that may exist in each membrane either do not all bind the antagonists (a proposition supported by electrophysiological studies, which have demonstrated that some voltage-dependent calcium channels are insensitive to the 1,4-dihydropyridines [Nilius et al., 1985]) or that the 1,4-dihydropyridines have the same affinity for two or more types of calcium channels. The importance of this concept to biochemical and pharmacological studies increases in the light of mounting evidence for the existence of more than one calcium channel in a particular membrane.

This review summarizes what is presently known about the molecular properties of calcium channel proteins. The 1,4-dihydropyridines have been utilized as high-affinity probes to identify the channel proteins subsequent to biochemical analysis. Such an approach restricts these molecular studies to those voltage-dependent calcium channels that possess a high-affinity binding site for the 1,4-dihydropyridines. The use of these antagonists per se does not necessarily distinguish between the intact calcium channel and a fragment of the channel protein which has retained the 1,4-dihydropyridine binding site, nor does it differentiate between multiple types of calcium channels possessing high-affinity 1,4-dihydropyridine binding sites.

Schwartz et al. [1985] have proposed that most of the 1,4-dihydropyridine binding sites may not be associated with functional voltage-dependent calcium channels. Other components have been found to bind some of these ligands with varying affinity. These include 1) the receptor operated calcium channel [reviewed by Schramm and Towart, 1985], which may be a different protein from the voltage-dependent channel, and 2) a voltage sensor, located in the membranes of transverse tubules of skeletal muscle, which has been shown to bind nifedipine [Rios and Brum, 1986]. The use of the 1,4-dihydropyridines per se as biochemical probes will not necessarily distinguish between the voltage-dependent calcium channel protein and various other proteins that bind these ligands.

However, there is considerable evidence to suggest that the 1,4-dihydropyridines bind selectively and with high affinity to voltage-dependent calcium channels. Thus, these ligands have been extensively characterized pharmacologically and shown to be potent voltage-dependent calcium channel antagonists in muscle membranes. In addition, when the calcium channel is solubilized and partially purified, it retains its ability to bind various structurally unrelated inhibitors of functional voltage-dependent calcium channels including the 1,4-dihydropyridines. These inhibitors are stereoselective, appear to bind to only one class of sites, and interact allosterically. The discrepancy between the dissociation constants of the 1,4-dihydropyridines obtained in biochemical as opposed to electrophysiological experiments has recently been explained by Borsotto et al. [1986], who reported that the affinity of the antagonist (+)PN200-100 was dependent upon the membrane potential. In electrophysiological experiments, the dissociation constant of this ligand for depolarized muscle cells (when most of the calcium channels are inactivated) was similar to that obtained from biochemical experiments using muscle membranes (0.15–0.3 nM). The affinity of the ligand decreased by a factor of 100 in electrophysiological experiments when measurements were made at the resting membrane potential.

There is, therefore, substantial evidence that the 1,4-dihydropyridines bind selectively to voltage-dependent calcium channels, and this property has been exploited in the molecular studies now discussed.

GENERAL PROPERTIES

The voltage-dependent calcium channel is composed of channel-forming proteins which transverse the lipid bilayer of the membrane. The channel is viewed as a large aqueous pore with a diameter at its narrowest point of no less than 6 Å [McCleskey and Almers, 1985]. Calcium ions move through the channel in single file, binding in succession to two calcium-specific sites. The results of Lee and Tsien [1983] suggest that one of these sites is on the outer surface where competition between calcium ions and other ions can occur, while the other is an inner site where competition with organic calcium channel antagonists occurs. Under physiologic conditions, calcium channels are very selective and exclude sodium and potassium cations [Fukushima and Hagiwara, 1985]. However, in the absence of extracellular calcium, the channels become freely permeable to many monovalent cations, such as sodium and lithium [Kostyuk et al., 1983; Hess and Tsien, 1984]. It appears as though the selectivity of the cal-

cium channel is only evident when a calcium ion occupies a specific high-affinity site on the channel protein. Interestingly, the binding of the 1,4-dihydropyridines to the channel antagonist site is also dependent upon the presence of calcium or magnesium [Glossmann et al., 1984]. Pumplin et al. [1981] have observed certain presynaptic membrane particles which they propose are the calcium channels. There were approximately 1,500 of these particles per μm^2 in the same vicinity in which transmitter release occurred by exocytosis from synaptic vesicles.

THE SOLUBILIZED CALCIUM CHANNEL ANTAGONIST BINDING SITES

Detergent solubilization is an important step in the molecular characterization of receptor proteins and ion channels. It permits such biochemical procedures as reconstitution, ion channel purification, and antibody cross-reactivity studies. Ideally, the detergent should free the calcium channel from the membrane and associated proteins, while maintaining the channel protein in a biologically active form.

Detergent Solubilization

Digitonin (0.2–2% w/v) has been the detergent of choice for the sodium channel and many receptor proteins, and it has been found to solubilize the calcium antagonist binding site from chick heart [Rengasamy et al., 1985], rat brain [Curtis and Catterall, 1983], and rabbit skeletal muscle [Curtis and Catterall, 1984]. Under optimum conditions, digitonin solubilized approximately 50% of the membrane protein and 7–38% [Curtis and Catterall, 1983, 1984; Glossmann and Ferry, 1983; Borsotto et al., 1984a] of the calcium antagonist binding sites.

3-[(3-Cholamidopropyl) dimethyl-ammonio] 1-propane sulfonate (CHAPS) at concentrations of 0.4–2% also solubilized the calcium channel antagonist binding site from the skeletal muscle of guinea pig [Glossmann and Ferry, 1983] and rabbit [Borsotto et al., 1984a,b], from bovine cardiac muscle [Ruth et al., 1986], but not from rat brain [Curtis and Catterall,

1983]. The addition of phospholipids or glycerol was found to stabilize the unlabelled antagonist binding sites and improve yields. CHAPS solubilized approximately 55–100% of the membrane protein and 17–70% of the calcium channel antagonist binding sites. The half-life of the binding sites at 4°C was found to be 34 hr.

Sodium deoxycholate has also been used to solubilize the antagonist binding sites from rabbit skeletal muscle [Kirley and Schwartz, 1984]. However, other detergents such as Triton X-100, Lubrol PX, Zwittergent 10, Nonidet P40, Tween 20, octylglucoside, etc., were unsuccessful [Borsotto et al., 1984a; Curtis and Catterall, 1983].

Pharmacology

The membrane-bound and detergent-solubilized calcium channel antagonist binding sites interact with the 1,4-dihydropyridines in a similar manner [Curtis and Catterall, 1983; Glossmann and Ferry, 1983; Borsotto et al., 1984a]. Binding of the 1,4-dihydropyridines to both forms of the binding site is specific, saturable, reversible, stereoselective, of high affinity, and antagonized by lanthanum and copper ions. The presence of either calcium or magnesium ions is essential for high-affinity 1,4-dihydropyridine binding to both membrane-bound and CHAPS-solubilized sites. A study of the equilibrium binding characteristics of the soluble antagonist site demonstrates that the 1,4-dihydropyridines bind to a single class of noninteracting sites.

Verapamil and diltiazem, which have an allosteric interaction with 1,4-dihydropyridine binding to membrane sites, were also found to interact with the binding of these ligands to the solubilized sites [Curtis and Catterall, 1983; Glossmann and Ferry, 1983; Borsotto et al., 1984a]. This indicates that the verapamil and diltiazem binding sites are solubilized in association with the 1,4-dihydropyridine binding site by both CHAPS and digitonin, supporting the hypothesis of Murphy et al. [1983] that these three separate binding sites are physically associated. Puri-

fication of the antagonist binding sites does not appear to alter these interactions [Campbell et al., 1984; Flockerzi et al., 1986].

The detergent-solubilized calcium channel antagonist binding sites are selectively adsorbed to immobilized lectins including concanavalin A and wheat germ agglutinin gels [Curtis and Catterall, 1983; Glossmann and Ferry, 1983; Borsotto et al., 1984b]. These data suggest that the calcium channel is a glycoprotein and possesses N-acetylglucosamine and/or sialic acid residues and D-glucose and/or mannose sugar residues.

Purification

There have been several reports in the literature concerning the partial purification of the calcium channel antagonist binding site to near homogeneity. These procedures have involved either the purification of the calcium antagonist binding site prelabelled with a 1,4-dihydropyridine or the purification of an unlabelled site which has been subsequently assayed by 1,4-dihydropyridine binding. Glossmann and Ferry [1983] solubilized the [³H]nimodipine-labelled binding site from guinea pig skeletal muscle membranes and, by using a variety of lectin-sepharose gels, were able to obtain a 17–40-fold purification of this protein. Curtis and Catterall [1984] reported a 330-fold purification of the [³H]nitrendipine-labelled binding site from rabbit skeletal muscle transverse tubule membranes. The [³H]nitrendipine-labelled binding sites were solubilized with digitonin and purified in a four-step process involving ion exchange chromatography, wheat germ agglutinin affinity chromatography, and sucrose gradient centrifugation. The authors reported a specific activity for the binding site in the final fraction of 1,950 pmol/mg protein. If the molecular weight of the calcium channel antagonist binding site is assumed to be approximately 178,000–278,000 (from radiation inactivation studies; see Table II), and if the binding site binds 1 mole of [³H]-nitrendipine, then the theoretical specific activity of the purified protein would be 3,597

−5,618 pmol/mg protein. This purification procedure, therefore, appears to yield a protein purity of 35–54%. SDS-PAGE of the purified fraction yields three protein bands (Table I).

Rengasamy et al. [1985] solubilized the $(+)[^3H]PN200$-110-prelabelled calcium channel antagonist binding site from chick heart muscle using digitonin and purified it by a four-step process. This involved ion exchange chromatography using DEAE-Sephadex, hexylamine agarose, wheat germ agglutinin affinity chromatography, and sucrose gradient centrifugation. A purification of approximately 600-fold was reported, with the purified fraction having a specific activity of 1,595 pmol/mg protein. SDS-PAGE of this fraction resulted in three protein bands (Table I). Two of these bands corresponded to the β and γ bands reported by Curtis and Catterall [1984].

Borsotto et al. [1984] solubilized the unlabelled calcium channel antagonist binding site from rabbit skeletal muscle transverse tubule membranes using CHAPS. The protein was purified by a two-step process involving filtration on an Ultrogel A_2 size exclusion column and wheat germ agglutinin affinity chromatography. The purified proteins bound the 1,4-dihydropyridine, $(+)[^3H]PN200$-110, and had a specific activity of 257 pmol/mg protein (5–7% pure). However, when correction was made according to the procedure of Curtis and Catterall [1984], these proteins had a specific activity of 2,100 pmol/mg protein, which represents a purity of 38–59%. SDS-PAGE of the purified fraction showed three bands (Table I). Two of these bands corresonded to the α and γ bands reported by Curtis and Catterall [1984].

More recently Borsotto et al. [1985] reported the further purification of the rabbit skeletal muscle calcium channel antagonist binding site by a three-step process utilizing ion exchange, wheat germ agglutinin chromatography, and gel filtration. The purified fraction gave the same three protein bands on SDS-PAGE as before, and although silver staining indicated that an extensive purifica-

tion had been achieved, the purified fraction only had a specific activity of 800 pmol/mg protein when assayed with $(+)[^3H]PN200$-110. This was an improvement on their previous purification procedure (which gave proteins having a specific activity of 257 pmol/mg protein), but only represents a purity of 14–22%. The authors suggest that the unlabelled calcium channel binding site loses it ability to bind ligands during the purification process and believe that at the end of their procedures they have a mixture of active and inactive calcium channel antagonist binding sites with very little other protein contaminants.

Recently, Biswas and Rogers [1986] reported the synthesis of a 1,4-dihydropyridine-affinity resin. Such an approach should facilitate the purification of the antagonist binding site.

MOLECULAR SIZE

Radiation Inactivation Target Size Analysis

Radiation inactivation target size analysis has been used to determine the molecular weight of receptors and enzymes (for a detailed methodology of this procedure, see Jung [1984] and Venter [1985]). It is the only known method for determining the molecular weight of a protein in situ in intact membranes. It has the advantage of being independent of protein purity and, therefore, of any artifacts produced as a result of the solubilization and purification procedures.

When tissues are exposed to ionizing radiation, such as high energy electrons, ionization occurs randomly throughout the tissue. The effects of ionizing radiation are localized to a spherical radius of 20 Å. If this volume is occupied by a protein, each primary ionization releases 66 eV of energy, which is sufficient to break several structural bonds, inducing a derangement in tertiary structure, and resulting in a loss of protein function. The inactivation of proteins increases exponentially as the radiation dose increases. Due to the small spherical radius of the direct

TABLE I. Purification and Subunit Composition of the Calcium Channel Antagonist Binding Site

Muscle type	[3H]Ligand	Detergent	Purification steps	Species	Apparent M_r^a ($\times 10^{-3}$)	Reference
Smooth (ileum)	Ortho-NCS[b]	SDS		Guinea pig	45; (35)[c]	Venter et al. [1983]
Cardiac	Ortho-NCS[b]	SDS		Guinea pig	45; (35)[c]	Venter et al. [1983]
	Nitrendipine	SDS		Dog	42; 33	Horne et al. [1984] Campbell et al. [1984]
				Dog	32	
	(+)PN200-110	Digitonin	DEAE- and hexylamine-ion exchange; WGA[d]-affinity; sucrose density gradients	Chicken	60; 54; 34[e]	Rengasamy et al. [1985]
Skeletal T-tubules	Nitrendipine	Digitonin	WGA-affinity (twice); DEAE-ion exchange; sucrose sedimentation gradients	Rabbit	130 (α); 50(β); 33(γ)[e]	Curtis and Catterall [1984]
	(+)PN200-110	CHAPS	Ultrogel A_2; WGA-affinity chromatography	Rabbit	142; 33; 32[e]	Borsotto et al. [1984b]
			DAE-ion exchange, WGA-affinity and gel filtration chromatography	Rabbit	142; 33; 32[e]	Borsotto et al. [1985]
				Chick	135; 31; 30[e]	
				Frog	141; 56[e]	
	Isothiocyanate-DHP[f]	SDS		Rabbit	110–150; 36	Kirley and Schwartz [1984]
Skeletal muscle microsomes	Azidopine	SDS		Rabbit	(240);[g] 158; (99)	Ferry et al. [1985]
				Frog	158	
				Chicken	158	
				Guinea pig	(240);[g] 158; (99); (55)	
				Guinea pig	145	Ferry et al. [1984]

[a] M_r (molecular weight) determined on reducing one-dimensional SDS-PAGE analysis.

[b] 2,6-Dimethyl-3,5-dicarbomethoxy-4-(2-isothiocyanatophenyl)-1,4,-dihydropyridine.

[c] Minor protein of $M_r = 35,000$ which was eliminated in the presence of protease inhibitors.

[d] Wheat germ agglutinin sepharose.

[e] All proteins are not necessarily associated with the calcium channel (see text).

[f] Dihydro-2,6-dimethyl-4-(2-isothiocyanatophenyl)-3,5-pyridinedicarboxylic acid dimethyl ester.

[g] M_r in parentheses represents proteins that were only observed on nonreducing SDS-PAGE analysis.

TABLE II. Molecular Size of the Intact Calcium Channel Antagonist Binding Site
as Determined by Radiation Inactivation Target Size Analysis

Species	Tissue	[^{3}H]Ligand	M_r^a ± SEM	Reference
Guinea pig	Ileum	Nitrendipine	278,000 ± 21,000	Venter et al. [1983]
	Skeletal muscle microsomes	(+)PN200-110	136,000 ± 12,000	Goll et al. [1983]
		Nimodipine	178,000 ± 7,000	Goll et al. [1983]
		Nitrendipine	210,000 ± 20,000	Goll et al. [1983]
		Verapamil	110,000 ± 7,000	Goll et al. [1984]
	Brain	Nimodipine	185,000 ± 26,800	Ferry et al. [1983]
	Cardiac	Nimodipine	184,000 ± 10,000	Glossmann et al. [1985]
Rat	Brain	Nitrendipine	210,000 ± 20,000	Norman et al. [1983]
Rabbit	Skeletal muscle T-tubules	Nitrendipine	210,000 ± 20,000	Norman et al. [1983]

^{a}M$_r$, molecular weight.

ionization and the random nature of ionizations produced throughout the membrane, larger proteins have a greater probability of being hit than smaller ones. Therefore, a relationship exists between the size of the protein molecule and the radiation dose required to inactivate it. Using enzymes or receptors of known molecular weight as internal standards, the unknown molecular weight of a protein can be determined.

For the calcium channel, inactivation is assayed by a decrease in [^{3}H]1,4-dihydropyridine binding. Therefore, this method will give the molecular weight of the intact protein in the membrane that is responsible for 1,4-dihydropyridine binding. Table II summarizes the data from three laboratories on the in situ molecular weight determinations of the calcium channel antagonist binding site in various tissues and species.

Venter et al. [1983] and Normal et al. [1983] were the first to report the molecular weight of the 1,4-dihydropyridine binding site (210,000–278,000). The results from these two laboratories suggest that the binding site has the same weight irrespective of the tissue and species examined. In all experiments, a simple exponential decay of 1,4-dihydropyridine binding activity was observed in each tissue with increasing doses of radiation, which is indicative of a single target size. These data suggest that the variety of calcium channels, which from electrophysiological

experiments have been shown to exist in neuronal and cardiac tissue, either have the same molecular weight, or those with different molecular weights do not bind the 1,4-dihydropyridines.

Norman et al. [1983] compared the calcium channel with the moleuclar weight of the sodium channel, as determined by this method. The sodium channel has a molecular weight of 260,000 when assayed with tetrodotoxin and scorpion toxin [Barhanin et al., 1983]. These findings suggest that the sodium and calcium channels are similar in size and that in these target size studies, the 1,4-dihydropyridine calcium channel antagonist binding site may represent the intact calcium channel.

Goll et al. [1983] reported that the molecular weight of the 1,4-dihydropyridine binding site in situ could be reduced by 60,000 in the presence of d-cis-diltiazem and suggested that a major rearrangement of the channel occurs when allosteric modulators are bound to the channel. The oligomeric nature of the calcium channel was demonstrated by Goll et al. [1984], who reported that the target size of the verapamil binding site was approximately 60,000 less than the nimodipine binding site. For a review of this work, see Glossmann et al. [1984, 1985].

Subunit Size

Table I summarizes data from several laboratories concerning the possible subunit composition of the 1,4-dihydropyridine labelled calcium channel antagonist binding site. The first study by Venter et al. [1983] made use of a newly developed covalent affinity label, ortho-NCS (synthesized by Dr. D.J. Triggle), to characterize the calcium channel in smooth and cardiac muscle. After specifically labeling the calcium channel with this radioactive ligand, the membrane proteins were solubilized in SDS and analyzed by SDS-PAGE under reducing conditions. Specifically labelled peaks of radioactivity on the gels were located and represent protein subunits associated with the calcium channel antagonist binding site. Subsequent studies have used a similar protocol but have relied upon specifically labelling the calcium channel with either a [3H] photoaffinity label (nitrendipine and azidopine) or a different [3H] covalent label (isothiocyanate-1,4-dihydropyridine).

The studies performed by Curtis and Catterall [1984, 1985], Borsotto et al. [1984b, 1985], and Rengasamy et al. [1985] first involved the partial purification of the solubilized calcium antagonist binding site to near homogeneity (Table I). Purified fractions were found to specifically bind [3H]1, 4-dihydropyridines, and SDS-PAGE of these fractions revealed that they are composed of several proteins, all of which may not necessarily possess the antagonist binding site.

The studies referenced in Table I have used membranes isolated from cardiac, smooth, and skeletal muscle. Different protocols, which have taken advantage of several detergents and various 1,4-dihydropyridines, have been utilized to determine the molecular weights of the subunits. It is possible that the 1,4-dihydropyridines may select for more than one type of the variety of calcium channels now known to exist and which may slightly differ in their molecular structure. On consideration of these variables, it is perhaps not surprising that so many subunits have been identified.

Despite the variability, however, several trends are evident (Table I). Regardless of muscle type and species and with the use of

all the 1,4-dihydropyridines except azidopine, a subunit with an apparent molecular weight of 32,000–36,000 is observed. This may represent the smallest subunit that contains the antagonist binding site. Campbell et al. [1984] demonstrated that a subunit of this size contained the verapamil binding site as well as the 1,4-dihydropyridine binding site, since verapamil was found to inhibit nitrendipine binding to this subunit.

A subunit of intermediate size (molecular weight 42,000–55,000) is common to all species and all muscle types when most of the 1,4-dihydropyridines listed in Table I are used as probes. A larger subunit (molecular weight 130,000–160,000) is only observed in skeletal muscle and may represent a subunit unique to this muscle type.

Curtis and Catterall [1984] have suggested that the calcium channel may be similar to the sodium channel [Catterall, 1982] in that it appears to be oligomeric in nature, being composed of several subunits. From Table I, it appears that more than one subunit of the calcium channel from each muscle tissue can bind the 1,4-dihydropyridines. Alternatively, it might be speculated that each subunit which specifically binds the 1,4-dihydropyridines might derive from more than one type of the several calcium channels now known to exist in muscle. However, reports by Venter et al. [1983] and Rengasamy et al. [1985] suggest that the smaller subunit (molecular weight 32,000–36,000) might represent a proteolytic fragment of a larger subunit, although it should be noted that the 32,000–36,000 subunit has been observed in experiments in which great care has been taken to prevent proteolysis [e.g., Campbell et al., 1984]. Proteolysis of the calcium channel antagonist binding site has been reported in other studies [Curtis and Catterall, 1984; Campbell et al., 1984] and would confuse the interpretation of these data. Further biochemical analysis of the subunits needs to be conducted to clarify these possibilities.

Recently, antibodies have been raised against the subunits of the antagonist binding site in skeletal muscle [Schmid et al., 1986] and against the 1,4-dihydropyridines [Campbell et al., 1986]. Purification studies by Borsotto et al. [1985] revealed that the binding site in skeletal muscle under reducing conditions is composed of a large glycoprotein of molecular weight 142,000 and two smaller subunits of molecular weight 33,000 and 32,000, as shown in Table I. Using antisera raised against the 142,000 and 32,000 proteins in skeletal muscle, this laboratory found that under nonreducing conditions, the 1,4-dihydropyridine binding site in skeletal muscle is a protein of molecular weight 170,000–176,000 and is composed of two subunits (140,000–145,000 and 32,000–34,000) covalently linked by disulfide bonds [Schmid et al., 1986]. The antagonist binding sites in both cardiac and smooth muscle membranes were also found to have a molecular weight of 170,000–176,000 under nonreducing conditions. A 32,000–36,000 protein was only identified in all three muscle types under reducing conditions, which indicates that this smaller protein is not a proteolytic fragment but a subunit of the calcium channel protein. However, the larger 140,000 subunit was not observed under reducing conditions when cardiac and smooth muscle membranes were analyzed immunochemically on SDS-PAGE, possibly because these muscle types, as opposed to skeletal muscle, have a lower density of antagonist binding sites which makes this large subunit difficult to detect [Schmid et al., 1986]. Alternatively, the large subunit could have different antigenic determinants depending upon the muscle type, or it may not even be present in cardiac and smooth muscle membranes.

In conclusion, the current information indicates that there is a high degree of structural homology among calcium channels that bind the 1,4-dihydropyridines in different tissues from various species. Only the skeletal muscle calcium channel appears to be different in that it has one large 130,000–160,000 subunit which is readily observed under reducing conditions. Recently, Schmid et al. [1986]

have suggested that the calcium channel in cardiac and smooth muscle may also possess this subunit.

PHOSPHORYLATION OF THE CALCIUM CHANNEL SUBUNITS

Many hormones, neurotransmitters, and drugs are known to affect the intracellular phosphorylation of proteins. For example, the phosphorylation of calcium channel proteins has been related to a β-adrenergic agonist effect in the heart (for reviews, see Reuter [1983]; Eckert and Chad [1984]). It has been postulated that phosphorylation may be involved in the regulation of calcium channels.

Horne et al. [1984] observed that nitrendipine induced a calcium-dependent cAMP-independent phosphorylation of three protein bands in cardiac membranes (Fig. 1), possibly as a result of an endogenous protein C kinase or other protein kinases. One of these bands (molecular weight 42,000) co-migrated with the [^{3}H]1,4-dihydropyridine-labelled calcium antagonist binding site (Table I). Although it is not clear whether the proteins are identical in both cases, this finding supports the proposition that the calcium channel protein is phosphorylated. Isoproterenol, a β-adrenergic receptor agonist and known calcium channel activator, also induced the calcium-dependent, cAMP-independent phosphorylation of the same three proteins, an effect blocked by propranolol and carbachol. Muscarinic cholinergic agonists and β-adrenergic agonists are known to have opposing effects on cardiac contractile force and heart rate, which may be mediated through phosphorylation of the calcium channels. It might be expected that isoproterenol, which stimulates the heart, and nitrendipine, which antagonizes cardiac muscle contraction, would have opposing effects on calcium channel phosphorylation. However, it is possible that the calcium channel is phosphorylated at more than one site by independent protein kinases in response to a variety of "agonists" and "antagonists."

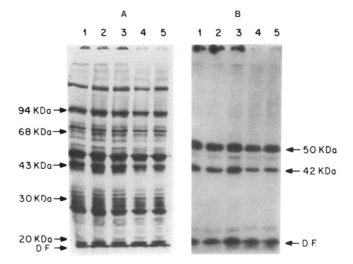

Fig. 1. *SDS-PAGE of nitrendipine-induced phosphorylation of cardiac membrane proteins. Membranes were suspended in 50 mM Tris (pH 7.4), 5 mM $MgCl_2$, 1 mM $CaCl_2$, and incubated in ice for 1 hr in the presence of 10 nM nitrendipine or BAY K8644. For calcium-free conditions, incubation was carried out in the presence of 1 mM EGTA. The phosphorylation reaction was initiated by the addition of 5 μM [γ-^{32}P]ATP ($\simeq$ 1 Ci/mmol) and stopped after 30 sec by addition of NaF and ATP to final concentrations of 0.2 M and 2 mM, respectively. A) Coomassie blue stained gel: Lane 1, control with 1 mM calcium; Lane 2, calcium with BAY K8644; Lane 3, calcium with nitrendipine; Lane 4, nitrendipine with EGTA; Lane 5, EGTA. B) Autoradiograph of the same gel. (From Horne et al., 1984, with permission.)*

Curtis and Catterall [1985] demonstrated that both the α and β proteins in their purified fraction (see Table I) were phosphorylated by a cAMP-dependent protein kinase in vitro. However, phosphorylation of intact transverse tubule membranes revealed that only the β subunit (molecular weight 50,000) is a substrate for phosphorylation in situ. Drug effects on this cAMP-dependent phosphorylation have not been determined. Therefore, the subunit of intermediate molecular weight 42,000–55,000 is a substrate for both drug-induced, cAMP-independent phosphorylation and cAMP-dependent phosphorylation mediated by a protein kinase.

Recently, it has been reported [Hosey et al., 1986; Flockerzi et al., 1986] that the large subunit (protein molecular weight 142,000) of the calcium channel antagonist binding site can be efficiently phosphorylated in its membrane-bound state, in the presence of either a cAMP-dependent or a calcium/calmodulin-dependent protein kinase. In addition, this subunit was found to be dephosphorylated by the calcium/calmodulin-dependent phosphoprotein phosphatase, calcineurin [Hosey et al., 1986].

Flockerzi et al. [1986] demonstrated that phosphorylation of the reconstituted, purified calcium channel by cAMP-dependent protein kinase prolongs the open-channel life times and shortens the shut intervals between channel openings and/or groups of openings.

Taken together, the results suggest that the calcium channel is modulated by multiple mechanisms. Phosphorylation of both the intermediate and large subunits could be important regulatory mechanisms of calcium channel function.

RECONSTITUTION

There have been several reports in the literature which have demonstrated that calcium channels in membrane vesicles can be incorporated into planar lipid bilayers [Nelson et al., 1984; Ehrlich et al., 1986]. In addition, detergent-solubilized, voltage-dependent calcium channels from skeletal muscle transverse tubule membranes have been partially purified [Curtis and Catterall, 1984], reconstituted into phospholipid bilayer membranes, and found to be modulated by cAMP-dependent protein kinases [Flockerzi et al., 1986; Talvenheimo et al., 1986]. Two types of calcium channels were observed by Talvenheimo et al. [1986] in electrophysiological experiments, which were distinguished by their slope conductances (8 psec and 15–20 psec in 60 mM barium). Thus, these two channels have co-purifed and may, therefore, be structurally related.

CONCLUSIONS

A combination of electrophysiological and biochemical techniques has provided convincing evidence that active voltage-dependent calcium channels are being purified from skeletal muscle. Protein phosphorylation studies indicate that the regulatory mechanisms for voltage-dependent calcium channel function may be known in the near future. The development of antibodies should continue to provide useful information on the structure and function of the calcium channels, including their subunit composition.

Most of the biochemical studies have focused on skeletal muscle since it is a rich source of calcium antagonist binding sites. However, there appear to be significant differences between this binding site and the antagonist binding sites in smooth and cardiac muscle membranes. Not only are the dissociation constants of the 1,4-dihydropyridines different, but it has been consistently reported that the skeletal muscle 1,4-dihydropyridine binding site has a large unique subunit (molecular weight 130,000–160,000).

Future biochemical studies should address the possibility that the use of the 1,4-dihydropyridines as probes may identify one or several of the variety of calcium channels that have been characterized by electrophysiological experiments. It is not known what, if any, molecular differences exist between such channels. In addition, the possibility that the 1,4-dihydropyridines may not be entirely specific for the voltage-dependent calcium channel proteins, but that they may bind other proteins with high affinity, needs to be explored.

In conclusion, substantial progress has already been made toward the biochemical characterization and isolation of the voltage-dependent calcium channel proteins. Our understanding of calcium channel structure and function has been greatly enhanced by these molecular studies. Purification of the voltage-dependent calcium channel with a concomitant retention of all its 1,4-dihydropyridine binding activity would be an important development in these studies.

ACKNOWLEDGMENTS

S.M.S is a recipient of a grant from the American Heart Association (Vermont chapter).

REFERENCES

Barhanin J, Schmid A, Lombet A, Wheeler KP, Lazdunski M (1983): Molecular size of different neurotoxin receptors on the voltage-sensitive Na$^+$ channel. J Biol Chem 258:700–702.

Bean BP (1985): Two kinds of calcium channels in canine atrial cells. J Gen Physiol 86:1–30.

Biswas CJ, Rogers TB (1986): Synthesis of carboxynifedipine and its use in the preparation of an affinity resin for the 1,4-dihydropyridine receptor. Biochem Biophys Res Commun 134:922–927.

Borsotto M, Barhanin J, Fosset M, Lazdunski M (1985): The 1,4-dihydropyridine receptor associated with the skeletal muscle voltage-dependent Ca^{2+} channel. J Biol Chem 260:14255–14263.

Borsotto M, Barhanin J, Norman RI, Lazdunski M (1984b): Purification of the dihydropyridine receptor of the voltage-dependent Ca^{2+} channel from skeletal muscle transverse tubules using (+)[^{3}H]PN200-110. Biochem Biophys Res Commun 122:1357–1366.

Borsotto M, Norman RI, Fosset M, Lazdunski M (1984a). Solubilization of the nitrendipine receptor from skeletal muscle transverse tubule membranes. Eur J Biochem 142:449–455.

Campbell KP, Lipshutz GM, Denney GH (1984): Direct photoaffinity labeling of the high affinity nitrendipine-binding site in subcellular membrane fractions isolated from canine myocardium. J Biol Chem 259:5384–5387.

Campbell KP, Sharp A, Strom M, Kahl SD (1986): High affinity antibodies to the 1,4-dihydropyridine Ca^{2+} channel blockers. Proc Natl Acad Sci USA 83:2792–2796.

Catterall WA (1982): The emerging molecular view of the sodium channel. Trends in Neurosci 5:303–306.

Curtis BM, Catterall WA (1983): Solubilization of the calcium antagonist receptor from rat brain. J Biol Chem 258:7280–7283.

Curtis BM, Catterall WA (1984): Purification of the calcium antagonist receptor of the voltage-sensitive calcium channel from skeletal muscle transverse tubules. Biochemistry 23:2113–2118.

Curtis BM, Catterall WA (1985): Phosphorylation of the calcium antagonist receptor of the voltage-sensitive calcium channel by cAMP-dependent protein kinase. Proc Natl Acad Sci USA 82:2528–2532.

Ebashi S, Endo M (1968): Calcium ion and muscle contraction. Prog Biophys Molec Biol 18:123–183.

Eckert R, Chad JE (1984): Inactivation of calcium channels. Prog Biophys Molec Biol 44:215–267.

Ehrlich BE, Schen CR, Garcia ML, Kaczorowski GJ (1986): Incorporation of calcium channels from cardiac sarcolemmal membrane vesicles into planar lipid bilayer. Proc Natl Acad Sci USA 83:193–197.

Ferry DR, Goll A, Glossmann H (1983): Putative calcium channel molecular weight determination by target size analysis. Naunyn Schmiedeberg's Arch Pharmacol 323:292–297.

Ferry DR, Rombusch M, Goll A, Glossmann H (1984): Photoaffinity labelling of Ca^{2+} channels with [³H]azidopine. FEBS Lett 169:112–118.

Ferry DR, Kämpf K, Goll A, Glossmann H (1985): Subunit composition of skeletal muscle transverse tubule calcium channels evaluated with the 1,4-dihydropyridine photoaffinity probe, [³H]azidopine. EMBO J 4:1933–1940.

Fleckenstein A (1971): Specific inhibitors and promoters of calcium action in the excitation-contraction coupling of the heart muscle and their role in the prevention or production of myocardial lesions. In Harris P, Opie L (eds): "Calcium and the Heart." New York: Academic Press, pp 135–188.

Fleckenstein A (1977): Specific pharmacology of calcium in myocardium, cardiac pacemakers and vascular smooth muscle. Ann Rev Pharmacol Toxicol 17:149–166.

Flockerzi V, Oeken H-J, Hofmann F, Pelzer D, Cavalié A, Trautwein W (1986): Purified dihydropyridine-binding site from skeletal muscle t-tubules is a functional calcium channel. Nature (Lond) 323:66–68.

Fukushima Y, Hagiwara S (1985): Currents carried by

monovalent cations through calcium channels in mouse neoplastic B lymphocytes. J Physiol (Lond) 358:255–284.

Glossmann H, Ferry DR (1983): Solubilization and partial purification of putative calcium channels labelled with [³H]-nimodipine. Naunyn Schmiedeberg's Arch Pharmacol 323:279–291.

Glossmann H, Ferry DR, Goll A, Rombusch M (1984): Molecular pharmacology of the calcium channel: Evidence for subtypes, multiple drug-receptor sites, channel subunits, and the development of a radioiodinated 1,4-dihydropyridine calcium channel label, [¹²⁵I]iodipine. J Cardiol Pharmacol 6:S608–S621.

Glossmann H, Ferry DR, Goll A, Striessnig J, Zernig G (1985): Calcium channels and calcium channel drugs: Recent biochemical and biophysical findings. Arzneim-Forsch 35(II):1917–1935.

Goll A, Ferry DR, Glossmann H (1983): Target size analysis of skeletal muscle Ca^{2+} channels. FEBS Lett 157:63–69.

Goll A, Ferry DR, Glossman H (1984): Target size analysis and molecular properties of Ca^{2+} channels labelled with [³H]verapamil. Eur J Biochem 141:177–186.

Gould RJ, Murphy KMM, Snyder SH (1984): Tissue heterogeneity of calcium channel antagonist binding sites labeled by [³H]nitrendipine. Mol Pharmacol 25:235–241.

Hagiwara S, Byerly L (1981): Calcium channel. Ann Rev Neurosci 4:69–125.

Hess P, Tsien RW (1984): Mechanism of ion permeation through calcium channels. Nature (Lond) 309:453–456.

Horne P, Triggle DJ, Venter JC (1984): Nitrendipine and isoproterenol induce phosphorylation of a 42,000 dalton protein that co-migrates with the affinity labelled calcium channel regulatory subunit. Biochem Biophys Res Commun 121:890–898.

Hosey MM, Borsotto M, Lazdunski M (1986): Phosphorylation and dephosphorylation of dihydropyridine-sensitive voltage-dependent Ca^{2+} channel in skeletal muscle membranes by cAMP- and Ca^{2+}-dependent processes. Proc Natl Acad Sci USA 83:3733–3737.

Jung C (1984): Molecular weight determination by radiation inactivation. In Venter JC, Harrison LC (eds): "Receptor Biochemistry and Methodology," Vol 3. New York: Alan R. Liss, pp 193–208.

Katz B (1969): "The Release of Neural Transmitter Substances." Liverpool, England: Liverpool University Press.

Katz B, Miledi R (1964): The effect of calcium on acetylcholine release from motor nerve terminals. Proc R Soc Lond B Biol Sci 161:496–503.

Kirley TL, Schwartz A (1984): Solubilization and affinity labeling of a dihydropyridine binding site from skeletal muscle: Effects of temperature and diltiazem on [^{3}H]dihydropyridine binding to transverse tubules. Biochem Biophys Res Commun 123:41–49.

Kostyuk PG, Mironov SL, Shuba YM (1983): Two ion-selecting filters in the calcium channel of the synaptic membrane of mollusc neurons. J Membr Biol 76:83–93.

Lee KS, Tsien RW (1983): Mechanism of calcium channel blockade by verapamil, D600, diltiazem and nitrendipine in single dialysed heart cells. Nature (Lond) 302:790–794.

McCleskey EW, Almers W (1985): The Ca channel in skeletal muscle is a large pore. Proc Natl Acad Sci USA 82:7149–7153.

Murphy KMM, Gould RJ, Largent BL, Snyder SH (1983): A unitary mechanism of calcium antagonist drug action. Proc Natl Acad Sci USA 80:860–864.

Nelson MT, French RJ, Krueger BK (1984): Voltage dependent calcium channels from brain incorporated into planar lipid bilayer. Nature 308:77–80.

Nilius B, Hess P, Lansman JB, Tsien RW (1985): A novel type of cardiac calcium channel in ventricular cells. Nature (Lond) 316:443–446.

Norman RI, Borsotto M, Fosset M, Lazdunski M, Ellory JC (1983): Determination of the molecular size of the nitrendipine-sensitive Ca^{2+} channel by radiation inactivation. Biochem Biophys Res Commun 111:878–883.

Nowycky MC, Fox AP, Tsien RW (1985): Three types of neuronal calcium channel with different calcium agonist sensitivity. Nature (Lond) 316:440–443.

Pumplin DW, Reese TS, Llinas R (1981): Are the presynaptic membrane particles the calcium channels? Proc Natl Acad Sci USA 78:7210–7213.

Rengasamy A, Ptasienski J, Hosey MM (1985): Purification of the cardiac 1,4-dihydropyridine receptor/calcium channel complex. Biochem Biophys Res Commun 126:1–7.

Reuter H (1983): Calcium channel modulation by neurotransmitters, enzymes and drugs. Nature (Lond) 301:569–574.

Rios E, Brum G (1986): Nifedipine and the voltage sensor of skeletal muscle excitation-contraction (E-C) coupling. J Gen Physiol 88:50a.

Ruth P, Flockerzi V, Oeken H-J, Hofmann F (1986): Solubilization of the bovine cardiac sarcolemmal binding sites for calcium channel blockers. Eur J Biochem 155:613–620.

Schmid A, Barhanin J, Coppola T, Borsotto M, Lazdunski M (1986): Immunochemical analysis of subunit structures of 1,4-dihydropyridine receptors associated with voltage-dependent Ca^{2+} channels in skeletal, cardiac and smooth muscles. Biochemistry 25:3492–3495.

Schramm M, Towart R (1985): Modulation of calcium channel function by drugs. Life Sci 37:1843–1860.

Schwartz LM, McCleskey EW, Almers W (1985): Dihydropyridine receptors in muscle are voltage-dependent but most are not functional calcium channels. Nature 314:747–751.

Talvenheimo JA, Worley JF, Nelson MT (1986): Purified calcium channels from transverse-tubule membranes incorporated into planar lipid bilayers. J Gen Physiol 88:58a.

Triggle DJ, Swamy VC (1983): Calcium antagonists. Some chemical-pharmacologic aspects. Circ Res 52(Suppl I):17–28.

Venter JC (1985): Size of neurotransmitter receptors as determined by radiation inactivation-target size analysis. In Conn PM (ed): "The Receptors," Vol II. New York: Academic Press, pp 245–280.

Venter JC, Fraser CM, Schaber JS, Jung CY, Bolger G, Triggle DJ (1983): Molecular properties of the slow inward calcium channel. J Biol Chem 258:9344–9348.

Yousif F, Triggle DJ (1985): Functional interactions between organic calcium channel antagonists in smooth muscle. Can J Physiol Pharmacol 63:193–195.

Structure and Physiology of the Slow Inward Calcium Channel, pages 123–140
© 1987 Alan R. Liss, Inc.

7

Skeletal Muscle Ca^{2+} Channels

G.N. Beaty, G. Cota, L. Nicola Siri, J.A. Sánchez, and E. Stefani

*Department of Physiology, Biophysics, and Neurosciences, Centro de
Investigación y de Estudios Avanzados del Instituto Politécnico
Nacional, 07000 Mexico, D.F.*

Ca^{2+} channels are widely distributed among different cell types (see this volume). We shall describe in this paper the presence of voltage-dependent slow Ca^{2+} channels in mammalian and frog skeletal muscle fibers. The ionic conditions necessary to record Ca^{2+} currents (I$_{Ca}$), the localization of Ca^{2+} channels, the kinetic properties, and the effects of temperature on I$_{Ca}$ will be discussed. Finally, the possible physiological role of the channel will be considered. Ultimately, a fast-activated Ca^{2+} current, recently found, will be described.

Ca^{2+} ACTION POTENTIAL

Slow Ca^{2+} action potential can be elicited in twitch muscle fibers of frogs and mammals by blocking K$^+$ channels with tetraethylammonium (TEA) and by removing the Cl$^-$ shunt using an impermeant anion as sulphate (SO$_4^-$) or methanesulphonate (CH$_3$SO$_3^-$) [Beaty and Stefani, 1976a; Chiarandini and Stefani, 1983; Kerr and Sperelakis, 1983].

Figure 1A and B shows a Na$^+$ action potential recorded in a Cl$^-$-free solution; in B a long current pulse was delivered. After the initial Na$^+$ spike, there is a plateau which corresponds to the voltage passive response

associated with the current pulse. In Figure 1C and D, in addition to removal of Cl$^-$, 40 mM Na$^+$ of the external solution was replaced by 40 mM TEA to block K$^+$ currents. In this ionic condition, the Na$^+$ spike is prolonged (C). In records taken at a slower sweep speed, after the initial Na$^+$ spike, the cell remained depolarized and the membrane potential slowly creeps until a second slow action potential is being fired, with a threshold of approximately -30 mV. The second slow action potential is Ca^{2+}-dependent and is blocked by conventional Ca^{2+} antagonists such as Co^{2+}, Cd^{2+}, Mn^{2+}, D-600, nifedipine, etc. In addition, it is insensitive to 1 μM

Dr. Beaty's present address is Departamento de Ciencias de la Salud, Universidad Autónoma Metropolitana-Iztapalapa, Apartado Postal 55-535, 09340 México, D.F.

Dr. Cota's present address is Department of Physiology, School of Medicine, University of Pennsylvania, Philadelphia, PA 19104 USA.

Dr. Nicola Siri's present address is Instituto de Biología, Facultad de Medicina, Universidad de Buenos Aires, Paraguay 2155, Buenos Aires 1425, Argentina.

Dr. Sánchez's present address is Departamento de Farmacología, Centro de Investigación-IPN, Apartado Postal 14-740, 07000 México, D.F.

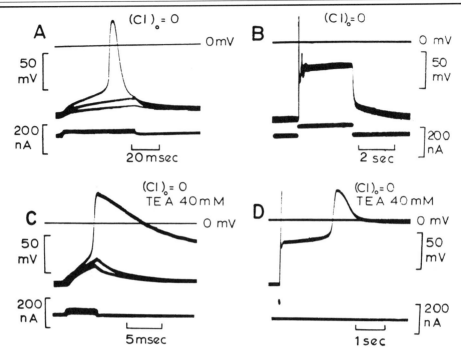

Fig. 1. Na^+ and Ca^{2+} action potential recorded from sartorius muscle fibers from Rana pipiens. Two-microelectrode current clamp technique. In A and B, the recording saline was (mM/l): Na_2SO_4 40, $CaSO_4$ 10, sucrose 113. In C and D, the recording saline was (mM/l): Na_2SO_4 20, $CaSO_4$ 10, sucrose 463, TEA_2SO_4 20. Temperature: 23.0°C. (Unpublished results from Beaty and Stefani.)

tetrodotoxin (TTX). A similar response can be recorded in mammalian and frog skeletal muscle fibers in the absence of Na^+ and with TTX added [Nicola Siri et al., 1980; Chiarandini and Stefani, 1983].

In fast twitch muscle fibers of mammals of the extensor digitorium longus muscle, the Ca^{2+} response was sustained during the duration of the depolarizing pulse and was not affected by repetitive stimulation. In contrast, in soleus muscles, which contain slow twitch muscle fibers, the first evoked response was generally sustained, but after repetitive stimulation, the responses were followed by a hyperpolarization. This is consistent with the presence of a functional Ca^{2+}-dependent K^+ conductance [Meech and Standen, 1975]. The entry of Ca^{2+} during the response would be followed by the opening of the Ca^{2+}-activated K^+ channel, which would tend to hyperpolarize the cell and, thus, shortens the duration of response; this is consistent with the after-hyperpolarization blockade by nifedipine and by Ca^{2+} replacement by Ba^{2+} [Chiarandini and Stefani, 1983].

An equivalent Ca^{2+}-dependent response, but smaller in amplitude, was recorded in tonic muscle fibers of mammals and frogs [Stefani and Uchitel, 1976; Huerta and Stefani, 1983; Chiarandini and Stefani, unpublished observations). Tonic fibers do not normally fire action potentials and are polyneurally innervated at multiple sites along their length by small motor axons.

VOLTAGE-DEPENDENT I_{Ca}

I_{Ca} can be recorded in frog and mammalian skeletal muscle fibers using the three-microelectrode voltage clamp technique in intact fibers, the vaseline gap technique in the cut fiber preparation, and the double-sucrose gap method [Stanfield, 1977; Beaty and Stefani, 1976b; Sánchez and Stefani, 1978; Almers et al., 1981; Potreau and Raymond, 1980a,b; Donaldson and Beam, 1983; Ríos et al., 1985].

In frog muscle, the I_{Ca} has a slow time course. For a depolarization near 0 mV, it has a peak time of 100–200 msec with a maximum value of -50 to -100 $\mu A/cm^2$ in the presence of 10 mM Ca^{2+} in the external recording solution. It spontaneously decays during the maintained pulse, with a time constant of about 0.5 to 1 sec (20–23°C). The I_{Ca} can be detected with pulse depolarizations close to -40 mV.

Figure 2A shows an example of I_{Ca} recorded in frog skeletal muscle fibers in TEA methanesulphonate with 5 mM 3,4-diaminopyridine (3,4-DAP). Each trace is the membrane current recorded with the three-microelectrode voltage clamp during 1-sec depolarizing steps to different potentials. The membrane potential of the cell was maintained at -90 mV. Record 1 is the membrane current associated with a subthreshold voltage pulse of +20 mV in amplitude. Records 2–9 were subtracted for linear resistive and capacitive components. Records 2 and 3 show transient outward and inward current at the beginning and at the end of the pulse, which corresponds to the described charge movement [Schneider and Chandler, 1973]. Record 3 shows a small sustained inward I_{Ca}. In record 4, there is a slow development of inward current which was followed abruptly by a faster one. This discontinuity in the current record, which becomes more evident in the region of negative slope of the voltage current relationship, suggests that the current is originated from membrane areas which are not adequately voltage-controlled. Thus, it suggests the possibility that the Ca^{2+} channels are located in the tubular system.

Records 5–7 show that the inward current becomes faster for larger depolarization and that it is not maintained during the pulse. It decays spontaneously after reaching a maximum. The decay of I_{Ca} can be explained by a voltage or current-dependent inactivation mechanism, by remaining K^+ outward currents, and/or by Ca^{2+} depletion from the tubular network. These possibilities will be discussed in detail. For larger pulses (records 7–9), I_{Ca} is contaminated by outward K^+ currents which are not blocked by TEA and 3,4-DAP. Figure 1B shows the I-V curves normalized for three different muscle fibers.

The slow inward current was identified as I_{Ca} on the following basis: 1) it was not recorded when external Ca^{2+} is replaced by Mg^{2+} [Sánchez and Stefani, 1978]; 2) its magnitude increases when external Ca^{2+} is raised; and 3) it was blocked by the addition of Ca^{2+} channel blockers such as Cd^{2+}, Ni^{2+}, Mn^{2+}, Co^{2+}, nifedipine, and D-600 [Stanfield, 1977; Sánchez and Stefani, 1978, 1983; Almers and Palade, 1981; Donaldson and Beam, 1983]. In addition, Ba^{2+} can permeate through this channel [Potreau and Raymond, 1980b; Almers et al., 1981; Donaldson and Beam, 1983; Cota and Stefani, 1984b].

In conclusion, Ca^{2+} and remaining K^+ currents are recorded in skeletal muscle fibers after partially blocking K^+ channels with TEA and 3,4-DAP in a Cl^--free solution. The current records show clamp inhomogeneities, which suggests the tubular localization of the channels. In order to do a detailed kinetic analysis of these currents, it becomes necessary to further block K^+ currents and to obtain uniform clamp records.

TUBULAR LOCALIZATION OF Ca^{2+} CHANNELS

Different experiments indicate that Ca^{2+} channels are located in the membrane of the tubular system. After muscle fiber detubulation with the glycerol treatment, I_{Ca} amplitude is reduced [Nicola Siri et al., 1980; Potreau and Raymond, 1980a,b]. In addition, in the cut fiber preparation, the decline of the current arises from Ca^{2+} depletion from an extracellular compartment which was identified as the lumen of the transverse tubules [Almers et al., 1981].

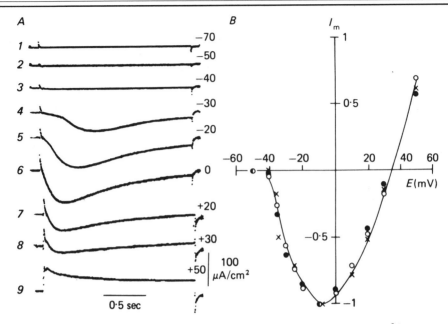

Fig. 2. *A) Membrane current recorded with the three-microelectrode current clamp technique in intact fibers from sartorius muscle of* Rana temporaria. *In this, and following figures, membrane current is recorded as* $V_2 - V_1$, *and pulse potential as* V_1. *Holding potential -90 mV. The recording saline was* *(mM/l): TEA(CH_3SO_3) 115, Ca^{2+} (CH_3SO_3)_2 10, K(CH_3SO_3) 2.5, sucrose 350, 3,4-DAP 5. Temperature 22–26°C. B) Normalized I-V curves for three different fibers in the same ionic conditions as A. (Data from Sánchez and Stefani, 1983, printed with permission of the publisher.)*

Figure 3A shows I_{Ca} records and Figure 3B shows the corresponding I-V curves during the glycerol treatment in frog skeletal muscle fibers. Records were obtained in the presence of 400 mM glycerol before the detubulation procedure was initiated. The left record corresponds to leakage current while the right one to I_{Ca} which has normal characteristics. Thus, the addition of glycerol to the recording saline does not greatly modify I_{Ca}. Records *b–d* show remaining I_{Ca} in fibers with different degrees of detubulation. The fraction of the expected tubular capacitive (FTC) was taken as an indication of the degree of the detubulation (numbers to the right of the leakage current). In fiber *d* there is no indication of I_{Ca} with an FTC of 0.16; only a remaining outward current was recorded. Fibers *b* and *c* show initial outward currents which are followed by small inward (b) and ingoing (c) currents. In Figure 3B, the corresponding I-V current for the four fibers in A are shown

after subtracting K^+ and leakage currents. It can be noticed that the voltage dependence of I_{Ca} was not greatly modified by the detubulation procedure and that there is a correlation between the degree of detubulation and the value of remaining I_{Ca}.

These results indicate that Ca^{2+} channels are located in the membranes of the tubular system. However, due to errors involved in the measurements of membrane currents and to the fact that the total surface area of tubular membranes is much larger than the corresponding external membrane area, we cannot rule out that a small fraction of the total I_{Ca} recorded may originate from channels located in the external membrane.

IMPROVEMENT OF I_{Ca} RECORDINGS

To make a kinetic study of I_{Ca}, it becomes necessary to further reduce outward K^+ cur-

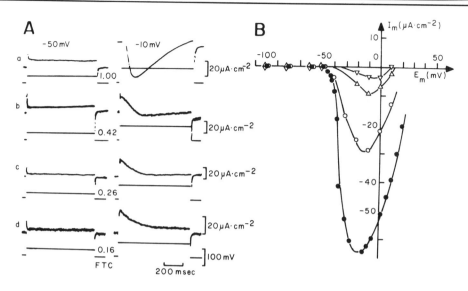

Fig. 3. *Glycerol effects on I_{Ca}. A) Left records correspond to leakage currents to -50 mV, while right records correspond to active current recorded at -20 mV. The recording solution was (mM/l): TEA_2SO_4 40, $CaSO_4$ 10, K_2SO_4 1.25. In a, 400 mM glycerol and 200 mM sucrose were added. Records b, c, and d are fibers after glycerol treatment with different degree of detubulation. The fraction of the expected tubular capacitive (FTC) was .42 in b, .26 in c, and .16 in d. B) The corresponding I-V curves of peak current. ●, a; ○, b; ▲, c; ▽, d. Sartorius muscle of Rana pipiens, at 22°C. The holding potential was -90 mV. (Data modified from Nicola Siri et al., 1980.)*

rents and to improve voltage-clamp uniformity. To this end, I_{Ca} records were obtained from fibers of small diameters after incubating the muscles overnight in a Cs^+- and TEA-containing solution [Cota et al., 1983]. The incubation procedure replaced most of the intracellular K^+ by cesium and/or TEA [Chiarandini and Stefani, 1983]; thus outward current during depolarizing pulses was almost abolished [Cota et al., 1983]. I_{Ca} in fresh muscles decays following a complex time course due to the remaining outward currents [see Fig. 1; Cota et al., 1983]. On the other hand, in incubated muscles, the decay of I_{Ca} follows a single exponential (Fig. 4). The decline of I_{Ca} in incubated muscle fibers cannot be explained by an increase of outward current with time. This is in agreement with the observation of Ca^{2+} tail-current amplitude at the K^+ equilibrium potential, measured with pulses of different durations. It was found that the envelope of tail current amplitudes declined with a time course similar to the decay of the I_{Ca} during a maintained depolarization [Sánchez and Stefani, 1983].

In addition to the incubation procedure, I_{Ca} records became more reliable by selecting small fibers (20–30 μm radius), which improved tubular space clamp. In this condition, clamp inhomogeneities, as demonstrated in Figure 2A (record 4), were not observed [Cota et al., 1983].

DECAY of I_{Ca}

Experimental Observations

Experiments performed in the cut fiber preparation equilibrated intracellularly with isotonic (tetraethylammonium)$_2$-ethylenglycol-bis(β-aminoethyl-ether) N,N'-tetraacetate (TEA$_2$-EGTA), indicate that the decay of I_{Ca} during a maintained depolarization can be explained by tubular Ca^{2+} depletion [Almers et al., 1981]. It was found in two-pulse experiments that the I_{Ca} during the second pulse was

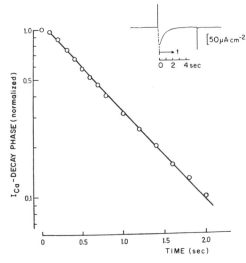

Fig. 4. *Decay of I_{Ca} in an incubated muscle. Recording solution (mM/l): TEA(CH₃SO₃) 120, Ca(CH₃SO₃)₂ 10, sucrose 350. The holding potential was -100 mV; voltage pulse to 0 mV. The decay of I_{Ca} was fitted to a single exponential with a time constant of 0.83 sec. Cutaneous pectoris muscle from* Rana moctezuma. *Temperature 23°C. (Unpublished data of Cota, Nicola Siri, and Stefani.)*

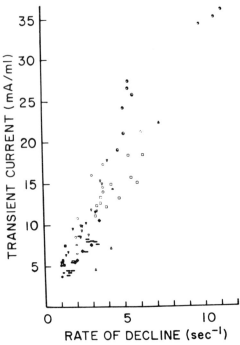

Fig. 5. *Relationship between the amplitude of the inward current through Ca^{2+} channels and its rate of decline in cut muscle fibers. The ordinate plots the means peak final current referred to unit fiber volume. The abscissa plots the reciprocal time constant of an exponential fitted to the final portion of decline. Each symbol shape refers to one fiber. Open symbols: standard 10 mM Ca^{2+} or 10 mM $CaCl_2$; filled symbols: results in presence of nifedipine, D-600, Ni^{2+}, tetracaine, or with Mn^{2+} instead of Ca^{2+}; half-filled symbols: Sr^{2+} or Ba^{2+} instead of Ca^{2+}. Experiments performed in the cut fiber preparation with the cut ends equilibrated in isotonic TEA₂-EGTA. Muscle fibers from* Rana temporaria. *(Data from Almers et al., 1981, with permission of the publisher.)*

reduced in size only if the prepulse elicited I_{Ca}. Moreover, the decline of I_{Ca} was a current-dependent process. The rate constant of decay was always proportional to the peak amplitude of I_{Ca}, no matter whether this amplitude was varied as a function of the membrane potential, by applying different Ca^{2+} channel blockers, or by changing the permeant ion (Fig. 5). Furthermore, the I_{Ca} decline was greatly slowed when an external Ca^{2+} buffering system was used (Ca-malate).

In this section, we shall present observations obtained in the intact muscle fiber preparation with the three-microelectrode voltage-clamp technique, which favors a voltage-dependent inactivation mechanism for the decay of I_{Ca}. In these experiments the external recording saline was made hypertonic by adding 350 mM sucrose to abolish contraction.

A) Effect of temperature. Figures 6 and 7 show that the time course of I_{Ca} is strongly dependent upon temperature. The time constant of decay (τ_d) was measured at 0 mV and

-20 mV between 12.5°C and 23°C. In all cases, the decay followed a single exponential. The Arrhenius plot (Fig. 7) gave a linear relationship. The values for the activation energy (E) and the corresponding Q_{10} (calculated for a 10–20°C transition) were respectively: 17.5 ± 1.0 kcal/mol and 2.9 ± 0.2 at 0 mV, and 18.0 ± 1.5 kcal/mol and 3.0 ± 0.3 at -20 mV. These high values of Q_{10} are similar to those reported for gating processes.

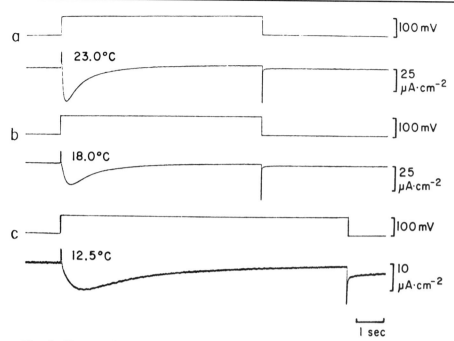

Fig. 6. *Kinetics of I_{Ca} at different temperatures. Records of voltage pulses and membrane currents in the same fiber. Cutaneous pectoris muscle from* Rana moctezuma *after incubation procedure. Recording solution as in Figure 4. The holding potential was -100 mV. Voltage pulses to 0 mV. (Unpublished data from Cota, Nicola Siri, and Stefani.)*

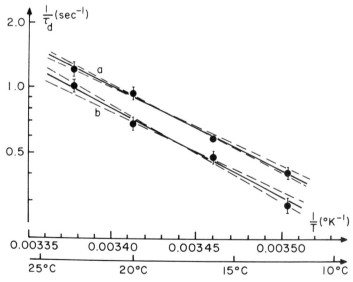

Fig. 7. *Dependence of the rate constant of decay of I_{Ca} with temperature. Arrhenius plots for different fibers of incubated muscles from* Rana moctezuma. *Recording solution as in Figure 4. Holding potential -100 mV. Voltage pulse to 0 mV in a and to -20 mV in b. Activation energy (kcal/mol) 17.5 ± 0.9 in a, and 18 ± 2 in b; Q_{10} (10–20°C) 2.9 ± 0.2 in a, and 3.0 ± 0.3 in b. (Data modified from Cota et al., 1983.)*

The temperature dependence of the time course activation of I_{Ca} was also determined at 0 mV. For this purpose I_{Ca} was described following the Hodgkin and Huxley equation using the m^3h relationship [Sánchez and Stefani, 1983]. For example, in one fiber the time constant of activation was 120 msec at 20.0°C and 210 msec at 15.0°C which gives a Q_{10} of 3.2. The fitted E for all data was 18.0 ± 1.5 kcal/mol with a corresponding Q_{10} of 3.0 ± 0.3 between 10 and 20°C [Cota et al., 1983].

In conclusion, the activation and the decay phases of I_{Ca} show similar temperature dependences, with Q_{10} values consistent with a gating mechanism. In similar experiments, the limiting Ca^{2+} permeability had a lower Q_{10} value of about 1.6, which is similar to that reported for the permeability of ionic channels.

B) Effect of a Ca^{2+} buffering system. The absence of intratubular Ca^{2+} depletion during I_{Ca} under our experimental conditions can be confirmed by recording in the presence of a high concentration of a Ca^{2+} buffering system in the external medium. It was found that 126 mM Ca-maleate in the recording solution does not modify the rate of decay of I_{Ca} during a maintained depolarization [Stefani and Cota, 1984].

C) Two-pulse experiments with I_{Ca}. In experiments carried out in muscles of *Rana temporaria* and *Rana pipiens*, it was difficult to detect inactivation with prepulses which did not elicit I_{Ca}, since in these frog species the membrane potentials for half-activation and inactivation had similar values. In the present experiments, activation and inactivation were analyzed in muscles of *Rana moctezuma*. In these frogs, the main advantage is that the inactivation curve is located at more negative membrane potential.

Figure 8 shows one of these experiments in *Rana moctezuma*. Seven-sec prepulses of different amplitudes were delivered prior to a test pulse to 0 mV. Records *a* and *f* show control currents at the beginning and at the end of the experiment. Records *b–e* show the effect of different prepulse amplitudes on the test I_{Ca}. It can be clearly seen in records *c* and *d* that the test I_{Ca} is reduced in size without any detectable current during the prepulse. Figure 9 shows the steady-state inactivation curve with 7-sec prepulses (filled and half-filled symbols) and the normalized I-V curve for I_{Ca} during the prepulses (open symbols). There is a broad range of prepulse potentials (-80 to -40 mV) which induce inactivation of I_{Ca} (up to about 50%) during the test pulse, without producing any detectable Ca^{2+} entry.

In two-pulse experiments with large positive conditioning prepulses, the degree of I_{Ca} inactivation remained practically unchanged, although Ca^{2+} influx during the prepulse greatly decreased as the Ca^{2+} equilibrium potential was approached [Stefani and Cota, 1984].

D) Rate of decay and I_{Ca} amplitude. Figure 10 shows that the rate of decay of inactivated I_{Ca} is independent of the degree of inactivation. Reduction of 70% in the amplitude of I_{Ca} did not produce any significant change in the rate constant of decay ($1/\tau_d$). Figure 11 shows the relation between $1/\tau_d$ and the peak amplitude of I_{Ca} measured at 0 mV. This amplitude varies due to changes in the control current between different fibers (filled circles) or due to different inactivation degrees (open circles; h_∞ from 1.00 to 0.20). It can be seen that the independence between I_{Ca} peak amplitude and $1/\tau_d$ is maintained over an amplitude range from -8 to -62 mA/cm^3.

The rate constant of decay of I_{Ca} is voltage-dependent and not current-dependent in the intact fiber preparation. The peak amplitude of I_{Ca} becomes smaller for larger depolarizations than 0 mV; in contrast, $1/\tau_d$ tends to become faster [Cota and Stefani, 1984a].

E) Effect of Ca^{2+} replacement by Ba^{2+}. The substitution of Ba^{2+} for Ca^{2+} in the external recording solution shifted to more negative potentials the voltage dependence of both peak current amplitude and steady-state inactivation degree [Cota et al., 1982]. These voltage shifts can be explained by surface charge effects [Cota and Stefani, 1984b]. The replacement of Ca^{2+} by Ba^{2+} did not result in slowing the rate of decay of the inward current nor reduce

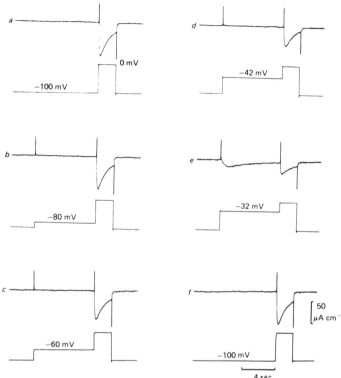

Fig. 8. *Two-pulse inactivation experiment in incubated cutaneous pectoris muscle of* Rana moctezuma. *Recording solution as in Figure 4. Prepulses of 7 sec; test pulses of 2 sec. Note the absence of I_{Ca} during the prepulse in b (h_∞ = 0.32), a prepulse to* -32 mV produced an I_{Ca} of -12 μA cm^{-2}. Control current (a and f) -68 μA cm^{-2}. Temperature 23°C. (Data from Cota et al., 1984, printed with permission of the publisher.)

the degree of steady-state inactivation, after correcting for the reported voltage shifts [G. Cota and E. Stefani, unpublished results].

F) Intracellular Ca^{2+} release and I_{Ca} inactivation. Ca^{2+} is released from the sarcoplasmic reticulum (SR) upon depolarization. Thus, I_{Ca} inactivation could be an intracellular Ca^{2+}-dependent mechanism. To investigate this possibility, we studied the effects of drugs that modify the intracellular Ca^{2+} movements on I_{Ca} properties. It was found that dantrolene sodium, which reduces Ca^{2+} release from SR, does not significantly modify the rate constant of decay of I_{Ca} nor the steady-state inactivation curve [Cota and Stefani, 1984b]. These results indicate that Ca^{2+} released from SR does not significantly contribute to inactivate Ca^{2+} channels under our experimental conditions. Further support for this idea is the fact

that caffeine, which increases the myoplasm Ca^{2+} concentration, does not reduce the I_{Ca} amplitude [Cota and Stefani, 1984b].

Discussion

The previous results in the intact muscle fiber preparation under hypertonic sucrose make unlikely an intratubular Ca^{2+} depletion process as the principal mechanism underlaying the decay of I_{Ca} during a maintained depolarization and favor the presence of a voltage-dependent inactivation mechanism.

We can consider two possibilities to explain why tubular Ca^{2+} is not reduced during I_{Ca} although Ca^{2+} channels are located in the tubular system: 1) a large tubular volume fraction, and 2) an active transport of Ca^{2+} ions into the tubular lumen from the my-

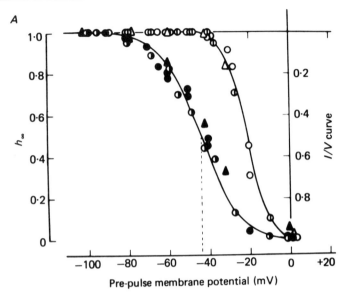

Fig. 9. *Steady-state I_{Ca} inactivation (filled and half-filled symbols) and normalized I/V (open symbols) curves for* Rana moctezuma. *Recording solution as in Figure 4. The normalized I/V curves for I_{Ca} were obtained during the prepulses. Data from three different fibers. Inactivation could be obtained without detection of I_{Ca} during the prepulse. The I/V curves were fitted by eye. The dashed lines indicate the midpoint of the inactivation curve. The experimental points of the inactivation curve were fitted to $h_{\infty} = (1 + exp(E_m - V_h)/k_h)^{-1}$, with $V_h = -44 \pm 3$ mV, and $k_h = 9.5 \pm 1.0$ mV. Temperature 23°C. (Data from Cota et al., 1984, printed with permission of the publisher.)*

oplasm [Cota et al., 1983, 1984]. Hypertonic sucrose is known to produce swelling of the tubular system, leading to an increase in the tubular volume fraction [Freggang et al., 1964]. The pump hypothesis is consistent with the reported Ca^{2+} ATPase in transverse tubular membrane vesicles (Lau et al., 1977; Scales and Sabaddini, 1979; Rosemblatt et al., 1981; Hidalgo et al., 1983] and with the fact that in muscles fatigued by repetitive stimulation, the tubular concentration of Ca^{2+} would be raised, probably by the action of such ATPase [Bianchi and Narayan, 1982].

If the source of the Ca^{2+} pumped into the tubular space during a depolarizing pulse is the sarcoplasmic reticulum (SR), it is expected that the inward current through Ca^{2+} channels in the presence of Ba^{2+} ions in the recording solution should be carried by both Ba^{2+} and Ca^{2+} ions. However, the amount of Ca^{2+} released from SR and pumped into the tubule probably is not significant under

our experimental conditions. This conclusion is supported by the following observations: 1) the inward current is greatly reduced or is abolished after substitution of Mg^{2+} for Ca^{2+} in the recording solution [Sánchez and Stefani, 1978; Cota et al., 1983]; and 2) dantrolene sodium, which reduces Ca^{2+} release from SR [Taylor et al., 1979a], does not modify the rate of decay of I_{Ca} (see above). The small amount of Ca^{2+} ions released from SR and pumped into the tubule may indicate a low pumping rate and/or a small Ca^{2+} release from SR under hypertonic external solutions. In fact, hypertonicity reduces Ca^{2+} release from SR, as it is inferred from measurements of Ca^{2+} transients by using a equorin [Taylor et al., 1979b]. Alternatively, the Ca^{2+} pumped from the myoplasm into the tubule could originate from the Ca^{2+} influx into the fiber. Under this hypothesis, the Ca^{2+} pump should be able to transport Ba^{2+} ions as well, in order to explain the fact that the rate con-

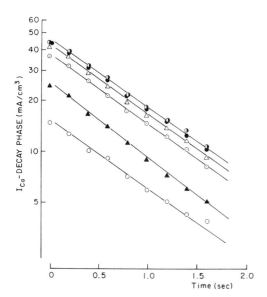

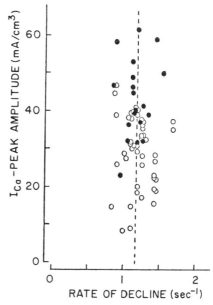

Fig. 10. *Rate of decay of I_{Ca} during the test pulse in two-pulse inactivation experiments. Semilog plots of the decay of the I_{Ca} for the experiment of Figure 7. Records a, ●; b, △; c, ☉; d, ▲; e, ○; and f, ◑. In each case, I_{Ca} (t) - c_{Ca} (∞) vs. time (t) is plotted, where I_{Ca} (∞) is the steady-state value of I_{Ca} determined with pulses of 3-sec duration. In this fiber, I_{Ca} (∞) was 4–6% of the peak value of the control current (records a and f in Figure 7). In all cases, the initial 90% of decay can be adequately described by a single exponential. The values of the time constant of decay (τ_d) were (sec): 1.18 (●), 1.17 (△), 1.16 (☉), 1.12 (▲), 1.20 (○) and 1.18 (◑). The mean value of τ_d for all records was 1.17 ± 0.01 sec. Temperature 23°C. (Unpublished data of Cota, Nicola Siri, and Stefani.)*

Fig. 11. *Relationship between the peak amplitude of I_{Ca} and the rate constant of decay of the current in intact muscle fibers. Open symbols are inactivated currents from five different fibers; filled symbols correspond to individual values of peak amplitude of control I_{Ca} for 19 other fibers. The mean value of the rate constant of decay ($1/\tau_d$) is 1.18 ± 0.02 sec^{-1} (n = 66). I_{Ca} was recorded during test pulses to 0 mV. Recording solution as in Figure 4. Incubated muscle fibers from Rana moctezuma. Temperature 23°C. (Data from Cota et al., 1984, printed with permission of the publisher.)*

stant of decay of the inward current remains practically unchanged after the replacement of Ca^{2+} by Ba^{2+} in the recording solution (see above).

Our results contrast with those of Almers et al. [1981] in cut muscle fibers whose interior was equilibrated with isotonic EGTA to block contraction. In this experimental condition, tubular Ca^{2+} depletion during I_{Ca} was clearly shown. It is likely that in such high intracellular concentration of EGTA, the Ca^{2+} pump could not transport Ca^{2+} into the tubular lumen. In addition, the tubular volume fraction is smaller than in our experimental conditions. Another discrepancy is the near

absence of Ca^{2+} channel inactivation reported in cut fibers in the presence of a high concentration of a Ca^{2+} buffering system or 100 mM Ca^{2+} in the external medium. Under these conditions, the upper limit for the sum of rate constants of all processes other than tubular Ca^{2+} depletion, which may cause current to decline, is 0.172–0.090 sec^{-1} for depolarizations between -10 and +20 mV [Almers et al., 1981]. On the other hand, in our experimental conditions $1/\tau_d$ can be taken as the rate constant of inactivation and is about 1.10 sec^{-1} at 0 mV (data at about 23°C). Thus, it appears that the rate constant of Ca^{2+} channel inactivation should be at least 6–12 times slower in the cut fiber preparation than in intact fibers. These observations suggest that the inactivation mechanism of Ca^{2+} channels operates in a different way in cut fibers than in intact fibers. The possibility that Ca^{2+} channel inactivation is mediated by internal Ca^{2+} released from SR upon depolarization could explain this difference; under this hypothesis, a reduced myoplasmic Ca^{2+} transient by the presence of EGTA would give a lesser degree of Ca^{2+} channel inactivation. However, our results, in the present of dantrolene sodium and caffeine, make unlikely this possibility (see above).

An important point that remains open to future investigation is the time course of the current through Ca^{2+} channels and the role of Ca^{2+} released from SR in intact fibers under isotonic solutions. Indirect evidence suggests that in these conditions, depletion of intratubular Ca^{2+} may occur during a maintained depolarization [Lorkovíc and Rüdel, 1983; Miledi et al., 1983].

On the other hand, preliminary results indicate that both the activation phase and decay of I_{Ba} follow a faster time course in isotonic than in hypertonic conditions; in addition, in two-pulse experiments, inactivation of I_{Ba} during the test pulse can be obtained with prepulses that do not induce detectable Ba^{2+} entry as is the case in hypertonic solutions (G. Cota and E. Stefani, unpublished results). It is reasonable to assume that in these isotonic conditions, the active Ca^{2+} transport into the tubules would not by itself be sufficient to avoid tubular Ca^{2+} depletion and so, both processes, inactivation and tubular depletions may contribute to the decay of the current through Ca^{2+} channels.

KINETIC PARAMETERS OF I_{Ca}

The previous observations indicate that I_{Ca} activates and inactivates in a voltage-dependent manner. In this section, the kinetic parameters of I_{Ca} will be described, following the Hodgkin and Huxley model. A detailed analysis of the procedure was described by Sánchez and Stefani [1983]. The reported results correspond to experiments performed in *Rana temporaria* using the three-microelectrode voltage-clamp technique in intact muscle fiber and hypertonic solution. The notation and equation are described following Hodgkin and Huxley [1952].

Figure 12 shows the fitting procedure to experimental records of I_{Ca} using the following equation:

$$I_{Ca} = A(1 - \exp(-t/\tau_m))^a \quad (1)$$
$$(h_\infty - (h_\infty - 1)\exp(-t/\tau_h)),$$

where A is an amplitude factor; τ_m, τ_h, and h_∞ refer to the usual terminology introduced by Hodgkin and Huxley [1952] to describe Na^+ permeability of squid axons; and a is an integer constant.

We have assumed that at the holding potential (-90 mV), $h_0 = 1$ and $m_0 = 1$. To calculate the rate constants of activation, α_m and β_m, the steady-state parameter of activation (m_∞) has to be determined. m_∞ can be obtained from A in Equation (1) provided the current-voltage relation of open Ca^{2+} channels is known. We assumed that the Goldman-Katz equation also applies to the Ca^{2+} channels of skeletal muscle:

$$I_{Ca} = \frac{4F^2 E P_{Ca}}{RT} \frac{(Ca^{2+})_o (\exp(2F(E - E_{Ca})/RT) - 1)}{(\exp(2FE/RT) - 1)}, \quad (2)$$

where F, R, and T have the usual thermodynamic meanings, E is the membrane potential, $E_{Ca} = +150$ mV, and P_{Ca} is the Ca^{2+} permeability. To account for the voltage dependence of Ca^{2+} activation, P_{Ca} can be expressed as:

$$P_{Ca} = \overline{P}_{Ca} m_\infty^3, \quad (3)$$

where $\overline{P}_{Ca}$ is the limiting Ca^{2+} permeability. The amplitude factor A is determined by:

$$A = \frac{\overline{P}_{Ca} m_\infty^3 4F^2 E (Ca^{2+})_o (\exp(2F(E - E_{Ca})/RT) - 1)}{RT (\exp(2FE/RT) - 1)}. \quad (4)$$

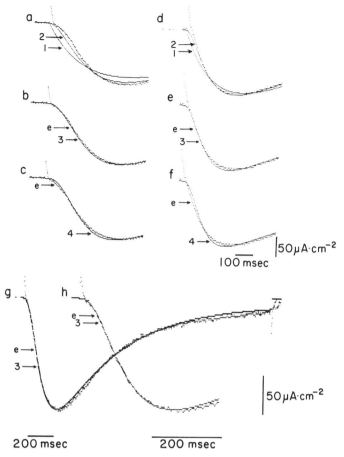

Fig. 12. *Superimposed I_{Ca} records (subtracted for linear capacity and leakage currents, e and fitted curves, with a = 1, a = 2, a = 3, and a = 4. In a), b), and c), pulse to -20 mV; in d)–h) pulse to 0 mV. The fitted curves were determined according to Equation 1. Fresh muscles from Rana temporaria. Recording saline as in Figure 2. Temperature 22–26°C. (Records g and h are from Sánchez and Stefani, 1983, printed with permission of the publisher.)*

The product $\bar{P}_{Ca}\, m_\infty^3$ was calculated according to Equation 4, and its cube root was fitted to the following equation:

$$\left(\bar{P}_{Ca} m_\infty^3\right)^{1/3} = \tag{5}$$

$$\bar{P}_{Ca}\left(1 + \exp((E_{m1/2} - E)/K_m)\right)^{-1},$$

where $E_{m1/2}$ is the midpoint, E is the test-pulse potential, and k_m is a measure of the steepness. The fitting provided values of $\bar{P}_{Ca}$, $E_{m1/2}$ and k_m. The calculated values of the left-hand side of Equation (5) were then normalized, averaged, and fitted again to Equation (5) to obtain the m_∞.

Figure 12 shows records of I_{Ca} (after subtraction of linear components) and the corresponding fitted curves of Equation (1). In this figure, e is experimental I_{Ca}, and the numbers are the values of a for the fitted curves. It is clearly seen that the best fit was obtained for a = 3. Records in g and h show another example at different sweep speeds, with a = 3. The value a = 3 might be overestimated because of clamp nonuniformities in the tubular system. For more negative potentials (-70 and 90 mV), τ_m was calculated from the relaxation time constant of tail currents multiplied by 3.

TABLE I. Activation and Inactivation Parameters of I^{Ca} in Intact Fibers in Hypertonic Solution with the Three-Microelectrode Voltage Clamp Technique*

Activation	Inactivation
m_∞ curve: k_m 9.9 mV	h_∞ curve: k_h 6.3 mV
$E_{m\frac{1}{2}}$ −35.2 mV	$E_{h\frac{1}{2}}$ −33.0 mV
$\bar{\alpha}_m$ 1.74 mV^{-1} sec^{-1}	$\bar{\alpha}_h$ 0.08 sec
$\bar{\beta}_m$ 0.12 sec^{-1}	$\bar{\beta}_h$ 1.4 sec^{-1}
E_m −43.0 mV	E_h −25.5 mV
$V_{\alpha m}$ 19.2 mV	$V_{\alpha h}$ 19.7 mV
$V_{\beta m}$ 23.1 mV	$V_{\beta h}$ 6.1 mV
$\bar{P}_{Ca}$ 1.4 ± 0.4 × 10^{-4} cm sec^{-1}	

The data were obtained from Sánchez and Stefani, 1983, printed with permission of the publisher.
*Sartorius muscle from *Rana temporalia*. Temperature 22–26°C.

Table I shows the obtained activation and inactivation parameters following the Hodgkin and Huxley model. The parameters of Table I were used to calculate the Ca^{2+} influx during a single normal action potential [Sánchez and Stefani, 1983]. The time integral of the calculated I_{Ca} corresponds to a Ca^{2+} entry of about 0.06 pmol/cm^2 of external surface per action potential. This value is much smaller than the previous ones of about 1 × 10^{-12} mol/cm^2 per twitch calculated by using repetitive stimulation and tracer flux measurements [Bianchi and Shanes, 1959; Curtis, 1966; Bianchi and Narayan, 1982). The Ca^{2+} entry we reported would not produce any significant change in the intracellular Ca^{2+} concentration. Similar values were obtained by Almers and Palade [1981] from Ca^{2+} tail current measurements.

PERMEATION AND SELECTIVITY OF SKELETAL MUSCLE Ca^{2+} CHANNELS

Ca^{2+} channels near physiological external Ca^{2+} are not permeable to Na^+ ions. However, when external Ca^{2+} is lowered below 1–10 μM, Na^+ and other small monovalent cations can flow through Ca^{2+} channels [Almers and McCleskey, 1984]. When external Ca^{2+} was increased from 10^{-10} M to 10^{-2} M, the Na^+ inward current first diminishes 10-fold at external Ca^{2+} = 60 μM, and then

increased as Ca^{2+} flows through the channel. The blockade of the channel at Ca^{2+} concentrations lower than 10^{-5} M could be described by the binding of a single Ca^{2+} to a site with a dissociation constant of 0.7 μM at -20 mV [Almers et al., 1984].

In addition, membrane currents in Ba^{2+}/Ca^{2+} mixtures show anomalous mole fraction behavior, suggesting that Ca^{2+} channels are single-file, multi-on pores. It was proposed that Ca^{2+} channel selectivity depends on the existence of high affinity Ca^{2+} binding sites located in the aqueous channel [Almers and McCleskey, 1984].

Ca^{2+} and Ba^{2+} currents and conductances tend to saturate as divalent cation concentration was increased [Cota and Stefani, 1984b]. The Michaelis Memten constants were 5.6 and 6.0 mM for Ca^{2+} and 12.5 and 8.0 mM for Ba, respectively. When external Ca^{2+} and Ba^{2+} concentrations were increased, the voltage-current relationships were shifted to more positive potentials. The shifts were more pronounced for Ca^{2+} than for Ba^{2+}. They were described following the Gouy-Chapman theory with a density of surface charges near Ca^{2+} channels of 0.20 e/nm^2 and including a specific site for Ca^{2+} with a binding constant of 45 M^{-1}.

The permeation of the Ca^{2+} channel was described in an initial attempt following the Eyring rate theory as a two-barrier model [Cota and Stefani, 1984b].

FAST Ca^{2+} CHANNEL

Since the reported slow Ca^{2+} channel cannot explain the extra ^{45}Ca^{2+} influx elicited by an action potential (see above), we performed experiments to search for fast Ca^{2+} channels which can be activated during a single twitch. The experiments were carried out with the three-microelectrode voltage clamp technique on intact fibers in hypertonic solution. It was found that Ca^{2+} currents recorded immediately after the addition of hypertonic solution showed a fast component which was followed by the already described slow I$_{Ca}$ [Cota and Stefani, 1984c, 1985].

Figure 13A and B shows membrane currents and the corresponding I-V curves obtained 7 minutes after the addition of hypertonic solution. A fast-activated inward current, associated with the second and first pulse, can be seen. During the largest pulse, the fast inward current is followed by the described slow I$_{Ca}$. This fast I$_{Ca}$ was detected at approximately -60 mV. At about 0 mV, the time constant of activation was 5 msec, while a value of 150 msec was measured for the slow component. The fast-activated current did not significantly decline during depolarization up to 2 sec of duration at membrane potential between -60 to -30 mV.

Fast I$_{Ca}$ tended to disappear as a function of the time to exposure to the hypertonic recording solution. Its maximum amplitude decreased from about -30 μA/cm^2 during the first 5 minutes to about -5 μA/cm^2 after 25 minutes, while the slow I$_{Ca}$ remained practically unchanged (maximum peak amplitude of about -60 μA/cm^2).

This rundown of fast I$_{Ca}$ may be due to a reduction of Ca^{2+} channel conductance by hypertonicity; however, it is not clear what mechanism is involved.

Fast I$_{Ca}$ is not recorded in intact fibers incubated for several hours in a TEA- and Cs$^+$-containing solution prior to experiments [Cota et al., 1983], nor in cut fibers loaded with TEA and EGTA [Almers and Palade, 1981]. The existence of functional fast-activated Ca^{2+} channels may depend on intracellular components that could be lost under

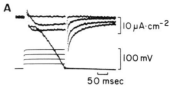

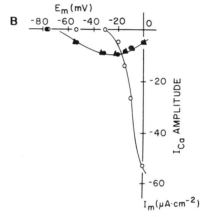

Fig. 13. *Slow- and fast-activated Ca^{2+} currents. A) I$_{Ca}$ records during 200-msec pulses obtained after 7 min of exposure to a hypertonic recording saline similar to that of Figure 2. Fresh muscle from* Rana moctezuma. *Temperature 18°C. B) I-V relationships obtained from the fiber in A). The amplitude of I$_{Ca}$ at the end of 200-msec pulses is plotted. Filled circles: fast-activated I$_{Ca}$; open circles: slow-activated I$_{Ca}$. (Unpublished results from Cota and Stefani.)*

these experimental conditions. Alternatively, the absence of fast I$_{Ca}$ in these cases may reflect an effect of intracellular TEA$^+$ accumulation. In fact, in the cut fiber preparation, the peak I$_{Ca}$ amplitude declines by 30–50% when intracellular K$^+$ is replaced by 160 mM TEA$^+$, suggesting that TEA$^+$ acts as a weak Ca^{2+} channel blocker [Almers and Palade, 1981]. Such reduction of I$_{Ca}$ by internal TEA$^+$ has also been observed in cardiac muscle [Lee and Tsien, 1982].

In view of the kinetic properties of fast-activated Ca^{2+} channels, one may expect that they significantly activate during a single twitch.

SLOW I$_{Ca}$ and CONTRACTION

The role of the slow I$_{Ca}$ on excitation-contraction remains controversial. It is well established that external Ca^{2+} plays a role in maintaining the tension during prolonged depolarization and K^+ contracture: the peak tension, the duration, and the time constant of spontaneous relaxation decrease progressively as external Ca^{2+} is reduced [Cota and Stefani, 1981]. It is clear that the slow I_{Ca} cannot play a significant role during a single twitch or during the initial phase of the K^+ contracture, since both mechanical events were not modified by the removal of external Ca^{2+} [Lüttgau, 1963; Caputo and Giménez, 1967; Armstrong et al., 1972; Stefani and Chiarandini, 1973; Lüttgau and Spiecker, 1979; Potreau and Raymond, 1980a,b; Cota and Stefani, 1981]. The fact that after replacing Ca^{2+} by Ni^{2+}, which does not flow through Ca^{2+} channels, the sustained phase of K^+ contracture is not modified, strongly indicates a lack of direct action of Ca^{2+} current on mechanical activation during K^+ contractures [Caputo, 1981]. Along this line, it was reported that after blocking I_{Ca} with 1×10^{-6} M diltiazem, K^+ contractures were not modified [González-Serratos et al., 1982]. However, the Ca^{2+} channel blockage with diltiazem is not convincing since a half-blockage concentration value of about 80×10^{-6} M was reported [Almers and McCleskey, 1984], and 1×10^{-6} M diltiazem has very little effect on I_{Ca} (Cota, Gamboa and Stefani, unpublished results).

In recent experiments, the time course of myoplasmic Ca^{2+} concentration was measured with antipyrylazo III, and intramembrane charge movement and I_{Ca} were simultaneously recorded [Ríos et al., 1985]. It was found that upon membrane depolarization to 0 mV, the initial fast phase of rise of intracellular Ca^{2+} concentration was independent of external Ca^{2+}. The intitial phase was followed by a prolonged increase in intracellular Ca^{2+}. When external Ca^{2+} was removed or 3 mM Cd^{2+} added, the I_{Ca} is abolished and the initial phase is followed by a decrease in intracellular Ca^{2+} concentration. In 2 mM external Ca^{2+}, the transmembrane I_{Ca} was about 30 nA which corresponds to a Ca^{2+} influx of 0.075

μM/msec. The voltage-dependent Ca^{2+} influx into the myoplasm is 1 μM/msec larger in 2 mM Ca^{2+} [Ríos et al., 1985]. A slight reduction in the Ca^{2+} signal measured with arsenazo III was also detected after reduction of extracellular free Ca^{2+} to low levels using EGTA [Miledi et al., 1984].

In conclusion, the inward I_{Ca} cannot account for the large increase in myoplasmic Ca^{2+} concentration, which must be originated by extra Ca^{2+} release from the SR. These observations, in agreement with mechanical experiments, indicate that external Ca^{2+} modulates Ca^{2+} release from the SR. This extra Ca^{2+} release can be induced by the reported I_{Ca} or by specific interactions of external Ca^{2+} with Ca^{2+} sites in the tubular membranes. Cd^{2+} could equally block Ca^{2+} channels and/or reduce the availability of Ca^{2+} sites to external Ca^{2+}. Further experiments will clarify this point.

ACKNOWLEDGMENTS

The authors are indebted to Josefina Quiroga and Cidia Urquiza for their skillful help in preparing the manuscript. This work was supported by grants PCCBBEU 020187 and PCCBBEU 022519 (CONACyT, México), grant 1R01 AM35085-01 (National Institute of Health, USA) to Dr. E. Stefani, and by the Guggenheim Foundation (E. Stefani is a Guggenheim Fellow).

REFERENCES

Almers W, Palade PT (1981): Slow calcium and potassium currents across frog muscle membrane: Measurements with a vaseline-gap technique. J Physiol (Lond) 312:159–176.

Almers W, McCleskey EW (1984): Non-selective conductance in calcium channels of frog muscle: Calcium selectivity in a single-file pore. J Physiol (Lond) 353:585–608.

Almers W, Fink F, Palade PT (1981): Calcium depletion in frog muscle tubules: The decline of calcium current under maintained depolarization. J Physiol (Lond) 312:177–207.

Almers W, McCleskey EW, Palade PT (1984): A nonselective cation conductance in frog muscle membrane blocked by micromolar external calcium ions. J Physiol (Lond) 353:565–583.

Armstrong CM, Benzanilla FM, Horowicz P (1972): Twitches in presence of ethyelene glycos bis(β-amino-ethyl ether)-N,N'-tetraacetic acid. Biochim Biophys Acta 267:605–608.

Beaty GN, Stefani E (1976a): Calcium dependent electrical activity in twitch muscle fibres of the frog. Proc R Soc B 194:141–150.

Beaty GN, Stefani E (1976b): Inward calcium current in twitch muscle fibres of the frog. J Physiol (Lond) 260:27P.

Bianchi PC, Narayan S (1982): Muscle fatigue and the role of transverse tubules. Science 215:295–296.

Bianchi CP, Shanes AM (1959): Calcium influx in skeletal muscle at rest, during activity and during potassium contracture. J Gen Physiol 42:803–815.

Caputo C (1981): Nickel substitution for calcium and the time course of potassium contractures of single muscle fibres. J Muscle Res Cell Motility 2:167–182.

Caputo C, Giménez M (1967): Effects of external calcium deprivation on single muscle fibers. J Gen Physiol 50:2177–2195.

Chiarandini DJ, Stefani E (1983): Calcium action potentials in rat fast- and slow-twitch muscle fibres. J Physiol (Lond) 335:29–41.

Cota G, Stefani E (1981): Effects of external calcium reduction on the kinetics of potassium contractures in frog twitch muscle fibres. J Physiol (Lond) 317:303–316.

Cota G, Stefani E (1984a): Effect of caffeine and dantrolene sodium on Ca channels in frog skeletal muscle fibers. Biophys J 45:179a.

Cota G, Stefani E (1984b): Saturation of calcium channels and surface charge effects in skeletal muscle fibres of the frog. J Physiol (Lond) 351:135–154.

Cota G, Stefani E (1984c): Search for an early Ca channel in frog skeletal muscle fibers. Abstract Soc. for Neuroscience, 14th Annual Meeeting, p 11.

Cota G, Stefani E (1985): Fast and slow Ca channels in twitch muscle fibres of the frog. Biophys J 47:65a.

Cota G, Nicola Siri L, Stefani E (1982): Current-independent inactivation of the calcium channel in frog skeletal muscle. Biophys J 37:316a.

Cota G, Nicola Siri L, Stefani E (1983): Calcium channel gating in frog skeletal muscle membrane: Effect of temperature. J Physiol (Lond) 338:395–412.

Cota G, Nicola Siri L, Stefani E (1984): Calcium channel inactivation in frog (Rana pipiens and Rana moctezuma) skeletal muscle fibres. J Physiol (Lond) 354:99–108.

Curtis BA (1966): Ca fluxes in single twitch muscle fibers. J Gen Physiol 50:255–267.

Donaldson, PL, Beam KG (1983): Calcium currents in a fast-twitch skeletal muscle of the rat. J Gen Physiol 82:449–468.

Freygan WH Jr, Goldstein DH, Hellam DC, Peachey LD (1964): The relation between the late after-potential and the size of the transverse tubular system of frog muscle. J Gen Physiol 48:235–263.

Gonzalez-Serratos H, Valle-Aguilera R, Lathrop DA, and Garcia MC (1982): Slow inward calcium currents have no obvious role in muscle excitation-contraction coupling. Nature 298:292–294.

Hidalgo C, González ME, Lagos R (1983A): Characterization of the Ca^{2+} or Mg^{2+}-ATPase of transverse tubule membranes isolated from rabbit skeletal muscle. J Biol Chem 258:13927–13945.

Hodgkin AL, Huxley AF (1952): A qualitative description of membrane current and its application to conduction and excitation in nerve. J Physiol (Lond) 117:500–544.

Huerta M, Stefani E (1983): Ca^{++} action potentials and Ca^{++} currents in tonic muscle fibers of the frog. Biophy J 41:60a.

Kerr LM, Sperelakis N (1983): Ca^{++}-dependent slow action potentials in normal and dystrophic mouse skeletal muscle. Am J Physiol 245:C415–C422.

Lau YH, Caswell AH, Brunschwig JP (1977): Isolation of transverse tubules by fractionation of triad junctions of skeletal muscle. J Biol Chem 252:5565–5574.

Lee KS, Tsien RW (1982): Reversal of current through calcium channels in dialysed single heart cells. Nature (Lond) 297:498–501.

Lorković H, Rúdel R (1983): Influence of divalent cations on potassium contracture duration in frog muscle fibres. Pflügers Arch 398:114–119.

Lüttgau HC (1963): The action of calcium ions on potassium contractures of single muscle fibres. J Physiol (Lond) 168:679–697.

Lüttgau HC, Spiecker W (1979A): The effects of calcium deprivation upon mechanical and electrophysiological parameters in skeletal muscle fibres of the frog. J Physiol (Lond) 296:411–429.

Meech RW, Standen NB (1975): Potassium activation in Helix aspersa neurons under voltage clamp: A component mediated by calcium influx. J Physiol (Lond) 249:211–239.

Miledi R, Parker I, Zhu PH (1983): Changes in threshold for calcium transients in frog skeletal muscle fibres owing to calcium depletion in the T-tubules. J Physiol (Lond) 344:233–241.

Miledi R, Parker I, Zhu PH (1984): Extracellular ions and excitation-contraction coupling in frog twitch muscle fibres. J Physiol (Lond) 351:687–710.

Nicola Siri L, Sánchez JA, Stefani E (1980): Effect of glycerol treatment on the calcium current of frog skeletal muscle. J Physiol 305:87–96.

Potreau D, Raymond G (1980a) Calcium-dependent electrical activity and contraction of voltage-clamped frog single muscle fibres. J Physiol (Lond) 307:9–22.

Potreau D, Raymond G (1980b): Slow inward barium current and contraction on frog single muscle fibres. J Physiol (Lond) 303:91–109.

Ríos E, Stefani E, Brum G, Goldman J (1985): Extracellular Ca modifies Ca release from the sarcoplasmic reticulum (SR) in skeletal muscle fibers. Biophys J 47:353a.

Rosemblatt M, Hidalgo C, Vergara C, Ikemoto N (1981): Immunological and biochemical properties of transverse tubule membranes isolated from rabbit skeletal muscle. J Biol Chem 256:8140–8148.

Sánchez JA, Stefani E (1978): Inward calcium current in twitch muscle fibres of the frog. J Physiol (Lond) 337:1–17.

Scales DJ, Sabbadini RA (1979): Microsomal T system: A stereological analysis of purified microsomes derived from normal and dystrophic skeletal muscles. J Cell Biol 83:33–46.

Schneider MF, Chandler WK (1973): Voltage dependent charge movement in skeletal muscle: A possible step in excitation contraction coupling. Nature (London) 242:244–246.

Stanfield PR (1977): A calcium dependent inward current in frog skeletal muscle fibres. Pflügers Arch 368:267–270.

Stefani E, Chiarandini DJ (1973): Skeletal muscle: Dependence of potassium contractures one extracellular calcium. Pflügers Arch 343:143–150.

Stefani E, Cota G (1984): Inactivation as a mechanism for Ca current decay in intact skeletal muscle fibers of the frog. Biophys J 45:37a.

Stefani E, Uchitel O (1976): Potassium and calcium conductance in slow muscle fibres of the toad. J Physiol (Lond) 255:435–448.

Taylor SR, López JR, Shlevin HH (1979a): Calcium movements in relation to muscle contraction. Proc West Pharmacol Soc 22:321–326.

Taylor SR, López JR, Shlevin HH (1979b): Calcium in excitation-contraction coupling of skeletal muscle. Biochem Soc Trans 7:759–764.

Structure and Physiology of the Slow Inward Calcium Channel, pages 141–159

8

Biochemical Characterization of the Skeletal Muscle Ca^{2+} Channel

Michel Fosset and Michel Lazdunski

Centre de Biochimie du Centre National de la Recherche Scientifique,
Parc Valrose, 06034 Nice Cedex, France

INTRODUCTION

The voltage-dependent calcium channel allows the passive movement of Ca^{2+} across plasma membrane of a variety of excitable cells. Such a mechanism has been shown to be important for excitation-contraction coupling in invertebrate muscle and in vertebrate heart and smooth muscle [Lakshminarayanaiah, 1981; Fleckenstein, 1977; Reuter, 1979; Cauvin et al., 1983]. It is also important in secretory processes [Baker and Knight, 1984]. Conversely, in mammalian skeletal muscle, contractile force is often considered to be independent of Ca^{2+} influx [Lüttgau and Spiecker, 1979]. The Ca^{2+} involved in skeletal muscle contraction is believed to come mainly, if not entirely, from stores in sarcoplasmic reticulum, although during sustained depolarizations a sizable amount of Ca^{2+}, enough to trigger tension, may enter the muscle cell [Stefani and Chiarandini, 1982; Almers et al., 1981].

The skeletal muscle cell presents a unique and highly differentiated membrane system with at least two morphologically identifiable membranes in contact with the extracellular fluid, the sarcolemma, and the transverse tubule (T-tubule) system. Electrophysiological experiments have shown that Ca^{2+} channels are present in frog skeletal muscle and have suggested that most if not all calcium conductances are localized in the (T-tubule) system [Stefani and Chiarandini, 1982; Potreau and Raymond, 1980a,b; Almers et al., 1981].

The existence of several types of voltage-dependent Ca^{2+} channels has now been demonstrated in neurons as well as in cardiac, skeletal, and smooth muscle cells [Carbone and Lux, 1984; Bossu et al., 1985; Bean, 1985; Nowycky et al., 1985; Nilius et al., 1985; Cognard et al., 1986a; Huerta and Stefani, 1986; Friedman et al., 1986]. These Ca^{2+} channels differ in their voltage dependence, in their kinetics, and in their pharmacology. One class of Ca^{2+} channel in mammalian skeletal muscle activates and inactivates slowly, the threshold for activation being -30 mV [Cognard et al., 1986b]. Both the kinetics [Cognard et al., 1986b; Rosenberg et al., 1986] and the voltage dependence of inactivation of this class of slow Ca^{2+} channels are different in skeletal and cardiac muscle.

Inhibition of Ca^{2+} entry through long-lasting, voltage-dependent Ca^{2+} channels by spe-

TABLE I. Binding Characteristics and Rate Constants for Ca^{2+} Channel Effectors to Skeletal Muscle Membranes*

Ligand	Temp. (°C)	K_D (nM)	B_{max}	B_{max} with d-cis-diltiazem	Rate constants k_1 and k_{-1}	References
(±)[³H]Nitrendipine	10	1.8 (TT)	50 (R)	—	$k_1 = 1.8 \times 10^6$	Fosset et al., 1982
	10	0.7 (TT)	20 (F)	—	$k_{-1} = 1.7 \times 10^3$	Fosset et al., 1983
	37	3.6 (M)	7 (G)	14.7	—	Ferry et al., 1983b
	25	2.2 (M)	1.1 (G)	—	—	Gould et al., 1984
	10 and 37	1.7–4.3 (TT)	12 (R)	18		Kirley and Schwartz, 1984
(±)[³H]Nimodipine	37	1.5–3.6 (M)	2.1–8 (G)	8–14	$k_{-1} = 2.2 \times 10^{-2}$	Ferry and Glossmann, 1982; Ferry et al., 1983a,b
	37	1.3 (TT)	12 (G)	30–65	—	Glossmann et al., 1983b
	10 and 37	2.3–3.1 (TT)	12 (R)	18	—	Kirley and Schwartz, 1984
(±)Nifedipine	37	4.9 (M)	3.9 (G)	8.6	—	Ferry et al., 1983b
	2	4.7 (TT)	16.9 (G)	20.6	—	Goll et al., 1984a
(±)[³H]PN 200–110	37	1.4 (M)	20 (G)	25	$k_{-1} = 5 \times 10^{-3}$	Ferry et al., 1983b; Goll et al., 1983
(+)[³H]PN 200–110	10	0.2 (TT)	50–90 (R)		—	Borsotto et al., 1984b
(±)[¹²⁵I]Iodipine	25	0.35 (M)	3.9 (G)		$k_1 = 1.7 \times 10^6$ $k_{-1} = 4.6 \times 10^{-4}$	Ferry and Glossmann, 1984
(±)[³H]Azidopine	25	0.35 (M)	28 (G)		$k_1 = 6.3 \times 10^6$ $k_{-1} = 2.5 \times 10^{-3}$	Ferry et al., 1984
(±)[³H]Bay K8644	20	1.8 (TT)	2.1 (F)		—	Ildefonse et al., 1985

*F, frog; G, guinea pig; R, rabbit; M, microsome membranes; TT, T-tubule membranes; B_{max}, maximum binding capacity in pmol/mg protein; K_{max}, equilibrium dissociation constant; k_1 is the association constant in $M^{-1}s^{-1}$, and k_{-1} is the dissociation constant in s^{-1}.

cific organic calcium channel inhibitors represents one of the most important therapeutic means in the treatment of many cardiovascular disorders such as angina, hypertension, and tachycardia [Fleckenstein, 1977; Nayler and Horowitz, 1983]. Some of these Ca^{2+} channel inhibitors have been used to block Ca^{2+} currents and Ca^{2+}-dependent slow action potentials [Sanchez and Stefani, 1978; Almers et al., 1981; Almers and McCleskey, 1984; Schwartz et al., 1985; Gonzales-Serratos et al., 1982; Ildefonse et al., 1985; Kerr and Sperelakis, 1982] in frog skeletal muscle or to alter contractions in rat and frog skeletal muscle [Kaumann and Uchitel, 1976; Eisenberg et al., 1983; Walsh et al., 1984; Ildefonse et al., 1985].

The organic calcium channel modulators used in biochemical experiments with skeletal muscle include (1) the 1,4-dihydropyridine series comprising the inhibitors nifedipine, nimodipine, nitrendipine, nisoldipine, PN 200-110, azidopine, and iodipine, and activators of the voltage-dependent Ca^{2+} channel such as Bay K8644 and CGP 28392; (2) a chemically heterogenous group of compounds comprising verapamil and its analogs methoxy-verapamil (D600) and desmethoxy-verapamil (D888), bepridil, and the benzothiazepine diltiazem; (3) diphenylbutyl-piperazine compounds such as prenylamine, lidoflazine, cinnarizine, flunarizine, and neuroleptics of the diphenylbutylpiperidine series (fluspirilene, pimozide, and penfluridol) [see Gould et al., 1983; Spedding, 1985].

The following review will describe several aspects of the molecular properties (molecular pharmacology, affinity labeling, purification and subunit structure, phosphorylation, immunology, in vivo and in vitro development, and physiopathology) of the skeletal muscle Ca^{2+} channel.

MOLECULAR PHARMACOLOGY
Specific Binding Sites for 1,4-Dihydropyridines

Data obtained with commonly used [^{3}H]1,4-dihydropyridines are summarized in Table I.

The most utilized compound of this series has been nitrendipine because it was the first one to be commercially available. The binding of compounds belonging to this series to microsomes or T-tubule membranes from frog, rat, guinea pig, or rabbit skeletal muscle is of high affinity, with equilibrium dissociation constants K_D of 0.2–3 nM. At present (+)PN 200-110 seems to be the most useful radiolabeled ligand for binding studies because it has the best affinity for the skeletal muscle dihydropyridine receptor (K_D = 0.2 nM). This affinity is in excellent agreement with results obtained in electrophysiology. The blockade by (+)PN 200-110 of Ca^{2+} currents measured by the voltage-clamp technique in skeletal muscle myoballs (prepared from newborn rats) [Fukuda et al., 1976] is voltage-dependent and the concentration to block 50% of maximum current is $K_{0.5}$ = 0.15 nM under depolarizing conditions [Cognard et al, 1986b]. The apparent affinity for PN 200-110 varies by a factor of 86 depending on the state of the Ca^{2+} channel. It is high when the Ca^{2+} channel is in the inactivated form.

Maximum binding capacities, B_{max}, for the association of dihydropyridine inhibitors to extensively purified rabbit T-tubule membranes are 50–80 pmol [^{3}H]1,4-dihydropyridine bound/mg protein. These values are 50–100 times higher than binding capacities found for other excitable membranes prepared from brain, heart, or smooth muscle [Janis and Triggle, 1984]. Binding is rapid, saturable, and reversible. This binding is also stereospecific, as will be shown below. One single population of high affinity binding sites has been found. Rates of association and dissociation for different dihydropyridine ligands have been measured and are summarized in Table I. Kinetic results are in good agreement with equilibrium binding data derived from saturation isotherms or from competition studies at equilibrium. Two reports [Glossmann et al., 1983a; Kirley and Schwartz, 1984] have shown that [^{3}H]nitrendipine and [^{3}H]nimodipine binding are temperature-dependent, the binding capacity decreasing with increasing temperatures between 2 and 37°C.

TABLE II. Binding Characteristics and Rate Constants for Ca^{2+} Channel Inhibitors*

Ligand	Temp. (°C)	K_D (nM)	B_{max}	Rate constants k_1 and k_{-1}	References
d-cis-[³H]Diltiazem	10	45–55 (TT)	45–55 (R)	$k_1 = 8 \times 10^3$ $k_{-1} = 3.2 \times 10^{-4}$	Galizzi et al., 1986a
	2	39 (M)	11 (G)	$k_1 = 8.8 \times 10^3$ $k_{-1} = 3.3 \times 10^{-4}$	Glossmann et al., 1983a
	30	37 (M)	2.9 (G)	—	Glossmann et al., 1983a
(±)[³H]Verapamil	10	27 (TT)	50 (R)	$k_1 = 3.3 \times 10^4$ $k_{-1} = 1.6 \times 10^{-3}$	Galizzi et al., 1984b
	25	37.6 (M)	(Rt)	—	Reynolds et al., 1983
	2	45 (M)	37 (G)	$k_1 = 1.6 \times 10^4$ $k_{-1} = 6 \times 10^{-4}$	Goll et al., 1984a
(−)[³H]Desmethoxy-verapamil	25	1.2 (M)	18 (G)	$k_1 = 9 \times 10^5$ $k_{-1} = 5.3 \times 10^{-4}$	Goll et al., 1984b
	10	1–2 (TT)	70 (R)	$k_1 = 3 \times 10^5$ $k_{-1} = 3.5 \times 10^{-4}$	Galizzi et al., 1986a
(±)[³H]Bepridil	10	15–25 (TT)	80 (R)	$k_1 = 4.2 \times 10^5$ $k_{-1} = 7 \times 10^{-3}$	Galizzi et al., 1986a
[³H]Fluspirilene	25	0.1 (TT)	80 (R)	—	Galizzi et al., 1986b

*Rt, rat; G, guinea pig; R, rabbit; M, microsome membranes; TT, T-tubule membranes; B_{max}, maximum binding capacity in pmol/mg protein; K_D, equilibrium dissociation constant; k_1 is the association constant in $m^{-1}s^{-1}$, and k_{-1} is the dissociation constant in s^{-1}.

Binding studies with frog, rabbit, and guinea pig skeletal muscle from the hind legs have shown that most of the [^{3}H]dihydropyridine binding sites are present in the T-tubule membranes [Fosset et al., 1982; Fosset et al., 1983; Glossmann et al., 1983b]. Little or no binding was found in sarcoplasmic reticulum membranes. Binding sites detected in sarcoplasmic reticulum membranes [Fairhurst et al., 1983] and in surface membranes [Fosset et al., 1983] may represent contamination of these membranes with T-tubule membranes. Binding of [^{3}H]nitrendipine to rabbit and guinea pig T-tubule or microsomal membranes is pH-dependent and reveals the presence of an essential ionizable group on the receptor with a $pK_a = 5.4$ (10°C) [Fosset et al., 1983]. [^{3}H]Nitrendipine binding to rabbit T-tubule membranes has been shown to be protease-sensitive. The binding is destroyed by trypsin, chymotrypsin, pronase, papain, and leucineaminopeptidase, indicating the protein nature of the Ca^{2+} channel [Fosset et al., 1983].

Specific Binding Sites for (±)[^{3}H]Verapamil, (−)[^{3}H]D888, D-cis-[^{3}H]Diltiazem, and (±)[^{3}H]Bepridil

Table II summarizes K_D and B_{max} values found for the binding of this new group of tritium-labelled calcium channel inhibitors to microsomes or T-tubule membranes from rat, guinea pig, or rabbit skeletal muscle. These ligands have affinity constants for their receptor in T-tubule membranes ranging from 1–60 nM. (−)D888 is the best radiolabelled ligand from this class. It has an affinity for its receptor ($K_D = 1.2$ nM) which is 20–60 times higher than that of any other drug in this group. Binding capacities of pure T-tubule membranes for the four tritiated drugs used range between 50 and 80 pmol/mg membrane protein. The number of binding sites for dihydropyridine inhibitors, for verapamil-like drugs, for diltiazem, and for bepridil in T-tubule membranes seems to be identical.

Rates of association and dissociation have been determined and are summarized in Table II. They provide K_D which are in good agreement with binding constants derived from equilibrium binding studies with ^{3}H-ligands.

A low affinity binding site for verapamil [Galizzi et al., 1984a; Goll et al., 1984a] and for bepridil and diltiazem [Galizzi et al., 1984a] has been detected by studies of dissociation kinetics of the [^{3}H]verapamil-receptor complex in the presence of high concentrations of verapamil, D600, bepridil, and diltiazem. Affinities at these sites correspond to $K_{0.5}$ values with rank order of potency: bepridil ($K_{0.5} = 0.7$ μM > (+)verapamil ($K_{0.5} = 2.5$ μM) > (±)verapamil ($K_{0.5} = 4$ μM) > (−)verapamil ($K_{0.5} = 5$ μM) > d-cis-diltiazem ($K_{0.5} = 50$ μM) >> l-cis-diltiazem [Galizzi et al., 1984a].

Two reports [Goll et al., 1984a; Glossman et al., 1983a] have suggested that [^{3}H]verapamil and d-cis-[^{3}H]diltiazem binding to guinea pig muscle microsomes are temperature-dependent. Maximal binding seems to decrease with increasing temperature over the range 2–37°C, without any change of K_D value. Other results showed that [^{3}H]verapamil binding to rat muscle microsomes was temperature-independent between zero and 25°C [Reynolds et al., 1983].

Binding studies with guinea pig skeletal muscle membranes have shown that most (±)[^{3}H]verapamil and (−)[^{3}H]D888 binding sites are present in T-tubule membranes [Goll et al., 1984a,b]. Binding of (±)[^{3}H]verapamil to rabbit and guinea pig T-tubule or microsomal membranes is pH-dependent and reveals the presence of an essential ionizable group on the receptor with a $pK_a = 6.5–7.6$ [Galizzi et al., 1984a; Goll et al., 1984a]. (±) [^{3}H]Verapamil binding to rat muscle microsomal membranes has been shown to be destroyed by trypsin [Reynolds et al., 1983].

Effect of Unlabelled Ca^{2+} Channel Inhibitors on [^{3}H]1,4-Dihydropyridine Binding to Skeletal Muscle Membrane

Radioligands which have been used in these studies are [^{3}H]nitrendipine, [^{3}H]nimodipine, [^{3}H]PN 200-110, [^{3}H]azidopine, and [^{125}I]iodipine.

Effect of unlabelled 1,4-dihydropyridines. The results are consistent with competitive inhibition between labelled and unlabelled drugs. Complete displacement of specific binding is observed with Hill coefficients close to one. Generally, the experimental conditions used (very low concentrations of [³H]1,4-dihydropyridine) give half-maximum inhibition constants which represent the true K_D for the unlabelled 1,4-dihydropyridine-receptor complex. All determined K_D values are in the range of 0.2–4 nM, in good agreement with equilibrium binding data determined from saturation studies with ³H-ligands. Rank order of potencies are: PY108–068 ($K_D = 0.65$ nM) > nitrendipine = nisoldipine ($K_D = 1.4$ nM) > nifedipine = nimodipine ($K_D = 4$ nM) [Fosset et al., 1983; Gould et al., 1984]. K_D values have also been determined for the Ca_{2+} channel activators Bay K8644 ($K_D = 37$ nM) and CGP 28392 ($K_D = 1,250$–1,800 nM) [Gould et al., 1984; Ferry and Glossmann, 1984].

This type of approach has allowed a detailed study of the stereoselectivity of association of the dihydropyridine binding sites using enantiomers of PN 200-110, nicardipine, Bay e 6927, and nimodipine. Rank order of potencies are: (+)PN 205033 ($K_D = 0.3$–2 nM) > (−)PN 205034 ($K_D = 198$–343 nM) [Ferry and Glossmann, 1982; Ferry and Glossmann, 1984; Ferry et al., 1984], (+)nicardipine ($K_D = 7$ nM) > (−)nicardipine ($K_D = 42$ nM) [Ferry and Glossmann, 1984], (−)Bay e 6927 ($K_D = 3$ nM) > (+)Bay e 6927 ($K_D = 420$ nM) [Ferry and Glossmann, 1984], and (−)nimodipine($K_D = 3$ nM) > (+)nimodipine ($K_D = 17$ nM) [Striessnig et al., 1985].

Effect of verapamil, D600, bepridil, diltiazem, and drugs in the diphenylbutylpiperazine series. These unlabelled drugs are noncompetitive inhibitors of [³H]dihydropyridine binding to its own sites [Fosset et al., 1983; Gould et al., 1984]. Only partial inhibition of specific [³H]1,4-dihydropyridine binding is generally found for this class of drugs. Half-maximum inhibition constants, $K_{0.5}$, are in the range of 17–1,000 nM, with a rank order of potency: prenylamine ($K_{0.5} = 17$ nM) > lidoflazine ($K_{0.5} = 28$ nM) > flunarizine ($K_{0.5} = 60$ nM) > (±)verapamil ($K_{0.5} = 48$–200 nM) > tiapamil (K = 240–292 nM) > cinnarizine (K $_{0.5}$ = 330 nM) > (±)bepridil ($K_{0.5} = 1,000$ nM) >> 1-cis-diltiazem [Fosset et al., 1983; Gould et al., 1984; Ferry and Glossmann, 1982]. Diphenylbutylpiperazines have been reported to be 3 to 10-fold more potent for inhibition of [³H]nitrendipine binding to skeletal muscle membranes than to heart membranes, smooth muscle membranes, or brain membranes [Gould et al., 1984]. Results obtained using different enantiomers of verapamil and D600 are confusing. For inhibition of [³H]nimodipine binding, the rank order of potency was: (+)D600 ($K_{0.5} = 1$ μM) > (−)D600 ($K_{0.5}$ > 10 μM) [Ferry and Glossmann, 1982]. For inhibition of [¹²⁵I]iodipine binding, the rank order of potency was: (−)D600 ($K_{0.5} = 21$ nM) > (+)D600 ($K_{0.5} = 190$ nM) [Ferry and Glossmann, 1984], and (+)verapamil ($K_{0.5} = 54$ nM) > (−)verapamil ($K_{0.5} = 98$ nM) [Ferry and Glossmann, 1984]. For inhibition of [³H]azidopine binding, the rank order of potency was: (−)verapamil ($K_{0.5} = 44$ nM) > (+)verapamil ($K_{0.5} = 350$ nM) [Ferry et al., 1984].

Verapamil, D600, 1-cis-diltiazem, prenylamine and analogs, function as negative heterotropic allosteric effectors of the dihyropyridine binding site. They increase the rate of dissociation of the preformed [³H]1,4-dihydropyridine-receptor complex induced by an unlabelled 1,4-dihydropyridine [Gould et al., 1984; Ferry et al., 1984]. Diltiazem stimulates binding (B_{max}) of most [³H]1,4-dihydropyridine ligands (Table I). This effect is 1) stereospecific; d-cis-diltiazem is the active enantiomer, while 1-cis-diltiazem is a weak inhibitor [Glossmann et al., 1984]; 2) concentration-dependent; the half-maximum stimulation of binding is $K_{0.5} = 0.3$-1 μM which is relatively low in comparison to the affinity constant of 37–55 nM measured directly (Table II) [Gould et al., 1984; Ferry and Glossmann, 1984; Ferry and Glossmann, 1982; Ferry et al., 1983a]; 3) temperature-dependent; stimulation of binding increases (20 to

100%) with increasing temperature over the range 4-37°C [Glossmann et al., 1983a; Kirley and Schwartz, 1984]. Diltiazem functions as a positive heterotropic allosteric effector of dihydropyridine binding, decreasing the rate of dissociation of the preformed complex induced by the unlabelled 1,4-dihydropyridine.

Effect of Unlabelled Ca^{2+} Channel Inhibitors on ($\pm$)[^{3}H]Verapamil, ($-$)[^{3}H]D888, d-cis-[^{3}H]Diltiazem, and ($\pm$)[^{3}H]Bepridil Binding to Skeletal Muscle Membranes

Inhibition by verapamil and analogs, bepridil, and diltiazem. Competitive inhibition is observed between labelled and unlabelled drugs [Galizzi et al., 1984b, 1986a]. Complete inhibition of specific binding of ^{3}H-ligands was observed with Hill coefficients close to one. K_D values for ^{3}H-ligand-receptor complexes are in the range of 20–900 nM. Rank order of potencies are ($\pm$)D600 (K_D = 28–70 nM) > ($\pm$)verapamil (K_D = 25–37 nM) > ($\pm$)bepridil (K_D = 40–120 nM) > tiapamil (K_D = 197–406 nM) > ($\pm$)diltiazem (K_D = 200–964 nM) [Galizzi et al., 1984b; Reynolds et al., 1983; Goll et al., 1984a; Glossmann et al., 1983a]. For enantiomers, the rank order of potency is: (+)verapamil (K_D = 10–43 nM) > ($-$)verapamil (K_D = 40–77 nM) [Galizzi et al., 1984a; Goll et al., 1984a; Glossmann et al., 1983a]; ($-$)D600 (K_D = 12-20 nM) > (+)D600 (K_D = 42-67 nM) [Galizzi et al., 1984a; Glossmann et al., 1983a; Goll et al., 1984a,b]; ($-$)D888 (K_D = 1.5-3 nM) > (+)D888 (K_D = 3-17 nM) [Goll et al., 1984b; Galizzi et al., 1986a]; d-cis-diltiazem (K_D = 50-215 nM) > 1-cis-diltiazem (K_D = 1,000-14,000 nM) [Galizzi et al., 1984a; Glossmann et al., 1983a; Goll et al., 1984a,b; Galizzi et al., 1986a]; and (+)bepridil (K_D = 16 nM) > ($-$)bepridil (K_D = 20 nM [Galizzi et al., 1986a].

The observation that diltiazem, bepridil, and D888 are mutually competitive in their binding to receptor sites in T-tubule membranes differs from the conclusions of other authors who have proposed noncompetitive interaction between verapamil and diltiazem [Glossmann et al., 1984]. These conclusions were based on experiments with high diltiazem concentrations (1–10 μM), which cannot be related to the high-affinity sites reported herein.

Inhibition by unlabelled 1,4-dihydropyridines. These drugs are noncompetitive inhibitors for the binding of compounds including verapamil, diltiazem, and bepridil to T-tubule membranes [Galizzi et al., 1984b; Goll et al., 1984a,b]. Partial inhibition of the binding of ^{3}H-ligands was found. Half-maximal inhibition constants, $K_{0.5}$, are between 1.4 and 3.5 nM, with a rank order of potency: ($\pm$)nitrendipine ($K_{0.5}$ = 1.4 nM) > ($\pm$)nimodipine ($K_{0.5}$ = 1.6 nM) > ($\pm$)nifedipine ($K_{0.5}$ = 3.5 nM) > ($\pm$)nisoldipine ($K_{0.5}$ = 5 nM) [Galizzi et al., 1984b]. $K_{0.5}$ values for Ca^{2+} channel activators are $K_{0.5}$ = 30–67 nM for Bay K8644, and $K_{0.5}$ = 700 nM for CGP 28392 [Galizzi et al., 1984b; Goll et al., 1984a]. Stereospecific inhibition has been found with PN 200-110, Bay e 6927, and nicardipine: (+)PN 200-110 ($K_{0.5}$ = 2–3.9 nM) > ($-$)PN 200-110 ($K_{0.5}$ = 76-300 nM) [Goll et al., 1984a,b]; ($-$)Bay e 6927 ($K_{0.5}$ = 3.8 nM) > (+)Bay e 6927 ($K_{0.5}$ = 102 nM) [Goll et al., 1984a]; (+)nicardipine ($K_{0.5}$ = 12 nM) > ($-$)nicardipine ($K_{0.5}$ = 90 nM) [Goll et al., 1984a]. Depending on experimental conditions, unlabelled 1,4-dihydropyridines can either stimulate (30°C) or inhibit (2°C) d-cis-[^{3}H]diltiazem binding to skeletal muscle microsome membranes [Glossmann et al., 1983a].

An Emerging New Pharmacology for Skeletal Muscle Ca^{2+} Channels

[^{3}H]Fluspirilene, a neuroleptic molecule of the diphenylbutylpiperidine series, binds to skeletal muscle T-tubule membranes with a high affinity, corresponding to a dissociation constant K_D = 0.11 $\pm$ 0.04 nM. A 1:1 stoichiometry was found between [^{3}H]fluspirilene binding and the binding of ($-$)[^{3}H]desmethoxyverapamil, one of the most potent Ca^{2+} channel inhibitors. Ca^{2+} channel inhibitors such as desmethoxyverapamil, verapamil, gallopamil, bepridil, or diltiazem antagonize [^{3}H]flusprilene binding as well as [^{3}H]desmethoxyverapamil binding. Neuroleptics, especially those of the diphenylbutylpiperidine family, antagonize (−)[^{3}H]desmethoxyverapamil binding as well as [^{3}H]fluspirilene binding. There is an excellent correlation between affinities found from [^{3}H]fluspirilene and from (−)[^{3}H]desmethoxyverapamil binding experiments.

Analysis of the properties of these cross-inhibitions indicates that [^{3}H]fluspirilene binds to a site which is not exactly the same as for phenylalkylamine derivatives (gallopamil, verapamil, diltiazem, bepridil).

Voltage-clamp experiments have shown that fluspirilene is a very efficient inhibitor of the voltage-dependent Ca^{2+} channel, with a half-maximum effect near 0.1–0.2 nM and a nearly complete blocking effect at a concentration of 1 nM. Fluspirilene blockade has very little voltage dependence [Galizzi et al., 1986b].

Effects of Inorganic Cations on the Binding of [^{3}H]Dihydropyridines, (±)[^{3}H]Verapamil, (−)[^{3}H]D888, d-cis-[^{3}H]Diltiazem, and (±)[^{3}H]Bepridil to T-Tubule or Microsomal Membranes

Ca^{2+} is essential for defining the ionic selectivity of the voltage-dependent Ca^{2+} channel in skeletal muscle [Almers et al., 1985] as it is for cardiac muscle [Hess and Tsien, 1984]. When external Ca^{2+} is removed, the ionic channel becomes permeable to monovalent cations such as Na^+, K^+, Li^+, Rb^+, and Cs^+. Ca^{2+} and several other divalent cations reversibly block this inward current of monovalent cations so that, in the presence of Ca^{2+} in the external medium, the channel is permeable to Ca^{2+} (or to Ca^{2+} analogs such as Ba^{2+}) but not to monovalent cations.

Inhibition of [^{3}H]1,4-dihydropyridine binding to T-tubule or microsomal membranes. Tri- and divalent cations inhibit binding. Half-maximum inhibition constants, $K_{0.5}$, are observed for cationic concentrations of 0.1–5 mM, with the following rank order of potency: La^{3+} ($K_{0.5}$ = 0.1–0.2 mM) > Ni^{2+} ($K_{0.5}$ = 1.8 mM) > Co^{2+} ($K_{0.5}$ = 2.7 mM)

> Mn^{2+} ($K_{0.5}$ = 4.8 mM). Ca^{2+} is a very poor inhibitor of binding, with a $K_{0.5}$ = 65 mM, while monovalent cations such as Na^+ and K^+ up to 100 mM, are without effects on binding [Fosset et al., 1983; Ferry and Glossmann, 1982, 1984; Ferry et al., 1984]. Ni^{2+} has been reported to be a noncompetitive inhibitor for the binding of [^{3}H]nitrendipine to its site [Fosset et al., 1983]. Affinities found for Ni^{2+}, Co^{2+}, and Mn^{2+} to inhibit of dihydropyridine to their receptor sites are similar to the ones found in electrophysiologic experiments for the block of Ca^{2+} channel currents in frog skeletal muscle [Almers et al., 1985]. Also, the rank order of affinities of Ni^{2+}, Co^{2+}, and Mn^{2+} at this site found by electrophysiology is the same as the one found in [^{3}H]dihydropyridine binding experiments.

Inhibition of (±)[^{3}H]verapamil, (−)[^{3}H]D888, d-cis-[^{3}H]diltiazem, and (±)[^{3}H]bepridil binding to T-tubule membranes. Binding of (−)[^{3}H]D888, d-cis-[^{3}H]diltiazem, and (±)[^{3}H]bepridil to T-tubule membranes is inhibited by Ca^{2+} with half-maximum inhibition constants which are similar for the three labelled molecules, $K_{0.5}$ = 5 μM [Galizzi et al., 1985]. Ca^{2+} is a noncompetitive inhibitor for the binding of diltiazem, D888, and bepridil to their common receptor site. Ca^{2+} binds to its own coordination site which is distinct from the receptor site for organic Ca^{2+} channel inhibitors. The order of potency for different divalent cations at this Ca^{2+} coordination site is: Ca^{2+} ($K_{0.5}$ = 5 μM) > Sr^{2+} ($K_{0.5}$ = 25 μM) > Ba^{2+} ($K_{0.5}$ = 50 μM) > Mg^{2+} ($K_{0.5}$ = 170 μM). The affinity for Ca^{2+} found from the three ^{3}H-ligand binding experiments, $K_{0.5}$ = 5 μM, is similar to the one that has been found for the Ca^{2+}-calcium channel complex in electrophysiological experiments, K_D = 0.7–2 μM [Almers et al., 1985; Hess and Tsien, 1984; Fukushima and Hagiwara, 1985]. Also, the order of affinity of Ca^{2+}, Sr^{2+}, Ba^{2+}, and Mg^{2+} at this site found by electrophysiology is nearly the same as the one found in (−)[^{3}H]D888 binding experiments. All these data taken together suggest that the Ca^{2+} binding site which allosterically prevents binding of verapamil-like molecules,

TABLE III. Molecular Size of Receptors of the Ca^{2+} Channel Inhibitors by Radiation Inactivation

Ca^{2+} channel inhibitor	M_r	M_r with d-cis-diltiazem	M_r with l-cis-diltiazem	References
$(\pm)[^3H]$Nitrendipine	210,000	—	—	Norman et al., 1983
$(\pm)[^{125}I]$Iodipine	207,000	—	—	Ferry and Glossmann, 1984
$(\pm)[^3H]$Nimodipine	180,000	111,000	158,000	Ferry et al., 1983a; Goll et al., 1984a,b
$(+)[^3H]$PN 200–110	138,000	75,000	123,000	Goll et al., 1983
d-cis-$[^3H]$Diltiazem	130,000	—	—	Goll et al., 1984b
$(\pm)[^3H]$Verapamil	110,000	—	—	Goll et al., 1984a,b
$(-)[^3H]$D888	107,000	—	—	Goll et al., 1984b

bepridil and diltiazem, to their sites is the same Ca^{2+} coordination site that regulates ionic selectivity of the Ca^{2+} channel.

$(\pm)[^3H]$Verapamil binding to T-tubule membranes is also sensitive to monovalent cations. $K_{0.5}$ values of inhibition are in the rank order of potency: $K^+ = Cs^+$ ($K_{0.5} = 30$ mM) $> Li^+$ ($K_{0.5} = 50$ mM) $> Na^+$ ($K_{0.5} = 80$ mM) [Galizzi et al., 1984a].

Determination of the Molecular Size of the Voltage-Sensitive Calcium Channel by Radiation Inactivation

With this technique, purified membrane samples are irradiated with high energy electrons; and the inactivation of the protein is assumed to be related to its size. The technique has given excellent results in the determination of the M_r of the voltage-sensitive Na^+ channel [Barhanin et al., 1983]. With all $[^3H]$-ligands of the Ca^{2+} channel used, simple exponential decay of the binding activity has been observed, indicative of a sole target size. The observed loss of binding activity is due to a loss of the number of functional binding sites, since irradiation has no significant effect on the value of equilibrium dissociation constants measured at different stages of inactivation. The molecular size was calculated using the empirical equation $M_r = 6.4 \times 10^5/D_{37}$ [Kepner and Macey, 1968], where D_{37} is the radiation dose which conserves 37% of the initial binding activity. Table III summarizes M_r obtained with the

different classes of calcium channel inhibitors. Two kinds of results have been obtained. Results obtained using 1,4-dihydropyridines such as nitrendipine, nimodipine, and iodipine gave M_r in the range of 180,000 to 210,000, which also correspond to values found for the dihydropyridine receptor in brain and heart [Norman et al., 1983; Glossmann et al., 1984]. Surprisingly, lower M_r of the dihydropyridine receptor, ranging from 75,000 to 158,000, have been obtained when preparations have been incubated before irradiation with the allosteric ligands/d-cis-diltiazem or l-cis-diltiazem.

Radiation inactivation experiments to determine the molecular size of receptors for $(\pm)$verapamil, $(-)$D888, and diltiazem gave M_r in the range of 107,000 to 130,000, which is 40 to 60% smaller in size than M_r found for the 1,4-dihydropyridine receptor.

The exact interpretation of these results is for the moment uncertain. It is probably safer at the present time to retain the highest M_r value as the best value, as for the (Na^+, K^+)ATPase [Ottolenghi and Ellory, 1983].

Identification by Photoaffinity Labelling Experiments of the Polypeptide Chains Bearing the Receptors for the Ca^{2+} Channel Inhibitors and Reconstitution of the Ca^{2+} Channel into Phospholipid Bilayers

1,4-Dihydropyridines, including azidopine, PN 200-110, and compounds such as d-cis-diltiazem and bepridil, are light-sensitive compounds. Because of this property they appeared to be potential photoaffinity ligands. This possibility has been borne out experimentally. After normal or high intensity irradiation, both classes of compounds are essentially and specifically incorporated into peptide bands of M_r 145,00–170,000 as shown in Table IV. Affinity labelling with an isothiocyanate dihydropyridine derivative gave covalent incorporation of radioactivity in a peptide band of $M_r = 36,000$. At present, affinity labelling experiments strongly suggest that receptors for dihydropyridines, diltiazem, and bepridil are located on the same polypeptide chain of M_r 170,000 ± 5,000.

T-tubule membranes reconstituted in bilayers have functional Ca^{2+} channels that can be identified after activation with Bay K8644 [Affolter and Coronado, 1985; Rosenberg et al., 1986]. Partially purified preparations of the Ca^{2+} channel protein have also been reconsituted successfully [Curtis and Catterall, 1986; Flockerzi et al., 1986]. Reconstitution of the Ca^{2+} channel activity has been followed by $^{45}Ca^{2+}$ flux studies [Curtis and Catterall, 1986] and by single channel recordings [Affolter and Coronado, 1985; Rosenberg et al., 1986; Flockerzi et al., 1986]. Electrophysiological recordings have shown that the partially purified preparations had all the properties of a normal Ca^{2+} channel. It could be activated by membrane potential variations and by the Ca^{2+} channel activator Bay K8644. It could be phosphorylated by cAMP-dependent processes [Flockerzi et al., 1986].

PURIFICATION AND SUBUNIT STRUCTURE OF THE PUTATIVE VOLTAGE-DEPENDENT Ca²⁺ CHANNEL IDENTIFIED AS THE DIHYDROPYRIDINE RECEPTOR

One of the difficulties in the purification of macromolecules that confer electrical excitability to biological membranes is that they are almost always present in very low amounts in the membranes. Purification of the Ca^{2+} channel from solubilized membrane is an important step toward the understanding of the

molecular aspects of the structure and mechanism of this channel. From the binding data with the different Ca^{2+} channel inhibitors in different tissues [Janis and Triggle, 1984], it is clear that the best source of receptors for Ca^{2+} channel inhibitors is the skeletal muscle T-tubule membranes [Fosset et al., 1983]. The solubilization of the native dihydropyridine receptor from guinea pig and rabbit and skeletal muscle microsomes or T-tubule membranes has been carried out successfully [Glossmann and Ferry, 1983; Borsotto et al., 1984a; Curtis and Catterall, 1984], and the pharmacological properties of the solubilized receptor have been studied using [³H]nimodipine [Glossmann and Ferry, 1983], [³H]nitrendipine [Borsotto et al., 1984a; Curtis and Catterall, 1984], and [³H]PN 200-110 [Borsotto et al., 1984b, 1985].

Among the various detergents assayed, digitonin [Glossmann and Ferry, 1983; Curtis and Catterall, 1984] and 3-[(3-cholamidopropyl)-dimethylammonio]-1-propanesulfonate (CHAPS) [Glossmann and Ferry, 1983; Borsotto et al., 1984a,b] have been reported to have the required qualities for solubilization of the dihydropyridine receptor. However, digitonin micelles give a very low recovery of the binding activity after solubilization [Glossmann and Ferry, 1983]. CHAPS has proved to be the most useful detergent in the solubilization procedure. This detergent provides a good yield of solubilization and a low, nonspecific component in binding studies with [³H]dihydropyridines [Borsotto et al., 1984a, b]. The most effective protein-to-detergent ratio was carefully investigated and found to be close to 0.28 (W/W). Adding glycerol (5 to 10%) and/or phospholipids (0.02%) during solubilization substantially increased the binding capacity of the extract [Borsotto et al., 1984a,b]. Glycerol and phospholipids also stabilized the dihydropyridine receptor in its active form, with a half-life of 34 hr at 4°C [Borsotto et al., 1984a].

Scatchard plots for specific binding of [³H]nimodipine, [³H]nitrendipine, and (+)-[³H]PN 200-110 to solubilized microsomes or

TABLE IV. Molecular Size of Ca^{2+} Channel Subunits in Photoaffinity Labelling Experiments

Ca^{2+} channel inhibitor	M_r	References
(+)[^{3}H]PN 200–110	170,000	Galizzi et al., 1986a
(±)[^{3}H]Azidopine	145,000	Ferry et al., 1984
d-cis-[^{3}H]Diltiazem	170,000	Galizzi et al., 1986a
(±)[^{3}H]Bepridil	170,000	Galizzi et al., 1986a
[^{3}H]Isothiocyanate dihydropyridine	36,000	Kirley and Schwartz, 1984

T-tubule membranes are linear, indicating the presence of a single class of noninteracting binding sites. The dissociation constants, K_D, are respectively 2.2 nM ([^{3}H]nimodipine), 7 nM ([^{3}H]nitrendipine); and 0.7 nM [(+)[^{3}H]PN 200-110]. These values are very close to the respective K_D values found for the membrane-bound receptor: 1.5 nM, 1.8 nM, and 0.2 nM [Glossmann and Ferry, 1983; Borsotto et al., 1984a,b]. Solubilized rabbit muscle T-tubule membranes have a maximal binding capacity, B_{max}, of 85 pmol/mg protein for (+)[^{3}H]PN 200-110, which is comparable to that of the starting native membranes (90 pmol/mg protein) [Borsotto et al., 1984b]. Different unlabelled calcium channel inhibitors have been tested for their ability to interfere with [^{3}H]1,4-dihydrodihydropyridine binding to the solubilized receptor [Glossmann and Ferry, 1983; Borsotto et al., 1984a]. These molecules not only include 1,4-dihydropyridines but also l- and d-cis-diltiazem, (+) and (−)verapamil, (+) and (−)D600, and (±)bepridil. The rank order of potencies to inhibit 50% of the specific binding ($K_{0.5}$) are: (+)PN 200-110 ($K_{0.5}$ = 0.7–9.8 nM) > nifedipine ($K_{0.5}$ = 7 nM) > nitrendipine ($K_{0.5}$ = 9 nM) > (−)PN 200-110 ($K_{0.5}$ = 1200 nM) for 1,4-dihydropyridines, and (+)D600 ($K_{0.5}$ = 480 nM) > (+)verapamil ($K_{0.5}$ = 500 nM) > (±)bepridil ($K_{0.5}$ = 4,000 nM) > (−)verapamil ($K_{0.5}$ = 50,000 nM) > l-cis-diltiazem ($K_{0.5}$ = 59,000 nM) > (−)D600 ($K_{0.5}$ = 65,000 nM). d-cis-Diltiazem has a potentiating effect in dihydropyridine binding with a $K_{0.5}$ = 500–3,600 nM, as for native membranes.

All these results taken together indicate that the ligand specificity and stereoselectivity of the solubilized receptor are very close to those known for the membrane-bound receptor. Solubilization not only preserves the dihydropyridine binding activity but also the binding activity for other Ca^{2+} channel inhibitors.

The dihydropyridine receptor has been purified from rabbit skeletal muscle microsomes and from purified T-tubule membranes. If the stoichiometry of binding is 1 mol [^{3}H]dihydropyridine per 1 mol receptor, the specific activity of a homogenous preparation can be calculated to be 5,000 pmol/mg protein, assuming a molecular weight of the dihydropyridine receptor of 200,000 (see Table III). One of the purifications was achieved using the following steps: solubilization with digitonin of T-tubule membranes followed by a combination of lectin affinity chromatography on wheat germ agglutinin (WGA), by ion exchange chromatography (DEAE), and by sucrose gradient centrifugation [Curtis and Catterall, 1984]. In this purification procedure, it was unfortunately not possible to measure the [^{3}H]nitrendipine binding activity after solubilization. Hence, purification was monitored only by following the bound [^{3}H]nitrendipine (dpm) which was added before solubilization. [^{3}H]dihydropyridine counts dissociate during purification, and the exact extent of the enrichment, as well as the quality of the purification, are difficult to assess. Gel electrophoresis of the purified material in reducing conditions gave a protein pattern suggesting a composition of the receptor involving at least three polypeptides of M_r

130,000, 50,000, and 33,000. Another purification scheme used a solubilization with CHAPS of pure T-tubule membranes. This solubilization was followed by a combination of gel filtration on a Ultrogel A_2 column and WGA chromatography. Glycerol, phospholipids, and protease inhibitors were added as stabilizing agents. The purified material contained three polypeptides with M_r of 142,000, 32,000, and 33,000. These three polypeptides components copurified with [^{3}H]PN 200-110 binding activity [Borsotto et al., 1984b]. More recently, starting from rabbit muscle microsomal membranes (10–15 pmol [^{3}H]PN 200-110 bound/mg protein of CHAPS-solubilized material), an improved purification has been described [Borsotto et al., 1985], which used a combination of DEAE chromatography, WGA affinity column, and gel filtration on sephacryl S400 chromatography. (+)[^{3}H]PN 200-110 was used not only as a marker associated with the solubilized receptor, but also in direct binding experiments performed after each purification step. A specific activity of more than 800 pmol/mg protein was obtained. This specific activity is far from the theoretical maximal activity not because of a contamination of the purified material but because of the coexistence of active and inactivated receptors at the end of the purification procedure. The same purification procedure was applied to solubilized microsomal preparations of chick and frog skeletal muscle and has demonstrated the presence of a large polypeptide component of M_r 130,000 to 141,000 associated with the dihydropyridine receptor of these two other muscle sources. The doublet of small molecular weight at 32–33,000 was not found in the frog muscle preparation.

In order to explain some of the discrepancies between M_r values found from some affinity labelling experiments presented in Table IV and the M_r found after purification, we proposed that the Ca^{2+} channel protein is extremely sensitive to proteolysis and that the peptide of 140,000, which is the major peptide in extensively purified preparations, is a proteolytic product of the M_r 170,000 peptide

identified in T-tubule or microsomal membranes by photoaffinity labelling with [^{3}H]PN 200-110, [^{3}H]diltiazem, and [^{3}H]bepridil (Table IV). Proteolytic digestion has been one of the difficulties in establishing the exact M_r of the voltage-sensitive Na^+ channel of skeletal muscle [Casadei et al., 1984].

ANTI-CALCIUM CHANNEL ANTIBODIES
Polyclonal Antibodies

Since purification studies of the 1,4-dihydropyridine receptor associated with the calcium channel of rabbit skeletal muscle have shown that it is composed of a large glycoprotein of M_r 140,000–145,000 associated with a smaller component of M_r 32,000–34,000, specific antisera have been prepared against the large component (anti-140 serum) and the smaller one (anti-32 serum). The specificity of these two antisera has been analyzed by immunoblot assays with microsomal preparations of rabbit skeletal muscle. Under disulfide-reducing conditions, the anti-140 serum specifically labelled a polypeptide of M_r 140,000 while the anti-32 serum labeled three polypeptides of M_r 32,000, 29,000, and 26,000. Under nonreducing conditions, both the anti-140 and the anti-32 sera specifically recognized a single large polypeptide of M_r 170,000. The same type of approach showed that the dihydropyridine receptor in nerve tissue and in cardiac and smooth muscle has a polypeptide composition similar to that found in skeletal muscle, with a large polypeptide of M_r 170,000–176,000 made of two different chains of about 140,000 and 34,000-32,000 associated by disulfide bridges [Schmid et al., 1986a,b].

Monoclonal Antibodies

Monoclonal hybridoma cell lines secreting antibodies against the (+)PN 200-110 and the (−)desmethoxyverapamil binding components of the voltage-dependent calcium channel from rabbit T-tubule membranes have been isolated. The specificity of these monoclonal antibodies was established by their ability to co-immunoprecipitate (+)[^{3}H]PN 200-110 and (−)[^{3}H]desmethoxyverapamil receptors. Monoclonal antibodies cross-reacted with rat, mouse, chicken, and frog skeletal muscle Ca^{2+} channels, but not with crayfish muscle Ca^{2+} channels. Cross-reactivity was also detected with membranes prepared from rabbit heart, brain, and intestinal smooth muscle.

These antibodies were used in immunoprecipitation experiments with ^{125}I-labeled detergent (CHAPS and digitonin)-solubilized membranes. They revealed a unique immunoprecipitating component of molecular weight 170,000 in nonreducing conditions. After disulfide bridge reduction, the CHAPS-solubilized (+)PN 200-110-(−)desmethoxyverapamil binding component gave rise to a large peptide of M_r 140,000 and to smaller polypeptides of M_r 30,000 and 26,000, whereas the digitonin-solubilized receptor appeared with subunits at M_r 170,000, 140,000, 30,000, and 26,000 [Vandaele et al., 1987].

All these results taken together are interpreted as showing that both the 1,4-dihydropyridine and the phenylalkylamine receptors are part of a unique polypeptide chain of M_r 170,000.

DEVELOPMENT

Appearance of voltage-sensitive Ca^{2+} channels during in vitro (chick) and in vivo (chick and rat) myogenesis of skeletal muscle cells has been followed using both [^{3}H]nitrendipine binding and ^{45}Ca^{2+} flux measurements [Kazazoglou et al., 1983; Schmid et al., 1984a].*

In Vitro Development of Chick Skeletal Muscle Cells

Embryonic skeletal muscle differentiates spontaneously in cell culture from mononucleated myogenic cells (myoblasts) to multinucleated cross-striated muscle fibers (myotubes), displaying electrical and contractile activity [Yaffe, 1969]. The nitrendipine receptor is absent in the earliest, undifferentiated myoblasts. [^{3}H]Nitrendipine binding sites appear after 20 hr of culture. The number of [^{3}H]nitrendipine binding sites then increases rapidly to reach a plateau value of 150 fmol/mg of protein in 55-hr-old myotubes.

The time-course of appearance of [^{3}H]nitrendipine binding sites closely follows the onset of fusion. The K_D value for the nitrendipine receptor complex remains at 0.4±0.1 nM during all stages of the cell culture. This value is similar to that measured from inhibition of dihydropyridine-sensitive ^{45}Ca^{2+} flux with myotubes in culture. The nitrendipine-sensitive component of Ca^{2+} flux is undetectable in 20-hr-old myoblasts in culture, whereas it is present in 72-hr-old myotubes differentiated in culture [Schmid et al., 1984a]. Inhibition of fusion of myoblasts into myotubes by adding EGTA or the protein synthesis inhibitor cycloheximide prevents the appearance of [^{3}H]nitrendipine binding sites. These data indicate that the appearance of the nitrendipine receptor during myogenesis is strictly linked to the fusion process which is known to generate the formation of T-tubules [Ezerman and Ishikawa, 1967].

In Vivo Development of Chick and Rat Skeletal Muscle Cells

The in vivo appearance of the chick nitrendipine-sensitive Ca^{2+} channel shows the existence of two different phases [Schmid et al., 1984a]. A first phase starts near day 10 of in ovo development. The level of Ca^{2+} channels then remains stable between day 11 and day 17 in ovo. At this stage, the maximum level of nitrendipine receptors (124 ± 10 fmol/mg of protein) and the K_D value (0.4 nM) are very similar to the level attained in the course of the in vitro development. This first phase of development corresponds to the in vivo fusion of myoblasts into myotubes. The second phase of development starts a little before hatching, and the change in number of [^{3}H]nitrendipine receptors is particularly fast between hatching and 7 days postnatal, when another plateau phase is reached corresponding to 900 fmol/mg of protein. This change in number of nitrendipine receptors is accompanied by a change in the equilibrium disso-

---

*Ca^{2+} uptake is insensitive to nitrendipine when chick myotubes in culture are polarized. Depolarization reveals a new component of ^{45}Ca^{2+} influx which is inhibited by nitrendipine.

ciation constant of the nitrendipine receptor complex. K_D values increase by factors of 4 to 10 when passing from the first phase to the second phase of development. The appearance of [³H]nitrendipine binding sites during postnatal development of rat skeletal muscle has also been studied [Kazazoglou et al., 1983]. As for chick muscle, there is a continuous increase in the number of [³H]nitrendipine binding sites after birth. However, a plateau level is reached after about 6 days for chick muscle, while it is reached after about 20 days for rat muscle. These differences in time-course of development are probably related to the fact that very soon after birth the chick must feed, drink, and walk, whereas the rat is born helpless and develops mature behavioral patterns only after 2–3 weeks of postnatal life.

Surgical denervation was carried out in order to know whether innervation is responsible for the second phase of development of nitrendipine-sensitive Ca^{2+} channels. Denervation has biphasic effect on nitrendipine receptors of rat and chick muscle [Schmid et al., 1984a,b]. During the first phase of denervation there is a 2-fold increase in the number of nitrendipine receptors after 15 days, then the number of [³H]nitrendipine binding sites declines. These changes in number of sites occur without any change in affinity of nitrendipine for its receptor. Denervation produces different effects on voltage-dependent Na^+ channels. It decreases the level of Na^+ channels with a high tetrodotoxin affinity [Schmid et al., 1984a,b] and renders Na^+ channels resistant to tetrodotoxin in mammalian muscle [Redfern and Thesleff, 1971]. The initial increase in the number of [³H]nitrendipine receptors following denervation may be due to an overproduction of T-tubule membranes [Pellegrino and Franzini, 1963], where Ca^{2+} channels seem to be localized.

The β-adrenergic system seems to play an important role in the regulation of the level of the dihydropyridine receptor sites during chick skeletal muscle development after hatching. In vivo treatments of 7-day-old chicks with reserpine, which inhibits norepi-

nephrine and epinephrine synthesis, or with alprenolol, which is a potent β-adrenergic antagonist, produce a decrease in the number of skeletal muscle nitrendipine receptors. This decrease in receptor number is accompanied by a 4–5-fold decrease in the affinity of nitrendipine for its receptor. These effects on the nitrendipine receptor were prevented by simultaneous injection of isoproterenol. Therefore, skeletal muscle nitrendipine receptors in reserpine and alprenolol-treated animals are more similar to "fetal" nitrendipine receptors than to the postnatal nitrendipine receptors. These results are clearly in favor of the conclusion that the physiological stimulation of β-adrenergic receptors regulates both the number of specific nitrendipine receptors and the affinity of the receptor for dihydropyridine [Schmid et al., 1985]. Furthermore, long-term treatment of myotubes in culture with isoproterenol and other compounds that increase intracellular cAMP leads to a large increase in the number of nitrendipine receptors. Alprenolol inhibited the long-term effects of isoproterenol. This increase in the level of dihydropyridine receptors due to long-term effects of isoproterenol via cAMP was also accompanied by a 4–10-fold decrease in the affinity of the receptors for nitrendipine.

Recent work [Hosey et al., 1986] has shown that the major subunit of the Ca^{2+} channel (M_r 160,000–170,000) is phosphorylated both by cAMP and Ca^{2+}-calmodulin-dependent phosphatase. Other results have shown that a polypeptide of M_r 50,000 could also be phosphorylated by a cAMP-dependent protein kinase [Curtis and Catterall, 1985], but it seems that this 50,000 M_r polypeptide is a degradation product of the M_r 160–170,000 component [Hosey et al., 1986].

PHYSIOPATHOLOGY

Is There a Relationship Between Muscular Dysgenesis and a Deficiency of Voltage-Dependent Ca^{2+} Channels

Muscular dysgenesis (*mdg*) is a spontaneous, recessive, lethal mutation expressed in the mouse embryo as a total lack of muscle contractile activity (excitation-contraction un-coupling) [Gluecksohn-Waelsch, 1963]. In the mutant called *mdg/mdg*, the first abnormality concerns the internal structure of the myofi-ber: It is disorganized, and the T-tubule sys-tem is immature. An ultrastructural study of the embryonic diaphragm shows dilation of the sarcoplasmic reticulum (SR) and frag-mented and disorganized myofibrils as early as days 13–14 of gestation [Pinçon-Raymond et al., 1985]. Peripheral couplings of SR and plasma membrane occur to a similar extent in control +/*mdg* or mutant *mdg/mdg* develop-ing myotubes. However, structural coupling of sarcolemma and SR [diads, triads, and spaced densities (feet)] is not observed or is extremely immature in *mdg/mdg* myotubes. In contrast, these structures show consider-able development in control myotubes. This structural defect is accompanied by a large decrease in the number of specific binding sites for [^{3}H]PN 200-110 in mutant striated skeletal muscle such as diaphragm, limb, or tongue. Compared to control muscle, the mu-tant muscles contain 3–10 fold fewer recep-tors, depending on the type of calculation made (fmol/mg protein, fmol/embryo, or fmol/wet weight) and on the type of muscle considered [Pinçon-Raymond et al., 1985]. Interestingly, the functioning of the heart in these animals is normal, and mutant and con-trol hearts have the same amount of [^{3}H]PN 200-110 binding sites. Electrophysiological measurements using the patch-clamp tech-nique [Beam et al., 1986; Romey et al., 1986] have confirmed the quasi absence of slow Ca^{2+} channels in *mdg/mdg* mutants.

These observations suggest that: 1) the lack of a well-differentiated physical coupling be-tween sarcolemma and SR in *mdg/mdg* mus-cle is responsible for the fact that membrane depolarization is not efficiently transduced to the SR, and 2) the lack of voltage-dependent Ca^{2+} channels is tightly related to the molec-ular alteration of the excitation-contraction coupling system in mutant mice.

Is There an Abnormality of Ca^{2+} Channels in Duchenne Muscular Dystrophy?

Duchenne muscular dystrophy (DMD) is a well-defined clinical entity with X-linked in-heritance [Roses, 1984]. An increase in intra-cellular Ca^{2+} content has been observed as an early and significant abnormality of the disease [Bodensteiner and Engel, 1978]. Im-paired Ca^{2+} regulation has been thought to be responsible for the hallmarks of this dis-ease: progressive weakness and degeneration of muscle with concomitant biochemical and histological evidence for external membrane abnormalities. The use of inhibitors of volt-age-sensitive Ca^{2+} channels in DMD treat-ment is now widespread. This comes from observations that heart muscle fibers undergo severe functional and structural alterations, finally resulting in necrotization when an ex-cess of Ca^{2+} penetrates the myocardial cell through the sarcolemma membrane. This nec-rotization may be totally prevented by admin-istration of Ca^{2+} channel inhibitors. It is for these reasons that verapamil and nifedipine have been tried as treatments for DMD [Emery et al., 1982; Brooke et al., 1984].

The interaction of [^{3}H]nitrendipine with its specific receptor has been shown to be similar in skeletal muscle from both normal young boys and boys with DMD, suggesting that the number of nitrendipine-sensitive Ca^{2+} chan-nels is not significantly altered in Duchenne patients [Desnuelle et al., 1986]. A possibility exists that although the number of dihydro-pyridine receptors is the same in normal hu-man and in DMD patients, the functioning of the Ca^{2+} channel is altered in the dysgenic muscle (e.g., different kinetics of activation and inhibition, or different voltage-depen-ence).

CONCLUSIONS

Skeletal muscle Ca^{2+} channels have recep-tors for all Ca^{2+} channel inhibitors and Ca^{2+} channel activators that are active on cardiac and smooth muscle. Their electrophysiologi-cal properties are not identical to those found in heart muscle; both the voltage dependence and the kinetics are different. However, the cationic selectivity is the same in heart and skeletal muscle as well as the mechanism by which this selectivity is controlled by Ca^{2+} itself [Almers et al., 1985; Hess and Tsien, 1984].

For all these reasons, and because skeletal muscle is by far the richest source of receptors for Ca^{2+} channel effectors, it turns out that T-tubule Ca^{2+} channels can be considered at present as the best system with which to carry out biochemical studies.

Future directions of research will of course focus on 1) application of monoclonal and polyclonal antibodies for immunocytolocalization studies, 2) isolation of cDNA(s) for the Ca^{2+} channel subunits in order to obtain the protein sequence of this channel, and 3) ways to study synthesis, expression, or repression of Ca^{2+} channels in development and physiopathological studies. Antibodies and cDNAs will provide an easier access to molecular properties of Ca^{2+} channels from nerve, cardiac, and smooth muscle.

ACKNOWLEDGMENTS

We wish to thank Dr. Busch (CERM, Riom and the CEA, France) for a gift of ($\pm$)[^{3}H]bepridil. (+) and (−)Bepridil are also gifts from Dr. Busch. (−)[^{3}H]D888 and (+) and (−)D888 were generously supplied by Knoll AG, FRG (Dr. Hollmann and Dr. Traut). d- and l-cis-Diltiazem were gifts from Synthelabo, Paris. 1,4-Dihydropyridines were a gift from Bayer AG, FRG.

Thanks are due to M. Hosey for reading the manuscript, to M. Tomkowiak and C. Roulinat-Bettelheim for expert technical assistance. This work was supported by the Association des Myopathes de France, the Centre National de la Recherche Scientifique, the Fondation sur les Maladies Vasculaires and the Ministère de l'Industrie et de la Recherche (grant No. 83.C.0696).

REFERENCES

Affolter H, Coronado R (1985): Agonists Bay K8644 and CGP 28392 open calcium channels reconstituted from skeletal muscle transverse tubules. Biophys J 48:341–347.

Almers W, Fink R, Palade PT (1981): Calcium depletion in frog muscle tubules: The decline of calcium current under maintained depolarization. J Physiol 312:177-207.

Almers W, McCleskey EW (1984): Non-selective conductance in calcium channels of frog muscle: Calcium selectivity in a single-file pore. J Physiol 353:585–608.

Almers W, McCleskey EW, Palade PT (1985): Calcium channel in vertebrate skeletal muscle. In Rubin RP, Weiss GB, Putney Jr JW (eds): "Calcium in Biological Systems." Plenum Publishing Corporation, pp 321-330.

Baker PF, Knight DE (1984): Calcium control of exocytosis in bovine adrenal medullary cells. Trends Neurosci 7:120-126.

Barhanin J, Schmid A, Lombet A, Wheeler KP, Lazdunski M (1983): Molecular size of different neurotoxin receptors on the voltage-sensitive Na^+ channel. J Biol Chem 258:700-702.

Beam KG, Knudson CM, Powell J (1986): A lethal mutation in mice eliminates the slow calcium current in skeletal muscle cells. Nature 320:168–170.

Bean BP (1985): Two kinds of calcium channels in canine atrial cells. Differences in kinetics, selectivity and pharmacology. J Gen Physiol 86:1-30.

Bodensteiner JB, Engel AG (1978): Intracellular calcium accumulation in Duchenne dystrophy and other myopathies: A study of 567,000 muscle fibers in 114 biopsies. Neurology 28:439-446.

Borsotto M, Barhanin J, Fosset M, Lazdunski M (1985): The 1,4-dihydropyridine-receptor associated with the skeletal muscle voltage-dependent Ca^{2+} channel: Purification and subunit composition. J Biol Chem 260:14255-14263.

Borsotto M, Barhanin J, Norman RI, Lazdunski M (1984b): Purification of the dihydropyridine receptor of the voltage-dependent Ca^{2+} channel from skeletal muscle transverse tubule using (+)[^{3}H]PN 200-110. Biochem Biophys Res Commun 122:1357-1366.

Borsotto M, Norman RI, Fosset M, Lazdunski M (1984a): Solubilization of the nitrendipine receptor from skeletal muscle transverse tubule membranes. Interactions with specific inhibitors of the voltage-dependent Ca^{2+} channel. Eur J Biochem 142:449-455.

Bossu JL, Feltz A, Thomann JM (1985): Depolarization elicits two distinct calcum currents in vertebrate sensory neurons. Pflügers Arch 403:360-368.

Brooke MH, Fenichel GM, Griggs RC, Mendell JR, Miller JP, Moxley R (1984): A trial of nifedipine in Duchenne muscular dystrophy. Neurology 34(suppl 1):290.

Carbone E, Lux HD (1984): A low voltage-activated, fully inactivating Ca channel in vertebrate sensory neurons. Nature 310:501-502.

Casadei JM, Gordon RD, Lampson LA, Schotland DL, Barchi RL (1984): Monoclonal antibodies against the voltage-sensitive Na$^+$ channel from mammalian skeletal muscle. Proc Natl Acad Sci USA 81:6227-6231.

Cauvin C, Loutzenhiser R, Van Breemen C (1983): Mechanism of calcium antagonist-induced vasodilatation. Ann Rev Pharmacol Toxicol 23:373-396.

Cognard C, Lazdunski M, Romey G (1986a): Different types of Ca^{2+} channels in mammalian skeletal muscle cells in culture. Proc Natl Acad Sci USA 83:517-521.

Cognard C, Romey G, Galizzi JP, Fosset M, Lazdunski M (1986b): Dihydropyridine-sensitive Ca^{2+} channels in mammalian muscle cells in culture: Electrophysiological properties and interactions with Ca^{2+} channel activator (Bay K8644) and inhibitor (PN 200-110). Proc Natl Acad Sci USA 83:1518-1522.

Curtis BM, Catterall WA (1984): Purification of the calcium antagonist receptor of the voltage-sensitive calcium channel from skeletal muscle transverse tubules. Biochemistry 23:2113-2118.

Curtis BM, Catterall WA (1985): Phosphorylation of the calcium antagonist receptor of the voltage-sensitive calcium channel by cAMP-dependent protein kinase. Proc Natl Acad Sci USA 82:2528-2532.

Curtis BM, Catterall WA (1986): Reconstitution of the voltage-sensitive calcium channel purified from skeletal muscle transverse tubule. Biochemistry 25:3077-3083.

Desnuelle C, Renaud JF, Delpont E, Serratrice G, Lazdunski M (1986): [^{3}H]Nitrendipine receptors as markers of a class of putative voltage-sensitive Ca^{2+} channels in normal human skeletal muscle and in muscle from Duchenne muscular dystrophy patients. Muscle and Nerve 9:148-151.

Eisenberg RS, McCarthy RT, Milton RL (1983): Paralysis of frog skeletal muscle fibres by the calcium antagonist D600. J Physiol 341:495-505.

Emery AEH, Skinner R, Howden LL, Matthews MB (1982): Verapamil in Duchenne muscular dystrophy. Lancet 26:559-563.

Ezerman BE, Ishikawa H (1967): Differentiation of the sarcoplasmic reticulum and T system in developing chick skeletal muscle in vitro. J Cell Biol 35:405-420.

Fairhurst AS, Thayer SA, Colker JE, Beatty DA (1983): A calcium antagonist drug binding site in skeletal muscle sarcoplasmic reticulum: Evidence for a calcium channel. Life Sci 32:1331-1339.

Ferry DR, Glossmann H (1982): Identification of putative calcium channels in skeletal muscle microsomes. FEBS Lett 148:331-337.

Ferry DR, Glossmann H (1984): [^{125}I]Iodipine, a new high affinity ligand for the putative calcium channel. Naunyn-Schmiedeberg's Arch Pharmacol 325:186-189

Ferry DR, Goll A, Glossmann H (1983a): Calcium channels: Evidence for oligomeric nature by target size analysis. EMBO J 2:1729-1732.

Ferry DR, Goll A, Glossmann H (1983b): Differential labelling of putative skeletal muscle calcium channels by [^{3}H]nifedipine, [^{3}H]nitrendipine, [^{3}H]nimodipine and [^{3}H]PN 200-110. Naunyn-Schmiedeberg's Arch Pharmacol 323:276-277.

Ferry DR, Rombusch M, Goll A, Glossmann H (1984): Photoaffinity labelling of Ca^{2+} channels with [^{3}H]azidopine. FEBS Lett 169:112-118.

Fleckenstein A (1977): Specific pharmacology of calcium in myocardium, cardiac pacemakers, and vascular smooth muscle. Ann Rev Pharmacol Toxicol 17:149-166.

Flockerzi V, Oeken HJ, Hofmann F, Pelzer D, Cavalié A, Trautwein W (1986): Purified dihydropyridine-binding site from skeletal muscle T-tubules is a functional calcium channel. Nature 323:66-68.

Fosset M, Jaimovich E, Delpont E, Lazdunski M (1982): [^{3}H]Nitrendipine labelling of the Ca^{2+} channel in skeletal muscle. Eur J Pharmacol 86:141-142.

Fosset M, Jaimovich E, Delpont E, Lazdunski M (1983): [^{3}H]Nitrendipine receptors in skeletal muscle. Properties and preferential localization in transverse tubules. J Biol Chem 258:6086-6092.

Friedman ME, Suarez-Kurtz G, Kaczorowski GJ, Katz GM, Reuben JP (1986): Two calcium currents in a smooth muscle cell line. Am J Physiol 250:H699-H703.

Fukuda J, Henkart MP, Fischbach GD, Smith TG (1976): Physiological and structural properties of colchicine-treated chick skeletal muscle cells grown in tissue culture. Dev Biol 49:395-411.

Fukushima Y, Hagiwara S (1985): Currents carried by monovalent cations through calcium channels in mouse neoplastic β lymphocytes. J Physiol 358:255-284.

Galizzi JP, Borsotto M, Barhanin J, Fosset M, Lazdunski M (1986a): Characterization and photoaffinity labelling of receptor sites for the Ca^{2+} channel inhibitors d-cis-diltiazem, ($\pm$)bepridil, ($-$)desmethoxyverapamil and ($+$)PN 200-110 in skeletal muscle transverse tubule membranes. J Biol Chem 261:1393-1397.

Galizzi JP, Fosset M, Lazdunski M (1984a): Properties of receptors for the Ca^{2+} channel blocker verapamil in transverse-tubule membranes of skeletal muscle. Stereospecificity, effect of Ca^{2+} and other inorganic cations, evidence for two categories of sites and effect of nucleoside triphosphates. Eur J Biochem 144:211-215.

Galizzi JP, Fosset M, Lazdunski M (1984b): [^{3}H]Verapamil binding sites in skeletal muscle transverse tubule membranes. Biochem Biophys Res Commun 118:239-245.

Galizzi JP, Fosset M, Lazdunski M (1985): Characterization of the Ca^{2+} coordination site regulating binding of Ca^{2+} channel inhibitors d-cis-diltiazem, ($\pm$)bepridil and ($-$)desmethoxyverapamil to their receptor site in skeletal muscle transverse tubule membranes. Biochem Biophys Res Commun 132:49-55.

Galizzi JP, Fosset M, Romey G, Laduron P, Lazdunski M (1986b): Neuroleptics of the diphenylbutylpiperidine series are potent calcium channel inhibitors. Proc Natl Acad Sci USA 83:7513-7517.

Glossmann H, Ferry DR (1983): Solubilization and partial purification of putative calcium channels labelled with [^{3}H]nimodipine. Naunyn-Schmiederberg's Arch Pharmacol 323:279-291.

Glossmann H, Ferry DR, Boschek CB (1983b): Purification of a putative calcium channel from skeletal muscle with the aid of [^{3}H]nimodipine binding. Naunyn-Schmiedeberg's Arch Pharmacol 323:1-11.

Glossmann H, Ferry DR, Goll A, Rombusch M (1984): Molecular pharmacology of the calcium channel: Evidence for subtypes, mutliple drug-receptor sites, channel subunits, and the development of a radioiodinated 1,4-dihydropyridine calcium channel label, [^{125}I]iodipine. J Cardiovasc Pharmacol 6:S608-S621.

Glossmann H, Linn T, Rombusch M, Ferry DR (1983a): Temperature-dependent regulation of d-cis-[^{3}H]diltiazem binding to Ca^{2+} channels by 1,4-dihydropyridine channel agonists and antagonists. FEBS Lett 160:226-232.

Glueksohn-Waelsch S (1963): Lethal genes and analysis of the differentiation. Science 142:1269-1276.

Goll A, Ferry DR, Glossmann H (1983): Target size analysis of skeletal muscle Ca^{2+} channels. Positive allosteric heterotropic regulation by d-cis-diltiazem is associated with apparent channel oligomer dissociation. FEBS Lett 157:63-69.

Goll A, Ferry DR, Glossmann H (1984a): Target size analysis and molecular properties of Ca^{2+} channels labelled with [^{3}H]verapamil. Eur J Biochem 141:177-186.

Goll A, Ferry DR, Striessnig J, Schober M, Glossmann H (1984b): ($-$)[^{3}H]Desmethoxyverapamil, a novel Ca^{2+} channel probe. Binding characteristics and target size analysis of its receptor in skeletal muscle. FEBS Lett 176:371-377.

Gonzalez-Serratos H, Valle-Aguilera R, Lathrop DA, del Carmen Garcia M (1982): Slow inward calcium currents have no obvious role in muscle excitation-contraction coupling. Nature 298:292-294.

Gould DJ, Murphy KMM, Snyder SH (1983): Studies on voltage-operated calcium channels using radioligands. Cold Spring Harbor Symp Quantitative Biol 48:355-362.

Gould RJ, Murphy KMM, Snyder SH (1984): Tissue heterogeneity of calcium channel antagonist binding sites labelled by [^{3}H]nitrendipine. Mol Pharmacol 25:235-241.

Hess P, Tsien RW (1984): Mechanism of ion permeation through calcium channels. Nature 309:453-456.

Hosey MM, Borsotto M, Lazdunski M (1986): Phosphorylation and dephosphorylation of dihydropyridine-sensitive voltage-dependent Ca^{2+} channel in skeletal muscle membranes by cAMP- and Ca^{2+}-dependent processes. Proc Natl Acad Sci USA 83:3733-3737.

Huerta M, Stefani E (1986): Calcium action potentials and calcium currents in tonic muscle fibers of the frog (Rana pipiens). J Physiol (Lond) 372:293-301.

Ildefonse M, Jacquemond V, Rougier O, Renaud JF, Fosset M, Lazdunski M (1985): Excitation-contraction coupling in skeletal muscle: Evidence for a role of slow Ca^{2+} channels using Ca^{2+} channel activators and inhibitors in the dihydropyridine series. Biochem Biophys Res Commun 129:904-909.

Janis RA, Triggle DJ (1984): 1,4-Dihydropyridine Ca^{2+} channel antagonists and activators: A comparison of binding characteristics with pharmacology. Drug Dev Res 4:257-274.

Kaumann AJ, Uchitel OD (1976): Reversible inhibition of potassium contractures by optical isomers of verapamil and D600 on slow muscle fibers of the frog. Naunyn-Schmiedeberg's Arch Pharmacol 292:21-27.

Kazazoglou T, Schmid A, Renaud JF, Lazdunski M (1983): Ontogenic appearance of Ca^{2+} channels characterized as binding sites for nitrendipine during development of nervous, skeletal and cardiac muscle systems in the rat. FEBS Lett 164:75-79.

Kepner GR, Macey RI (1968): Membrane enzyme systems molecular size determinations by radiation inactivation. Biochim Biophys Acta 163:188-203.

Kerr LM, Sperelakis N (1982): Effects of the calcium antagonists bepridil (CERM-1978) and verapamil on Ca^{2+}-dependent slow action potentials in frog skeletal muscle. J Pharmacol Exp Ther 222:80-86.

Kirley TL, Schwartz A (1984): Solubilization and affinity labelling of a dihydropyridine binding site from skeletal muscle: Effects of temperature and diltiazem on [^{3}H]dihydropyridine binding to transverse tubules. Biochem Biophys Res Commun 123:41-49.

Lakshminarayanaiah N (1981): Calcium channels in the Barnacle muscle membrane. In Weiss GB (ed): "New Perspectives on Calcium Antagonists." Bethesda: American Physiological Society, pp 19-34.

Lüttgau HCH, Spiecker W (1979): The effects of calcium deprivation upon mechanical and electrophysiological parameters in skeletal muscle fibers of the frog. J Physiol 296:411-429.

Nayler WG, Horowitz JD (1983): Calcium antagonists: A new class of drugs. Pharmacol Ther 20:203-262.

Nilius B, Hess P, Lansman JB, Tsien RW (1985): A novel type of cardiac calcium channel in ventricular cells. Nature 316:443-446.

Norman RI, Borsotto M, Fosset M, Lazdunski M, Ellory JC (1983): Determination of the molecular size of the nitrendipine-sensitive Ca^{2+} channel by radiation-inactivation. Biochem Biophys Res Commun 111:878-883.

Nowycky MC, Fox AP, Tsien RW (1985): Three types of neuronal calcium channel with different calcium agonist sensitivity. Nature 316:440-443.

Ottolenghi P, Ellory JC (1983): Radiation inactivation of (Na,K)-ATPase, an enzyme showing multiple radiation-sensitive domains. J Biol Chem 258:14895-14907.

Pellgrino C, Franzini C (1963): An electron microscope study of denervation atrophy in red and white skeletal muscle fibers. J Cell Biol 17:327-332.

Pinçon-Raymond M, Rieger F, Fosset M, Lazdunski M (1985): Abnormal transverse tubule system and abnormal amount of receptors for Ca^{2+} channel inhibitors of the dihydropyridine family in skeletal muscle from mice with embryonic muscular dysgenesis. Dev Biol 112:458-466.

Potreau D, Raymond G (1980a): Slow inward barium current and contraction on frog single muscle fibres. J Physiol 303:91-109.

Potreau D, Raymond G (1980b): Calcium-dependent electrical activity and contraction of voltage-clamped frog single muscle fibres. J Physiol 307:9-22.

Redfern P, Thesleff S (1971): Action potential generation in denervated rat skeletal muscle. II. The action of tetrodotoxin. Acta Physiol Scand 82:70-78.

Reuter H (1979): Properties of two inward membrane currents in the heart. Ann Rev Physiol 41:413-424.

Reynolds IJ, Gould RJ, Snyder SH (1983): [^{3}H]Verapamil binding sites in brain and skeletal muscle: Regulation by calcium. Eur J Pharmacol 95:319-321.

Romey G, Rieger F, Renaud JF, Pinçon-Raymond M, Lazdunski M (1986): The electrophysiological expression of Ca^{2+} channels and of apamin-sensitive Ca^{2+}-activated K$^+$ channels is abolished in skeletal muscle cells from mice with muscular dysgenesis. Biochem Biophys Res Commun 136:935-940.

Rosenberg RL, Hess P, Reeves JP, Smilowitz H, Tsien RW (1986): Calcium channels in planar lipid bilayers: Insights into mechanisms of ion permeating and gating. Science 231:1564-1566.

Roses AD (1984): Molecular genetics of myotonic and Duchenne muscular dystrophies. Trends Neurosci 7:190-193.

Sanchez JA, Stefani E (1978): Inward calcium current in twitch muscle fibres of the frog. J Physiol 283:197-209.

Schmid A, Barhanin J, Coppola T, Borsotto M, Lazdunski M (1986a): Immunochemical analysis of subunit structures of 1,4-dihydropyridine receptors associated with voltage-dependent Ca^{2+} channels in skeletal, cardiac and smooth muscles. Biochemistry 25:3492-3495.

Schmid A, Barhanin J, Mourre C, Coppola T, Borsotto M, Lazdunski M (1986b): Antibodies reveal the cytolocalization and subunit structure of the 1,4-dihydropyridine component of the neuronal Ca^{2+} channel. Biochem Biophys Res Commun 139:996-1002.

Schmid A, Kazazoglou T, Renaud JF, Lazdunski M (1984b): Comparative changes of levels of nitrendipine Ca^{2+} channels, of tetrodoxin-sensitive Na$^+$ channels and of ouabain-sensitive (Na$^+$,K$^+$)ATPase following denervation of rat and chick skeletal muscle. FEBS Lett 172:114-118.

Schmid A, Renaud JF, Fosset M, Méaux JP, Lazdunski M (1984a): The nitrendipine-sensitive Ca^{2+} channel in chick muscle cells and its appearance during myogenesis in vitro and in vivo. J Biol Chem 259:11366-11372.

Schmid A, Renaud JF, Lazdunski M (1985): Short-term and long-term effects of β-adrenergic effectors and cyclic AMP on nitrendipine-sensitive voltage-dependent Ca^{2+} channel of skeletal muscle. J Biol Chem 260:13041-13046.

Schwartz LM, McCleskey EW, Almers W (1985): Dihydropyridine receptors in muscle are voltage-dependent but most are non-functional calcium channels. Nature 314:747-751.

Spedding M (1985): Calcium antagonist subgroups. Trends Pharmacol Sci 6:109-114.

Stefani E, Chiarandini DJ (1982): Ionic channels in skeletal muscle. Ann Rev Physiol 44:357-372.

Striessnig J, Zernig G, Glossmann H (1985): Ca^{2+} antagonist receptor sites on human red blood cell membranes. Eur J Pharmacol 108:329-330.

Vandaele S, Fosset M, Galizzi JP, Lazdunski M (1987): Monoclonal antibodies that co-immunoprecipitate the 1,4-dihydropyridine and phenylalkylamine receptors and reveal the Ca^{2+} channel structure. Biochem 26 (in press).

Walsh KB, Bryant SH, Schwartz A (1984): Diltiazem potentiates mechanical activity in mammalian skeletal muscle. Biochem Biophys Res Commun 122:1091-1096.

Yaffe D (1969): Cellular aspects of muscle differentiation. Current Topics Dev Biol 4:37-77.

Structure and Physiology of the Slow Inward Calcium Channel, pages 161–246
© 1987 Alan R. Liss, Inc.

9

Calcium Channels in Neurones

Richard J. Miller

*Department of Pharmacological and Physiological Sciences,
University of Chicago, Chicago, Illinois 60637*

INTRODUCTION

The importance of Ca^{2+} ions as biological second messengers has been implied for many years. However, although the role of Ca^{2+} in certain events has been well defined, the fundamental cellular processes underlying the overall regulation of Ca^{2+} concentrations are only now becoming clear. This is true due to important breakthroughs in two areas. We now know that the normal resting concentrations of free Ca^{2+} in the cell are very low. In order to trigger many cellular events, these concentrations must rise considerably. This can occur in two general ways. It is clear that Ca^{2+} can be "mobilized" from intracellular bound stores associated with the endoplasmic reticulum. Regulation of this process can be achieved by several means including activation of cell surface receptors. A key development in our understanding of this process has been the production of novel methods for the convenient quantitation of free cytoplasmic Ca^{2+} concentrations using quin-2 [Tsien et al., 1982], fura-2 [Grynkiewicz et al., 1985], and related fluorescent probes. Another has been the identification of inositoltriphosphate (IP_3) as a second messenger link between the cell surface and bound intracellular Ca^{2+} pools [Berridge and Irvine, 1984]. These areas, which are outside the scope of this article, are currently the focus of enormous scientific endeavour.

A second mechanism for rapidly regulating the internal Ca^{2+} concentration is by increasing the Ca^{2+} permeability of the cell membrane. Normally this membrane is impermeable to Ca^{2+}. This fact, together with the operation of various pumps and exchange systems, serves to maintain a very large concentration gradient for Ca^{2+} across the cell membrane. This is normally about four or five orders of magnitude, much greater than that for Na^+, K^+, or Cl^-, for example. As in the case of other ions, specific channels exist through which Ca^{2+} can move into the cell at appropriate times [Reuter, 1983; Tsien, 1983; Hagiwara and Byerly, 1981]. Basically, two types of Ca^{2+} channel have been discussed in the literature. These have been designated "voltage-sensitive calcium channels" (VSCC) and "receptor-operated channels" (ROC) [Bolton, 1979]. Much experimental evidence directly demonstrating the existence of VSCC has been forthcoming, whereas ROCs have remained enigmatic. It is the voltage sensitive channel which is the subject of the present review. It should be noted that the distinction between VSCC and ROC may only be useful up to a point as there are now many potential examples of the regulation of VSCC by receptor mediated events.

It has now been known about 25 years that VSCC are found in neurones [Hagiwara, 1983; Hagiwara and Saito, 1959; Koketsu et al., 1959]. However, until recently they have remained purely biophysical concepts, their biochemical properties deduced by implication. This situation is now rapidly changing. Advances in pharmacology, biochemistry, and molecular biophysics are responsible for this turn of events. Thus, although it is clear that we know less about molecular aspects of VSCC than we do about sodium channels or nicotinic acetylcholine receptors, such knowledge will certainly be rapidly forthcoming. What are the particular issues that concern VSCC at this time? Some of these are as follows:

Heterogeneity

The situation with respect to VSCC appears complex [Miller, 1985]. Although it has been claimed that all VSCC are identical [Brown et al., 1982], this is clearly not the case. As will be discussed in detail below, at least three types of functional VSCC have been found in neurones. As we shall see, these are probably separate molecular entities. Indeed, if recent studies of K^+ channels can be taken as an example [Levitan, 1985; Latorre and Miller, 1983], further categories of VSCC may be anticipated. Clearly, therefore, the molecular characteristics of each type of VSCC are of interest, and as with any other protein, the relationship between structure and function must be analyzed.

Distribution

VSCC are found in a number of cell types. In some cells their functions seem quite straightforward. For example, an adrenal medullary cell does not do much except secrete bioactive amines and peptides. This is reflected by its relatively simple morphology. VSCC are found in the plasma membrane of adrenal medullary cells, and Ca^{2+} influx through them contributes to the hormone release process [Kidokoro and Ritchie, 1980; Brandt et al., 1976; Fenwick et al., 1982]. The functions of neurones are, however, altogether more complicated. Not only do they possess the secretory functions of an adrenal cell, but they must also integrate and communicate information. These facts are also reflected by their morphology which can

range from a simple soma and axon to something fantastically complex. The functions of different portions of the neurone may differ radically. Thus, although neurotransmitter release may occur from the axon terminal [Llinas and Walton, 1980], soma [Chow and Poo, 1985; Suetake et al., 1981] or dendrites [Mori et al., 1981] of a neurone, the requirements at each site may be quite different. There are indications that VSCC or at least some types of VSCC may be particularly prevalent in different regions of the neurone e.g., dendrites or terminals (vide infra) [Llinas, 1984; Llinas and Sugimori, 1980]. Clearly, this is an issue of great importance for neuronal function. Moreover, the microdistribution of VSCC or other membrane proteins is also an issue of great interest. There are indications that some VSCC may cluster into "hot spots" [Fox et al., 1985b; Pumplin et al., 1981]. The purposes and molecular basis of such an organization await study. In addition to all these considerations, it should also be realized that the distribution of VSCC in neurones appears to change during development (vide infra).

Function

What are the functions of the different VSCCs? Why does more than one type exist? In some cases, it has been observed that certain neurones can fire Ca^{2+} based action potentials ("spikes") under normal physiological conditions. Under such circumstances, it may be imagined that Ca^{2+} acts as a charge carrier in a similar fashion to Na^+. The action potential is the basic unit of neuronal communication. However, as we shall discuss in the majority of cases, neurones do not fire Ca^{2+} spikes under normal conditions, although VSCC are clearly present and can be revealed following various pharmacological manipulations. Influx of Ca^{2+} through such channels may still play a key role in the regulation of neuronal excitability. We know that several kinds of ion channels can be regulated by changes in the intracellular concentrations of Ca^{2+} as well as membrane potential. These include highly specific K^+ channels of various types [Latorre and Miller, 1983], nonspecific cation conducting channels [Yellen,

1982; Colquhoun et al., 1981], and at least one type of anion specific channel [Mayer, 1985; Owen et al., 1984]. Again, it is likely that further examples may be found. Following the entry of Ca^{2+} through VSCC, such channels may be activated. The often-observed phenomenon of an afterhyperpolarization (AHP) following a spike is the result of the activation by Ca^{2+} of a type of K$^+$ channel [Llinas and Walton, 1980; Thompson and Aldrich, 1980]. Activation of such channels subsequent to Ca^{2+} influx, therefore, alters the state of excitability of the neurone and is a major factor in determining spiking frequency. In some neurones, inactivation of VSCC by Ca^{2+} influx (vide infra) causes abrupt periodic cessations in spiking activity which results in a neurone firing action potentials in groups or "bursts" of various lengths [Adams, 1985; Adams and Levitan, 1985; Kramer and Zucker, 1985a,b]. This phenomenon, which has been investigated in detail in some cases [Llinas and Walton, 1980], is a mechanism by which neurones can encode information. Clearly, therefore, VSCC play a pivotal role in moulding the basic utterances of neuronal activity into the syntax of nerve communication.

Apart from the regulation of nerve excitability, there are numerous potential targets for Ca^{2+} entering the neurone. The role of Ca^{2+} as a trigger for neurotransmitter release is of course well known. In addition, Ca^{2+} dependent enzymes such as Ca^{2+} calmodulin-dependent kinases and protein kinase C have been implicated in many neuronal functions. Other possibilities include a role for Ca^{2+} in neuronal growth and development (vide infra). However, there are a host of possibilities.

Modulation

One of the most intriguing possibilities with respect to VSCC is that they can be biochemically modified, leading to alterations in their function. That this is so has been unequivocally demonstrated in cardiac tissue, for example [Reuter, 1983; Tsien, 1983; Siegelbaum and Tsien, 1983]. There are indications that similar mechanisms may occur

in neurones (vide infra). Indeed, the Ca^{2+} channel may itself be under the control of intracellular Ca^{2+} providing a convenient negative feedback system [Eckert and Chad, 1984]. Other possible illustrations of nerve VSCC modulation may be gleaned from phenomena such as VSCC "rundown" and the effects of neurotransmitters and second messengers. In addition to such biochemical modifications, VSCC may also be the locus of action of some importance classes of drugs. Of particular interest are the actions of the so-called organic calcium channel blockers of the dihydropyridine, phenylalkylamine, and benzothiazepine classes. The effects of such agents in the cardiovascular system have been well documented, but what of the nervous system?

In the present article, I shall discuss observations relating to our knowledge of these various aspects of VSCC structure and function. I shall consider VSCC in both vertebrate and invertebrate neurones. In addition, I shall also consider VSCC in adrenal medullary cells and the related clonal cell line PC12 [Greene and Tischler, 1982]. These interesting cells are often considered as "honorary" neurones, and indeed, they can be transformed into neurones by nerve growth factor under appropriate conditions.

MEASUREMENT AND DETECTION OF NEURONAL CALCIUM CHANNELS

VSCC in neurones can be analyzed in several different ways. These various methods all yield valuable information of different complementary types. Each method has its own advantages and drawbacks. It is not always obvious how the properties of a channel measured by one method relate to those obtained by another method. Clearly, one of the most important tasks that faces investigators at present is to attempt to sort out and correlate these various findings to produce a single all-encompassing picture. What are the basic ways in which the presence of VSCCs can be determined and their properties examined? I shall now briefly introduce these. Details of the experiments will be given in subsequent sections.

Electrophysiology

The most traditional manner for observing the presence of VSCC electrophysiologically is to observe a Ca^{2+} spike. In some cases, neurones will fire Ca^{2+} spikes or mixed Ca^{2+}/Na^+ spikes in normal physiological media. This appears to be particularly true for invertebrate neurones or vertebrate neurones early in development (vide infra). In the case of a mixed Ca^{2+}/Na^+ spike, the slower Ca^{2+} component is usually observed as a "shoulder" or "plateau" region. However, it should be noted that in some cases tetrodotoxin (TTX) insensitive, Na^+ conductances can also contribute to such aspects of spike morphology [Bossu and Feltz, 1984; Fukuda and Kameyama, 1980]. Because of the uneven distribution of VSCC in neurones, the presence of a Ca^{2+} spike may depend on the portion of the neurone under investigation. Thus, in the case of many (perhaps most) vertebrate neurones, Ca^{2+} spikes may be observed in the dendrites even though recording from the cell soma only reveals a Na^+ spike [Llinas, 1984; Llinas and Sugimori, 1979]. Another important consideration is the time of development of a particular neurone. As we shall discuss, there is considerable evidence for major changes in the contribution of Ca^{2+} to the normal action potential at different times of development.

In the vast majority of cases, however, Ca^{2+} spikes only become evident under abnormal ("nonphysiological") conditions. In such cases, opportunities for observing a Ca^{2+} spike can be increased by a variety of pharmacological manipulations. These manipulations have two major goals. One is to increase the size of the Ca^{2+} component itself. The second is to decrease the size of ionic currents which normally mask the Ca^{2+} component. Various combinations of these methods are often utilized. Some possibilities are as follows.

Na^+ currents. One possible manipulation involves the elimination of the Na^+ spike that may normally mask the presence of a Ca^{2+} component. The way this is normally done is by addition of tetrodotoxin (TTX) or saxitoxin (STX), which effectively blocks Na^+ channels in most neurones [Cahalan, 1980; Catterall, 1984]. However, this method is not infallible. It is now quite clear that neurones may possess Na^+ conductances that are essentially completely resistance to TTX. For example, in vertebrate sensory neurones the action potential often consists of a Ca^{2+} component and both a TTX-sensitive and insensitive Na^+ component [Bossu and Feltz, 1984; Fukuda and Kameyama, 1980]. Thus, the only way to be certain of suppressing all Na^+ conductances is to remove all external Na^+ and replace it with a nonpermeant cation.

K^+ currents. In order to obtain robust Ca^{2+} spikes, suppression of the K^+ conductances involved in spike repolarization and other phenomena is usually necessary. This may be achieved in a variety of ways. It should be noted that several types of K^+ channel exist, and the pharmacology of these channels may differ considerably. One type of K^+ channel, responsible for the Ca^{2+}-activated K^+ current, $I_{K(Ca)}$, is regulated by both membrane potential and cytoplasmic Ca^{2+} [Latorre and Miller, 1983]. The ability of incoming Ca^{2+} to activate this conductance helps to provide a negative feedback loop leading to the eventual turnoff of Ca^{2+} conductances in some cases.

The classical pharmacological manipulation used to suppress K^+ conductances is the addition of tetraethylammonium chloride (TEA) or a related quaternary amine. TEA is often but not invariably effective when added extracellularly [Latorre and Miller, 1983]. Consequently, intracellular administration is also often used. Other substances used to suppress K^+ currents (I_K) include 4-aminopyridine (4-AP) and related molecules and Ba^{2+}. Interestingly, both these substances (particularly Ba^{2+}) are able to increase Ca^{2+} currents (I_{Ca}) directly in addition to their ability to suppress I_Ks [Hagiwara and Byerly, 1981; Rogawski and Barker, 1983; Agoston et al., 1983; Riker et al., 1985]. Various toxins (e.g., apamin [Pennefather et al., 1985], charybdotoxin [Miller et al., 1985], dendrotoxin [Dolly et al., 1984]) are also available for the suppression of particular subclasses of I_Ks.

A further powerful method for eliminating I_Ks is to exchange all the intracellular K$^+$ for Cs$^+$ [Kostyuk, 1984]. This method is based on the fact that Cs$^+$ does not readily carry current through K$^+$ channels. Exchange of Cs$^+$ for K$^+$ can be achieved by permeabilizing neurones with nystatin, by dialysis, or by intracellular injection.

Intracellular introduction of EGTA has the effect of buffering the intracellular Ca^{2+} concentration and consequently removing the activation of $I_{K(Ca)}$ [Llinas and Walton, 1980]. Intracellular EGTA will also have the additional effect of removing I_{Ca} "inactivation" in many instances (vide infra) [Eckert and Chad, 1984].

Ca^{2+} currents. I_{Ca}s may themselves be directly enhanced in a variety of ways. The most direct way is to increase the external Ca^{2+} concentration. However, in virtually every case, Ba^{2+} (or Sr^{2+}) carry current through VSCC rather better than Ca^{2+} itself [see Bossu et al., 1985; Friedman et al., 1986 for data on the T channel]. The substitution of Ba^{2+} for Ca^{2+} can often boost I_{Ca}s sufficiently for Ca^{2+} spikes to be observed. Certain caveats should be noted with respect to these manipulations, however. In certain cases it can be shown that Ca^{2+} can carry sufficient current through Na$^+$ channels to produce an action potential [Watanabe et al., 1967a,b]. However, such events are rarely encountered and can be distinguished from true Ca^{2+} spikes as they can be blocked by TTX. The use of Ba^{2+} has certain advantages in addition to its ability to pass through VSCC easily. Once inside the cell, Ba^{2+}, unlike Ca^{2+}, does not activate $I_{K(Ca)}$ [Latorre and Miller, 1983]. Moreover, in many cases, I_{Ca}s have been shown to be self limiting due to a process mediated by increases in the cytoplasmic Ca^{2+} concentration (vide infra) [Eckert and Chad, 1984]. This process may involve the Ca^{2+} mediated biochemical modification of VSCC (possibly through a phosphorylation-dephosphorylation cycle) and is probably the basis of so-called "current-dependent" inactivation of Ca^{2+} conductances. (This term is used to distinguish it from "voltage-dependent" inactivation, as is classically observed with Na$^+$ currents. In such cases, channel inactivation is purely dependent on membrane potential and not on the movement of ions through the channel.) Ba^{2+} does not produce these effects on VSCC. Intracellular injection of EGTA will also buffer the intracellular Ca^{2+} concentration and block current-dependent inactivation as well as $I_{K(Ca)}$ activation as discussed above.

It is also possible to directly enhance some I_{Ca}s by using a variety of drugs. The reported effects of 4-AP have been mentioned, but more impressive are the effects of certain novel dihydropyridines (DHPs). These newly discovered VSCC "agonists" probably only act on a certain subtype of VSCC as will be discussed below. They seem to greatly increase the time that such VSCC remain open. This is a relatively new and unexplored area of great interest. A final possibility is the indirect modulation of neuronal Ca^{2+} currents by neurotransmitters or hormones. This type of modulation would be analogous to the β-adrenergic/cAMP-mediated enhancement of I_{Ca} in cardiac muscle. Indeed, a similar enhancement of I_{Ca} in the hippocampus by β-agonists has been recently reported [Gray and Johnston, 1985a,b].

Clearly, therefore, there are a number of ways in which neurones can be persuaded to exhibit Ca^{2+} spikes. Using various combinations of the above mentioned manipulations, Ca^{2+} spikes have now been observed in a very large number of neuronal types (Table I). The properties of such spikes can suggest a great deal about the properties of the underlying Ca^{2+} conductances. For example, characteristics such as spike threshold, refractoriness and drug sensitivity have often been interpreted (quite correctly!) as evidence for a multiplicity of VSCC types in different regions of the neurone [Llinas, 1984]. Although such insights are valuable and often correct, a much more direct method for the analysis of VSCC is to examine I_{Ca}s in isolation using voltage clamping or related techniques. However, although this is desirable, it is often difficult to achieve given the complex morphology of many neurones and the small size of the re-

TABLE I. Some Observations on Ca^{2+} Conductances in Vertebrate Neurones

Peripheral neurones
  Sensory neurones
    Chick DRG cells
      Bixby and Spitzer, 1983a
      Boll and Lux, 1985
      Brown et al., 1982
      Canfield and Dunlap, 1984
      Carbone and Lux, 1984a,b, 1985
      Deisz and Lux, 1985
      Dichter and Fischbach, 1977
      Dunlap, 1981, 1985
      Dunlap and Fischbach, 1978, 1981
      Forscher and Oxford, 1985a,b
      Fox et al., 1985a,b
      Hanada, 1977
      Hablitz et al., 1985
      Matsuda et al., 1978
      Nowycky et al., 1985a,b
      Rane and Dunlap, 1985a,b
    Rat DRG cells
      Carbone and Lux, 1984a
      Desarmenien et al., 1984
      Dolphin et al., 1985
      Fedulova et al., 1981, 1985
      Godfraind et al., 1981
      Kostyuk et al., 1981a,b,c
      McBurney and Neering, 1985
      Neering and McBurney, 1984
      Nerbonne and Gurney, 1985
      Schlichter et al., 1984
    Guinea pig DRG
      Fukuda and Kameyama, 1979, 1980
    Pigeon DRG
      Gorke and Pierall, 1980
    Mouse DRG
      Heyer and MacDonald, 1982
      Litzinger et al., 1985
      MacDonald et al., 1985a,b
      MacDonald and Werz, 1985
      Matsuda et al., 1976, 1978
      Pun and Litzinger, 1984
      Ransom and Holz, 1977
      Scott and Edwards, 1980
      Werz and MacDonald, 1984a,b,
      1985a,b,c
      Yoshida et al., 1978
      Yoshida and Matsuda, 1959, 1979, 1980
    Frog DRG cells
      Baccaglini, 1978
      Ishizuka et al., 1984
      Koketsu et al., 1963
    Petrose and nodose ganglia
      Baccaglini and Cooper, 1982
      Bossu and Felz, 1984
      Bossu et al., 1985
      Gallego, 1983
      Ito, 1982
      Ito et al., 1984
    Cat DRG
      Gallego and Eyzaguirre, 1978
    Lamprey sensory neurones
      Leonard and Wickelgren, 1984

Sympathetic and parasympathetic neurones
  Rat (usually SCG)
    Belluzzi et al., 1985
    Briggs et al., 1985a,b
    Brown and McAfee, 1982
    Freschi, 1983, 1984
    Galvan and Adams, 1982
    Henon and McAfee, 1983
    Horn and McAfee, 1980
    McAfee and Yarowsky, 1979
    Nerbonne and Gurney, 1985
    O'Lague et al., 1978
  Bullfrog
    Akasu and Koketsu, 1981
    Akasu et al., 1983a,b
    Koketsu and Akasu, 1982
    Koketsu and Nishi, 1968
    Koketsu and Nishi, 1969
    Minota and Koketsu, 1977
  Rabbit
    Greengard and Straub, 1959
    Hashiguchi, 1979
    Mo et al., 1985
  Chick (ciliary)
    Nerbonne and Gurney, 1985
Enteric neurones
  Guinea pig myenteric plexus
    Cherubini and North, 1984, 1985
    Hirst and Spence, 1973
    Hirst et al., 1985
    Nishi and North, 1973a,b
    North, 1973
    Slack, 1985
  Rat myenteric plexus
    Willard and Nishi, 1985
  Avian neural crest
    Bader et al., 1983
  Guinea pig submucous plexus
    Surprenant, 1984
Central neurones
  Spinal cord neurones
    Mouse
      Hedlund et al., 1985
      Heyer et al., 1981
      Ransom and Holz, 1977
      Ransom et al., 1977
    Rat
      Fulton and Walton, 1981
      Harada and Takahashi, 1983
      Murase and Randic, 1983
    Frog
      Alvarez-Leefmans and Miledi, 1980
      Baccaglini and Spitzer, 1977
      Barrett and Barrett, 1976
      Bixby and Spitzer, 1983a, 1984a,b
      Spitzer and Baccaglini, 1976
      Spitzer and Lamborghini, 1976
      Willard, 1980
    Cat
      Crill and Schwindt, 1983
      Krnjevic et al., 1978, 1979
      Schwindt and Crill, 1980a,b,c, 1982

—Continued

Hippocampus
  Pyramidal cells
    Benardo et al., 1982
    Brown and Griffiths, 1983a,b
    Brown et al., 1985, 1986
    Dingledine, 1983
    Gahwiler and Brown, 1985
    Hablitz and Johnston, 1981
    Halliwell, 1983
    Halliwell and Scholfield, 1984a,b
    Hotson and Prince, 1981
    Johnston et al., 1980
    Landfield and Pilter, 1984
    Masukawa and Prince, 1984
    Newberry and Nicoll, 1984
    Peacock and Walker, 1983
    Proctor and Dunwiddie, 1983
    Sah et al., 1985
    Schwartzkroin and Prince, 1978
    Schwartzkroin and Slawsky, 1977
    Segal and Barker, 1985
    Thompson et al., 1985
    Wong et al., 1979
    Wong and Prince, 1978, 1979, 1981
  Granule cells
    Gray and Johnston, 1985a,b
Other CNS neurones
  Inferior olive
    Llinas and Yarom, 1981a,b
  Red nucleus
    Kubota et al., 1985
  Locus coeruleus
    Williams and North, 1985
    Williams et al., 1984, 1985
  Substantia nigra
    Llinas et al et al., 1984
  Lateral geniculate
    Crunelli et al., 1985
    Deschenes et al., 1982
    Jahnsen and Llinas, 1984a,b
    Llinas, 1984
    Llinas and Jahnsen, 1982
  Cerebellum (Purkinje)
    Crepel et al., 1984
    Llinas and Hess, 1976
    Llinas and Sugimori, 1979, 1980a,b
    Mori-Okamoto et al., 1983
  Hypothalamus
    Bourque and Renaud, 1985
    Legendre et al., 1982
    Lemos et al., 1985
    Leng and Mason, 1984
    Obaid et al., 1985
    Salzberg et al., 1983, 1985
    Stuenkel et al., 1985
    Theodosis et al., 1983
  Cortex and olfactory bulb
    Connors et al., 1982

Dichter et al., 1983
Halliwell and Scholfield, 1984a,b
Jahr and Nicoll, 1980
Kuan et al., 1985
Mori et al., 1981, 1982
Nerbonne et al., 1985
Receptors
  Bader et al., 1982
  Clusin and Bennett, 1977
  Corey et al., 1984
  Fain et al., 1980
  Hudspeth and Corey, 1977
  Ito and Komatsu, 1979
  Ito et al., 1980, 1981, 1982a,b
  Kaneko and Tachibana, 1985
  Lewis and Hudspeth, 1983
  Zipser and Bennett, 1973
Neuroblastomas
  N1E-115
    Anglister et al., 1982
    Fishman and Spector, 1981
    Grinvald and Farber, 1981
    Moolenaar and Spector, 1978, 1979a,b
    Romey and Lazdunski, 1982
    Spector et al., 1973
    Tsunoo et al., 1985a,b
    Tuttle and Richelson, 1979
    Twombly and Narahashi, 1985
    Yoshii et al., 1984, 1985a,b
  NG108-15
    Atlas and Adler, 1981
    Bodewei et al., 1985
    Fishman and Spector, 1981
    Furuya and Furuya, 1983
    Furuya et al., 1983
    Herring et al., 1985
    Reiser et al., 1977
  Other
    Atlas and Adler, 1981
    Fox et al., 1984
    Kostyuk et al., 1978
    Platika et al., 1985
    Spector et al., 1973
    Vycklicky et al., 1985
Adrenal and PC12 cells
  Adrenal
    Biales et al., 1976
    Brandt et al., 1976
    Clapham and Neher, 1984
    Fenwick et al., 1982
    Hoshi et al., 1984
    Kidokoro and Ritchie, 1980
  PC12
    Brown et al., 1982, 1984a
    Kunze et al., 1985
    Ogura and Takahashi, 1984
    O'Lague and Huttner, 1980
    O'Lague et al, 1985
    Scholfield and Weight, 1984

gions of the neurone that may be of particular interest (e.g., the nerve terminal). Having said this, however, it is also true that recent advances in cell culture and molecular biophysical techniques have provided enormous advances in this area. Thus, using current patch clamp and related methodologies, it is possible not only to record I_{Ca}s from a variety of cells previously excluded from this type of analysis by size considerations but also to directly analyze currents flowing through single channels. Thus, the functioning of an individual channel can be observed on a moment-to-moment basis. In addition to these advances in molecular biophysics, there have been advances in cell culture and other in vitro methods for preserving functional neurones. It is now possible to gain convenient access to a large variety of neurones as they can be cultured or preserved in a brain slice. In other cases, small cells [O'Lague and Huttner, 1980] or even synaptosomes [Umbach et al., 1984] can be fused chemically to give giant structures suitable for recording purposes. These in vitro methods, combined with patch electrodes in one of their many configurations, have allowed virtually complete experimental control of the environment on both sides of the plasma membrane in many cases. In a further extension of these methods it is also possible to examine the functioning channel in a totally artificial environment. In such cases, membrane fragments containing the channel of interest or the purified channel itself can be inserted into an artificial lipid membrane. This may be a bilayer (black lipid membrane) [Affolter and Coronado, 1985; Ewald et al., 1985; Nelson et al., 1984], or alternatively, a liposome or bilayer situated at the end of a patch pipette [Tank et al., 1982, for CI—channels]. Following the incorporation of the channel, its properties may be monitored electrophysiologically or, in the case of liposomes, by using

$^{45}Ca^{2+}$ fluxes as well [Curtis and Catterall, 1985b]. Such combinations of molecular biophysics and biochemistry represent the current state of the art. Experiments of this type with VSCC from various sources including neurones have already been carried out (vide infra). It will be clear that the number of conditions under which VSCC function can be analyzed is now enormous. The various modifications in conditions used by different investigators may make a considerable difference to the actual results obtained. Sometimes this may lead to apparent discrepancies appearing in the literature. However, such discrepancies are really not surprising under the circumstances and are often more apparent than real.

In order to optimize the recording of I_{Ca}s under voltage clamp, similar considerations apply to those mentioned above when considering Ca^{2+} spikes. Contaminating currents can be removed and other manipulations can also be used to increase the visibility and viability of the I_{Ca}. Indeed, when observing single VSCCs using the patch clamp method, it is often necessary to utilize very high external Ba^{2+} concentrations in order to make the measurements feasible. Various criteria (discussed elsewhere in detail) are generally accepted for assessing whether an observed current is truly a Ca^{2+} current [Hagiwara and Byerly, 1981]. These include the ability of Ba^{2+} and Sr^{2+} to substitute for Ca^{2+}, blockade of the current by agents such as Cd^{2+} or La^{4+}, and insensitivity to TTX. However, many of these criteria were evolved before it was generally realized that VSCC were not a single entity. Indeed, some VSCC are clearly not blocked very well by Cd^{2+}, for example (vide infra). Thus, just how valuable these classical criteria will ultimately prove to be remains to be determined. However at present, they represent a useful starting point.

A particular phenomenon characteristic of at least some VSCCs is so-called VSCC "run-down". This phenomenon is usually evident when highly sophisticated voltage clamp configurations are used that involve the removal of the normal cytoplasmic contents of the cell. Under such circumstances I_{Ca}s are often found to steadily decrease with time until they are no longer apparent. Although this phenomenon is technically a nuisance, it is actually potentially very enlightening. It suggests (as does the phenomenon of current-dependent inactivation discussed above) that VSCCs are, indeed, modifiable by cytoplasmic factors. Moreover, it gives the experimenter the opportunity to identify such factors by adding back substances that may reverse "run-down" (vide infra). In summary, voltage clamp studies have certainly provided most of the best evidence thus far for VSCC heterogeneity and modifiability.

A final way of identifying the presence of VSCC electrophysiologically is somewhat round about, but is often used. As discussed above, most cells possess a K^+ conductance that is regulated by membrane potential and cytoplasmic Ca^{2+} (in fact, there is probably a whole family of such entities). Activation of this K^+ conductance tends to hyperpolarize the cell. If an I_{Ca} is activated during a spike, the influx of Ca^{2+} will often lead to an increase in the cytoplasmic Ca^{2+} concentration that is large enough to activate $I_{K(Ca)}$. This may result in an AHP. Thus, if an AHP can be blocked by a blocker of I_{Ca}s (e.g., Cd^{2+} or La^{3+} or a drug), then it is often postulated that it resulted from an influx of Ca^{2+} through VSCC. [Meech and Standen, 1975; Klein et al., 1980; Krnjevic et al., 1978, 1979]. In effect, activation of the $I_{K(Ca)}$ is used as a microbioassay for increases in cytoplasmic Ca^{2+} concentrations. (Activation of other Ca^{2+} sensitive conductances may potentially

also be used for this purpose.) It should be pointed out, however, that when cytoplasmic Ca^{2+} concentrations rise, the source of such Ca^{2+} is not necessarily extracellular. Thus, it is abundantly clear that many agonists [Berridge and Irvine, 1984] or even changes in membrane potential [Kendall and Nahorski, 1985; Veraga et al., 1985], can raise internal Ca^{2+} by mobilizing it from intracellular bound stores subsequent to PI breakdown and IP$_3$ synthesis. Thus, activation of $I_{K(Ca)}$ can only be considered indicative of the presence of VSCC if it can be blocked by manipulations that would also block VSCC.

When considering indirect methods for assessing VSCC in neurones, a further classical method should be noted. One extremely important function of VSCC in neurones is to provide Ca^{2+} for triggering the release of neurotransmitter. Thus, under appropriate conditions, measurement of the evoked release of neurotransmitter can reveal a great deal about the properties of VSCC in nerve terminals, and possibly in other portions of neurones as well. Thus, if a drug is found to block or increase evoked transmitter release, it may well do so by interacting with VSCC, although there are clearly alternative possibilities. At any rate, measurement of evoked transmitter release at the squid giant synapse, frog neuromuscular junction, or in other circumstances has provided much information concerning VSCC and also other important aspects of the transmitter release process [Katz and Miledi, 1971; Llinas and Walton, 1980]. It is anticipated that this method will continue to be of great use.

Optical Techniques

The presence of VSCC has also been indicated by using certain optical techniques.

These approaches are of two main types. In one kind of paradigm, dyes are used that are sensitive to membrane potential. In the second type of paradigm, substances which emit an optical signal subsequent to binding Ca^{2+} are introduced into cells.

Certain dyes of the cyanine and merocyanine type emit rapid optical signals in response to changes in membrane potential. Under appropriate conditions, these optical changes can reflect changes in membrane potential such as those occurring during the passage of an action potential. In most circumstances, it is only possible to actually record action potentials from the cell soma. Except for some invertebrate neurones [Lemos et al., 1985; Llinas et al., 1976a; Stuenkel et al., 1985], the nerve terminal is not amenable to direct recording techniques. However, a direct knowledge of the properties of action potentials in all portions of the neurone is certainly desirable. Voltage-sensitive dyes (e.g., the merocyanine dye NK2761) can therefore be sued in lieu of direct electrical recording techniques. Optical methods have been used, for example, to measure spikes in the terminals of isolated frog neurohypophyseal neurones [Obaid et al., 1985; Salzberg et al., 1983, 1985]. This action potential can be dissected into its various ionic components, as can a directly electrically measured spike. Indeed, a Ca^{2+} component is evident in the example mentioned.

A second type of paradigm utilizes substances that emit optical signals (fluorescent or phosphorescent) when they combine with Ca^{2+}. If such substances are introduced into neurones, then they are in a position to detect Ca^{2+} flowing into the cytoplasm following VSCC activation. To date, the most widely used substance has been the jellyfish-derived protein, aequorin, which emits a phosphorescent signal when it binds Ca^{2+}. Aequorin has been used successfully to monitor Ca^{2+} influx into squid axons (via both Na^+ and Ca^{2+} channels) [Baker et al., 1973; Llinas et al., 1972] and also into single dorsal root ganglion neurones (DRG) in culture [McBurney and Neering, 1985; Neering and McBurney, 1984]. Other dyes used to monitor Ca^{2+} influx mostly emit fluorescent signals when they combine with Ca^{2+}. Several studies with invertebrate neurones have utilized the dye arsenazo III to monitor the influx of Ca^{2+} into the cell soma [Ahmed and Connor, 1979; Gorman and Thomas, 1980; Gorman et al., 1982, 1984]. These sophisticated studies combine optical measurements with voltage clamping of the cell soma I_{Ca}, and even simultaneous measurement of soma Ca^{2+} concentrations using Ca^{2+}-sensitive microelectrodes. In this way, information can be obtained relating soma Ca^{2+} currents to changes in cytoplasmic Ca^{2+} concentrations at different positions within the cell body. Dyes such as arsenazo III are appropriate for neurones such as invertebrate giant cells where microinjection of the dye is a relatively simple affair. However, with many small cells, this is not easy to do. However, the recent introduction of the Ca^{2+}-sensing fluorescent dyes, quin-2 and fura-2, has substantially removed these problems [Grynkiewicz et al., 1985; Tsien et al., 1982]. These substances are analogues of EGTA which can freely permeate the cell membrane. Following their entry into the cytoplasm, they are enzymatically modified to produce polar molecules which are now trapped within the cell. These molecules can bind Ca^{2+} and emit a fluorescent signal. Thus, microinjection is unnecessary. It is certainly true to say that the introduction to quin-2 has completely revolutionized the measurement of free Ca^{2+} concentrations in many cell types. Thus, many hypotheses concerning the mobilization of intracellular Ca^{2+} are now being directly tested for the first time. Quin-2 has perhaps had less impact in neurobiology than in other fields, as neurobiologists had already become expert at microinjecting substances into cells due to their familiarity with microelectrode techniques. Nevertheless, quin-2 has been used to monitor Ca^{2+} influx into single cultured neuronal cells, and its further use in this field may be anticipated [Perney et al., 1984]. Indeed, very recently, several new reports have been published illustrating the use of quin-2 and fura-2 for measuring Ca^{2+} influx into cultured neurones [Connor, 1985; Hockberger and Connor, 1985; Koenig et al., 1985].

Calcium Flux Techniques

Intuitively, the most direct way to monitor VSCC would be to actually measure the influx of Ca^{2+} through the channels. Such an approach would be presumably be free of the various problems and uncertainties associated with electrophysiological identification of VSCC. Moreover, as radioactive Ca^{2+} (^{45}Ca^{2+}) is readily available, such studies should be relatively simple to carry out. In practice, however, the situation is not so simple. The advances in molecular biophysical techniques discussed above have really eliminated most of the ambiguities associated with the electrophysiological identification of I$_{Ca}$s. Moreover, such biophysical techniques have enormous advantages in terms of their sensitivity and also potentially in the number of different paradigms to which they can be applied. Direct measurement of Ca^{2+} flux through VSCC is conceptually easy to carry out. ^{45}Ca^{2+} influx into whole cells or a membrane vesicular fraction, such as a synaptosomal preparation, is measured under polarized and depolarized conditions, and the difference in the rate of influx represents Ca^{2+} influx through VSCC (provided other voltage-sensitive pathways are blocked). The specificity of the increment in uptake can be ascertained by examining the blocking effects of inorganic or other VSCC blockers, for example. Unfortunately, several problems may arise. Enough radioisotope must accumulate during the flux assay in order to be determined by scintillation counting or related techniques. Given the specific activity of Ca^{2+} isotopes, this means that, in practice, uptake into many cells or vesicles must be examined simultaneously. Moreover, under physiological conditions, VSCC, as other ion channels, may close rather rapidly after opening due to cell repolarization or channel in-

activation. This brief period of time may not belong enough to allow sufficient radioisotope to accumulate for detection. In other words, compared to biophysical techniques, radioisotope flux techniques usually require much larger quantities of tissue and more leisurely time periods to be carried out successfully. On the other hand, as we have discussed, the nerve terminal is usually unavailable for direct electrophysiological recording techniques. Electrophysiologists often measure Ca^{2+} conductances in the cell soma as a "model" for events occurring at the nerve terminal [Klein et al., 1980]. Although this may be true in some cases, the more we find out about the properties and distribution of VSCC, the more this assumption appears to be erroneous (vide infra). Ca^{2+} flux studies utilizing synaptosomal preparations, however, do provide a direct look at the properties of VSCC existing in nerve terminals. Indeed, the most complete information available about such VSCC comes from using these techniques. Flux techniques are also useful in channel reconstitution assays, for example, where purified or semi-purified channels are reconstituted into liposomes. In such cases, radioisotope flux studies are ideal for monitoring the reconstituted channel, particularly those functions such as ionic selectivity and drug sensitivity. The value of such techniques has been well illustrated in studies on the sodium channel [Catterall, 1984].

Ca^{2+} flux techniques have been successfully applied to the analysis of neuronal VSCC in a number of cases using synaptosomal preparations (vide infra). These studies have been interesting and informative. A further major disadvantage, however, is that the tissue source utilized is extremely heterogeneous. Synaptosomes in such preparations are derived from a number of neuronal types. Thus, it is all but impossible to characterize a particular type of Ca^{2+} conductance as coming from a particular type of neurone. The use of clonal cell lines can in some ways override such criticisms as these represent a homogeneous tissue source. However, the use of such cells are subject to other criticisms, as it can always be argued that they do not represent authentic neuronal tissue.

The introduction of stopped/flow techniques has increased the time resolution of flux methods into the subsecond range. However, even this may not be fast enough to detect some rapidly transient events. It should be noted, however, that some types of VSCC do appear to remain open for a relatively long period of time especially when compared to Na^+ channels, for example. Moreover, as in the case of Na^+ channels, drugs are currently available which allow some VSCC to remain open for increased periods of time (e.g., BAY K8644 and CGP 28392) (vide infra). The use of such agents can potentially increase the likelihood of detecting some VSCC in a flux assay. This type of manipulation is somewhat equivalent to the use of batrachotoxin in flux assays for Na^+ channels [Catterall, 1984]. Without the use of such a drug, flux assays with Na^+ channels would be extremely difficult to carry out. It should be pointed out that increased uptake of Ca^{2+} upon depolarization is not necessarily the result of Ca^{2+} influx through VSCC. Other voltage-sensitive processes, such as the Na^+/Ca^{2+} exchange system, may contribute to the uptake and even swamp the channel-mediated influx at longer incubation times [Turner and Goldin, 1985a]. That this is so has often not been recognized, and so the interpretation of much of the data in this field must be considered very critically. However, when such caveats are taken into account, measurement of depolarization-induced $^{45}Ca^{2+}$ influxes into synaptosomes or cultured cells has yielded a great deal of important data concerning the selectivity and pharmacology of VSCC in neurones. An adjunct to such techniques is the use of Ca^{2+} sensing dyes, as described above. In some cases, these can be used to measure voltage-sensitive Ca^{2+} influxes with a greater sensitivity than the use of radioisotope flux techniques, and moreover, influx into single cells or even portions of single cells can also be monitored (vide supra).

Biochemical Identification of Calcium Channels

Identification of the molecular characteristics of sodium channels [Catterall, 1984] and nicotinic receptors [Dolly and Barnard, 1984] from both the biochemical and biophysical points of view must be considered to be two of the greatest success stories in molecular neurobiology. The secret of this success is probably attributable to two major factors. One of these is the availability of a convenient tissue source, such as the electroplax. However, a more important factor from the biochemical point of view has been the availability of highly specific drugs and toxins which can be used to label the channel and to follow it during purification when it is no longer functional. For both the nicotinic receptor and the Na^+ channel, one is confronted with an embarrassment of riches. In both cases, different groups of drugs and toxins bind with high affinity to a variety of sites on the channel. These substances can be modified to produce affinity labels and other reagents that are invaluable for the biochemical detection and isolation of the channel proteins. Moreover, specific drugs and toxins are of great value in the identification of specific channels in situ, a good example being the use of TTX to define the major type of Na^+ channel.

Some progress of this type is being made with VSCC. At least one group of drugs, the dihydropyridines, appears to bind with very high affinity and specificity to one type of VSCC. That this is so has been amply demonstrated in many pharmacological and physiological investigations. Drugs such as nitrendipine, for example, can block VSCC in depolarized smooth muscle preparations in the subnanamolar range. One would predict, therefore, that labelled compounds of this type would be ideal tools for the biochemical identification of VSCC and essential aids in their purification. This has indeed proved to be the case. However, these studies have also raised several important and provocative issues.

Thus, [^{3}H] nitrendipine binding sites have been detected in a variety of tissues. Do all these binding sites represent VSCC, and if not, what are they [Miller and Freedman, 1984; Schwartz et al., 1985]? An analogy might be the use of α-bungarotoxin binding to study nicotinic receptors. Such binding sites clearly represent nicotinic receptors at the neuromuscular junction. However, what do such binding sites in the brain and sympathetic ganglia represent [Dolly and Barnard, 1984]? It is not clear that these are also nicotinic receptors. The importance of [^{3}H] dihydropyridine and other drug binding studies in relation to neuronal VSCC will be discussed in detail below.

Biochemical studies at the genetic level should also be of use in further studies of VSCC structure and function. In other cases, such as the nicotinic receptor [Mishina et al., 1984] and sodium channel [Noda et al., 1984], the genes that encode the channel proteins have been cloned. This has given much information concerning the structure of these channels, particularly through the use of site-directed mutagenesis and associated techniques [Mishina et al., 1985]. In a related paradigm, mRNA fractions from neuronal tissue can be injected into cells, such as oocytes, which will then translate channel proteins and incorporate them into the plasma membrane. In some recent reports, success has been claimed in expressing VSCC in oocytes following injection of brain mRNA [Miledi and Parker, 1984; Dascal et al., 1985a,b].

DEVELOPMENTAL ASPECTS OF NEURONAL CALCIUM CHANNELS

Before embarking on a basic description of Ca^{2+} currents in vertebrate and invertebrate neurones, I shall consider what is known about the developmental aspects of VSCC. In some types of neurones, it is clear that a precise developmental sequence occurs in which action potentials recorded from the cell soma show a developmental change from Ca^{2+} to Na$^+$ spikes [Spitzer, 1979; Spitzer,

1984b]. This sequence is best typified by the studies of Spitzer and his colleagues, using the Rohon-Beard neurones of the amphibian spinal cord. These are sensory cells that appear prior to dorsal root ganglion cells and later die [Spitzer and Baccaglini, 1976; Baccaglini and Spitzer, 1977]. The earliest form of excitability seen with these cells is a Ca^{2+} spike of fairly long duration ($>$ 100 msec). After about a day, the duration of the action potential shortens, and it becomes a mixed Na$^+$/Ca^{2+} spike. After still further development, the duration of the spike shortens to about 1 msec, and it becomes a pure Na$^+$ spike. Similar changes have been observed in amphibian DRG cells which develop following the death of Rohon-Beard cells [Baccaglini, 1978]. In addition, such events do not appear to be unique to vertebrate neurones as similar changes have also been recorded in the cell bodies of dorsal unpaired median (DUM) interneurones in grasshopper embryos [Goodman and Heitler, 1979; Goodman and Spitzer, 1981a,b]. In this case, Ca^{2+} becomes less able to support spike generation at later stages of development.

These developmental changes have also been extensively studied in cell culture [Bader et al., 1983]. In cells of the amphibian neural plate in culture, Spitzer and Lamborghini [1976] also described a change in action potential dependence from Ca^{2+} to Na$^+$ with time in culture. Willard [1980] found that the neurites of such cells initially fired Ca^{2+} spikes which later changed to Na$^+$ spikes, although neurites were still capable of producing Ca^{2+} spikes in Ba^{2+} solutions. Ultimately, even this latter capability was lost. The cell bodies of these same neurones also start by firing Ca^{2+} spikes and go through a developmental sequence where they end up producing Na$^+$ spikes. However in this case of the soma, the ability to fire Ca^{2+} spikes in Ba^{2+} is maintained. The developing axons of amphibian olfactory neurones also go through a similar Ca^{2+}-to-Na$^+$ dependent sequence [Strichartz et al., 1980]. Several studies have analyzed appearance of Ca^{2+} spikes on DRG and other sensory neurones in culture. It is quite clear that the cell bodies of DRG cells from many embryonic animals exhibit spikes with a Ca^{2+} component (Table I), although spikes in cell processes seem to depend solely on Na^+ [Dichter and Fischbach, 1977]. In the case of murine DRG cells in culture, Matsuda et al. [1978] observed that the number of cells exhibiting a Ca^{2+} component decreased with the maturity of the culture. In cultures from adult mice, only about 5% of cells showed mixed Na^+/Ca^{2+} spikes [Yoshida et al., 1978]. However, all cells were still able to produce Ca^{2+} spikes in TEA/Ba^{2+} solutions [Yoshida and Matsuda, 1980]. Indeed, it is clear that the somas of mature sensory neurones retain their ability to produce Ca^{2+} action potentials following pharmacological manipulations, whereas in immature cells, this intervention is often unnecessary (Table I). One study observed that cultures of adult mouse DRG cells produced predominantly Na^+ spikes, but that the number producing mixed Na^+/Ca^{2+} spikes actually increased with time. This process was attributed to "dedifferentiation" of cells in culture [Scott and Edwards, 1980]. In cultured rat cortical neurones, Dichter et al. [1983] found that younger cells possessed a larger Ca^{2+} component to their action potentials than older cells under physiological conditions. However, all cells could produce Ca^{2+} spikes in TEA/Ba^{2+} solutions.

Developmental changes are also seen in cultures of neuronal clonal cell lines. Many such clones do not proceed through a developmental sequence of their own accord, but morphological differentiation can be provoked by changes in culture conditions such as the addition of cyclic nucleotides or growth factors such as nerve growth factor (NGF). Under such conditions, cells may differentiate morphologically from round cells to cells with a neuronal morphology possessing many neurites. These neurites may reach lengths of several millimeters under appropriate conditions [Greene and Tischler, 1982; Nirenberg et al., 1983]. Miyake [1978] observed that in round undifferentiated N18 cells, Na^+ spikes could not be obtained. However, even in this undifferentiated state, small Ca^{2+} spikes could be produced if the membrane potential was preconditioned at -80 mV. This is particularly interesting as it suggests that in the undifferentiated state these cells already possess a low threshold type of Ca^{2+} conductance that is predominantly inactivated at resting membrane potentials [Bodewei et al., 1985; Herring et al., 1985]. Further evidence for the existence of such a VSCC will be presented below. Following differentiation, N18 cells exhibit compound Na^+/Ca^{2+} spikes with a large Ca^{2+} component. Preconditioning is now no longer necessary. In very mature cultures, Na^+ spikes begin to predominate. This sequence of events is similar to that observed wtih some authentic neurones (vide supra). Other investigators have shown that in a variety of other neuroblastomas, Ca^{2+} conductances as assessed by $^{45}Ca^{2+}$ flux assays [Freedman et al., 1984a; Nirenberg et al., 1983] or electrophysiologically are greatly increased following cell differentiation [Furuya et al., 1983; Vycklicky et al., 1985]. This is associated with the appearance of membrane particles in freeze-etch micrographs, which may represent VSCC [Furuya and Furuya, 1983]. Differentiated neuroblastomas possess high threshold Ca^{2+} conductances, which are activated by depolarizing from normal resting membrane potentials and therefore differ from the low threshold conductances activated in the undifferentiated N18 cells discussed above [Docherty and Miller, 1985; Fishman and Spector, 1981]. Actually, such low threshold Ca^{2+} conductances may also increase upon cell differentiation [Bodewei et al., 1985]. Much of this data could be taken as indicating the presence of different types of VSCC is neuronal cell lines at different stages of development. I shall discuss this further.

PC12 pheochromocytoma cells when grown in the absence of NGF strongly resemble adrenal chromaffin cells. The latter are known to produce Ca^{2+} spikes under appropriate conditions, and the VSCC underlying this process have been extensively characterized [Biales et al., 1976; Brandt et al., 1976; Fenwick et al., 1982]. PC12 cells can normally fire Ca^{2+} spikes, but Na^+ spikes are not observed. Interestingly, when differentiated with NGF, PC12 cells also develop the ability to produce Na^+ spikes in addition to Ca^{2+} spikes [O'Lague and Hutner, 1980].

There are some indications that VSCC may be particularly associated with areas of the neurone undergoing growth and regeneration. Following transection, lamprey reticulospinal neurones [MacVicar and Llinas, 1985] or adult cockroach giant axons [Meiri et al., 1981] produce Ca^{2+} spikes much more readily than normal cells. In both cases, the origin of such spikes can be traced to the tip of the neurone undergoing active growth/regeneration. This area can be shown to be associated with a specialized area known as a "growth cone." Ca^{2+} currents within this region have been studied in cultured cells and neuronal cell lines actively extending neurites. In N1E-115 cells, Ca^{2+} spikes can be recorded at the growth cone using either optical [Grinvald and Farber, 1981] or electrophysiological methods [Anglister et al., 1982] but not from the remainder of the axons. Similar observations have been made from the growth cones of PC12 cells actively extending neurites in response to NGF [O'Lague et al., 1985] or from the isolated growth cones of molluscan neurones [Marom and Dagan, 1985]. It appears that in addition, changes in VSCC may occur in other regions of a neurone which is actively growing. Ca^{2+} spikes recorded from the somas of adult guinea pig DRG cells in culture were observed to increase temporarily during the period after plating in which cells were actively extending processes. Na^+ spikes did not increase during the same period [Fukuda and Kameyama, 1979].

The above discussion gives an overall general impression that immature cells have a greater ability to produce Ca^{2+} spikes than more mature cells. Moreover, Ca^{2+} conductances may be actually increased, particularly in actively growing regions of a neurone such as the growth cone and also in the somas of cells actively extending neurites. However, the question remains as to why this should be. Presumably, larger internal Ca^{2+} concentrations are required during development or re-

generation. Indeed, it has been hypothesized that Ca^{2+} entry at the cell soma is one element that controls amino acid uptake and the axonal transport of proteins [Hammerschlag et al., 1975, 1977]. Moreover, it has also been argued that Ca^{2+} entry into the growth cone is necessary for this region to carry out its various functions such as the incorporation of new membrane [Anglister et al., 1982]. If this is so, then it should be possible to disrupt normal development or regeneration by blocking voltage-dependent Ca^{2+} entry. Bixby and Spitzer [1984b] grew frog embryonic spinal cord cells under normal conditions and in the presence of Mg^{2+}/TTX to block voltage sensitive Ca^{2+} and Na^+ conductances. These conditions still led to the normal developmental sequence observed for the action potential in these neurones (vide supra). Some changes were observed, however. Neurite outgrowth was *more* rapid than in control cultures (perhaps the opposite of what might have been expected). Secondly, the development of sensitivity to the electrophysiological actions of GABA was reduced. Anglister et al. [1982] using N1E-15 cells, however, observed that increasing Ca^{2+} influx into the growth cone using K^+ depolarization (or the Ca^{2+} ionophore A23187) considerably increased the area of these regions. The effects of K^+ were blocked by Cd^{2+}. Similar effects and conclusions were obtained by Suarez-Isla et al. [1984], suggesting that increased Ca^{2+} entry may indeed be important from some aspects of growth cone function. In general, however, the exact functions of the changes in Ca^{2+} conductances seen during the development of most neurones are not really clear.

ELECTROPHYSIOLOGICAL OBSERVATIONS ON NEURONAL CALCIUM CHANNELS

I shall now describe and discuss observations pertaining to the types and characteristics of VSCC in various neurones. I shall begin by discussing electrophysiological studies which certainly make up the majority of the data in this field. I shall then devote other sections to information obtained from biochemical, ion flux, and other techniques. Two important areas that will be discussed in particular will be the existence of multiple types of VSCC and the ability of drugs and neurotransmitters to modify channel function. Initially, observations on the effects of drugs and transmitters will only be mentioned in passing, but they will be discussed in greater detail later. To begin with, I shall discuss electrophysiological observations on VSCC in vertebrate and invertebrate neurones, separately.

Vertebrate Neurones

Peripheral neurones. Of all types of vertebrate neurones, sensory neurones have been by far the most intensively studied with respect to the characteristics and functions of VSCC. Indeed, studies on these cells have been extraordinarily revealing and informative particularly in the areas of VSCC modulation and heterogeneity. DRG cells are particularly convenient to study as they can be easily cultured and maintained. Moreover, from the historical point of view, voltage-dependent Ca^{2+} conductances in neurones were first described by Koketsu and his colleagues in frog DRG cells [Koketsu et al., 1959, 1963; see also Hagiwara, 1983]. Most studies on sensory neurones have for practical reasons concentrated on VSCC in the cell soma, although it should be noted that Ca^{2+} spikes have been recorded at the sensory nerve terminals of the frog muscle spindle and in other specialized endings such as hair cells and electroreceptors (Table I). Since the original observations by Koketsu et al., Ca^{2+} conductances have been identified in sensory neurones from a variety of species including cat, rabbit, rat, mouse chick, guinea pig, pigeon, and lamprey (Table I). As previously mentioned, Ca^{2+} components of the action potential are seen as "plateau" regions, "humps," or "inflexions" on the spike (Fig. 1). Such indications as to the presence of a Ca^{2+} component are more often found in neurones from young or embryonic animals in

normal physiological media (vide supra). In adult animals, they occur to more variable extents depending on the preparation. However, it is quite clear that even in such adult neurones, Ca^{2+} spikes are easily obtained following the appropriate suppression of Na^+ and K^+ currents and boosting of Ca^{2+} currents [Yoshida and Matsuda, 1980]. Indeed, under appropriate conditions, Ca^{2+} spikes with durations of up to 10 sec can be observed [Ishizuka et al., 1984]! It should be mentioned that the contribution of Na^+ to the DRG spike is quite complex, as it consists of a TTX-sensitive and a TTX-insensitive component [Gallego, 1983; Baccaglini and Cooper, 1982; Bossu and Feltz, 1984; Fukuda and Kameyama, 1980]. In certain conditions, some of the TTX-insensitive component may be due to movement of Na^+ through VSCC [Bossu and Feltz, 1984; Hablitz et al., 1985]. This can occur when external Ca^{2+} is removed, a phenomenon that has been observed in a number of cases and which has interesting implications for the mechanisms of ion permeability through the channel [Almers et al., 1984; Hess et al., 1986; McLesky et al., 1986a].

In comparison to other vertebrate neurones, a great deal is known from voltage clamp recordings about the Ca^{2+} conductances in sensory neurones. Because of this, it is worth examining the situation in some detail and using this as a basis for comparison with results from other cells. As things stand at present, it appears that DRG cells and other sensory neurones possess at least three operationally distinct Ca^{2+} conductances, which can be distinguished by various means. One of these conductances has so far only been identified by one group [Fox et al., 1985b; Nowycky et al., 1985a]. The other two have been observed by at least four groups [Carbone and Lux, 1984a,b; Forscher and Oxford, 1985a; Bossu et al., 1985; Fedulova et al., 1985; Nowycky et al., 1985a,b]. Because of this, it is possible to make some comparisons between the various sets of data. When this is done, a fairly consistent picture can be obtained. Comparison of the data in detail shows that there are, indeed, some differences in the

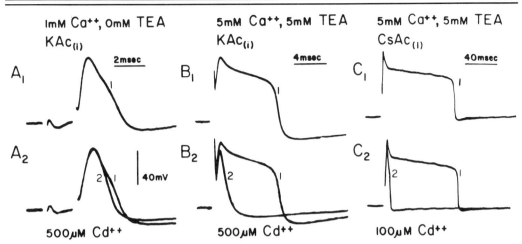

Fig. 1. *Action potentials of dorsal root ganglion neurons have sodium- and calcium-dependent components and have a potassium-dependent afterhyperpolarization. Action potentials were evoked from resting membrane potential at 15-sec intervals by 100–500 sec duration depolarizing stimuli. The action potentials illustrated in A_1 and A_2, however, were evoked by 2-sec depolarizing stimuli, while the modified Wheatstone bridge circuit was maintained in balance. Action potentials were evoked in medium containing 1 mM Ca^{2+} and 0 mM TEA$^+$ (A_1,A_2) or 5 mM Ca^{2+} and 5 mM TEA (B_1,B_2) during recording with KAc-filled micropipettes and in medium con-taining 5 mM Ca^{2+}, 5 mM TEA$^+$ during recording with CsAc-filled micropipettes (C_1,C_2). A_2, B_2, C_2: superimposed action potentials evoked prior to (1) and subsequent to (2) application of cadmium (Cd^{2+}), a calcium channel blocker. TEA at 5 mM partially blocked potassium conductance and augmented the calcium component of the action potential to a duration of about 10 msec (A,B). Intracellular cesium abolished substantial potassium conductance, thus abolishing the afterhyperpolarization and producing calcium-dependent action potentials with durations of 100–2,000 msec (C) [from Werz and MacDonald, 1985b].*

microbiophysical and pharmacological properties obtained in different labs. However, considering the differences in technique, internal and external solutions, temperatures, concentrations of ions, and so forth, these differences are hardly surprising. Some of the discrepancies may ultimately prove to be important. However, they may also prove to be trivial. Thus, at this point it is probably better just to concentrate on what is consistent in this rapidly developing field. The description I shall give, therefore, is a composite of data from several different studies.

The first Ca^{2+} conductance to be identified is similar to that described by Dunlap and Fischbach [1981] [Carbone and Lux, 1984a,b; Forscher and Oxford, 1985b; Bossu et al., 1985; Fedulova et al., 1985; Nowycky et al., 1985a,b; see also many other references in Table 1]. When cells are held around their resting potential (approximately -60 mV),

strongly depolartizing voltage steps to -10 mV or so elicit an I_{Ca} that peaks around 0 to 10 mV. Under appropriate conditions, this current inactivates only very slowly. Most authors have, in fact, described a half-time for inactivation in the second range. Because of this lack of inactivation, the current is not very sensitive to holding potential and can be elicited from positive holding potentials (-20 mV or even 0). This long-lasting current has been called various things, but in the present discussion, I shall use the designation L ("long lasting"), suggested by Nowycky et al. [1985a]. Observation of the L-current is very consistent and it can be recorded from virtually every cell. The L-current can be carried by Ba^{2+} and Sr^{2+}, as well as by Ca^{2+} [Carbone and Lux, 1984a; Bossu et al., 1985; Fedulova et al., 1985; Nowycky et al., 1985a,b] and weakly by Mn^{2+} and Zn^{2+} [Ishizuka et al., 1984]. There is some controversy as to whether Ca^{2+} or Ba^{2+} carry the current better, although most studies report that Ba^{2+} is superior. L-current can be blocked by Co^{2+}, being particularly sensitive to the latter [Nowycky et al., 1985a; see Bossu et al., 1985]. Organic VSCC modulators such as D-600, diltiazem, and particularly the dihydropyridines, appear to interact with the VSCC underlying L-currents (see Table VIII, below). The exact manner in which dihydropyridines modulate these channels is again controversial, and I shall return to this in a later section. Another finding of great interest is that L-currents can be modulated by a variety of neurotransmitters including GABA, catecholamines, 5-HT, adenosine, and dynorphin (see Table IX below). All of these block DRG L-currents. These observations are consistent with the effects of such agents on the duration of DRG Ca^{2+} spikes (Table IX). Two biochemical observations are also of considerable interest. As discussed above, Ca^{2+} currents may be subject to "rundown." This is clearly true for DRG L-currents [Forscher and Oxford, 1985b; Bossu et al., 1985; Fedulova et al., 1985]. Interestingly, however, L-current rundown can be reversed by the introduction of Mg-ATP and an ATP regenerating system (creatine phosphate and creatine phosphokinase) into the intracellular perfusing medium [Forscher and Oxford, 1985b]. It is possible that cAMP is also required although this is controversial [Forscher and Oxford, 1985b; Fedulova et al., 1985]. Such observations are most interesting as they suggest that, as in the heart for example, some neuronal VSCC (seemingly the dihydropyridine-sensitive variety in both cases) may be regulated by phosphorylating mechanisms. In contrast to the effects of ATP, L-currents can be blocked by raising the internal Ca^{2+} concentration [Bossu et al., 1985]. Clearly, this process may be the basis of the "current" or "Ca^{2+}"-dependent inactivation referred to previously [Eckert and Chad, 1984]. Internal perfusion with F^- will also block L-currents [Bossu et al., 1985]. Single channel recordings have identified the unitary current events underlying the L-conductance [Carbone and Lux, 1984a; Nowycky

et al., 1985a]. These L-channels have a slope conductance of 25 psec in 110 mM Ba^{2+}.

A second type of Ca^{2+} conductance observed in cultured DRG neurones has been designated T ("transient") [Carbone and Lux, 1984a,b; 1985; Bossu et al., 1985; Fedulova et al., 1985; Nowycky et al., 1985a]. T-conductances were not initially observed, as they are substantially inactivated at resting membrane potentials [Dunlap and Fischbach, 1981]. Moreover, T-conductances are apparently less reliably observed than L-conductances [Bossu et al., 1985]. Thus, there is less data available on this second system. In order to remove inactivation of T-channels, cells must be held at very negative potentials. If cells are held at -100 mV for example, depolarizing steps activate a transient I_{Ca} at about -60 mV. The current reaches its peak amplitude at about -40 mV. The T-current is observed as an obvious shoulder on the peak current-voltage curve. T-currents are substantially inactivated in the range of normal membrane potentials (complete inactivation at -40 mV, 90% at -60 mV). The reason for the transience of the T-current is not clear, but components of both current- and voltage-dependent inactivation have been suggested [Bossu et al., 1985]. The fact that the current is still transient when Ba^{2+} is used suggests, however, that voltage-dependent inactivation may be the major factor. This is consistent with data from other sources [e.g., Bean, 1985]. Ba^{2+} and Sr^{2+} both carry T-current, but it is not clear exactly what the relative permeability of these ions might be. It seems, however, that in this case, Ca^{2+} may be at least as permeable as Ba^{2+} [Bossu et al., 1985; Fedulova et al., 1985]. It should be noted, however, that results showing that Ca^{2+} carries T-currents better than Ba^{2+} could easily arise artifactually due to the superior ability of Ca^{2+} to screen charge. Inorganic blockers such as Cd^{2+} and Co^{2+} also block T-currents. Significantly, however, it appears that T-currents may be relatively resistance to blockade by Cd^{2+} in comparison to L-currents [Nowycky et al., 1985a]. Moreover, T-currents also do not appear to be altered by organic VSCC modulators (Table VIII, below). Again, these data from DRG cells is consistent with data from other sources. Thus, in addition to neuronal cells, both T and L-like currents have also been found in pituitary tumor cells [Armstrong and Matteson, 1985], and skeletal [Cognard et al., 1985], smooth [Hermsmeyer and Sturek, 1985; Sturek and Hermsmeyer, 1985], and cardiac muscle cells [Bean, 1985; Nilius et al., 1985]. In these cases, the properties of the currents involved seem very similar, if not identical, to those described for sensory neurones. A further distinction from L-currents is that T-currents do not run down, and they can be observed in cells long after L-currents have disappeared [Bossu et al., 1985]. Although the data are somewhat scanty at present, it appears that T-channels may also be subject to modification by neurotransmitters. GABA reduces T-currents but less effectively than L-currents, whereas the reverse is apparently true for norepinephrine [Deisz and Lux, 1985; Forscher and Oxford, 1985a]. Measurements by single channel analysis indicate that T-channels have a slope conductance of 8 psec in 110 mM Ba^{2+}, making them considerably smaller than L-channels [see Carbone and Lux, 1984a for an alternate view]. As mentioned previously, T and L-currents have also been recorded in a number of other neuronal and nonneuronal cells. However, T-currents do not appear to be found in all cases. Thus, it is claimed that they are not found in bovine adrenal medullary cells, sympathetic neurones, or some molluscan neurones [Carbone and Lux, 1984a; Bossu et al., 1985].

Nowycky and colleagues have, in addition, described a third type of Ca^{2+} conductance, at least in chick embryonic DRG cells in culture [Nowycky et al., 1985a; Fox et al., 1985b]. They have designated this third type of conductance N. As there are only two reports on this conductance, little data is available. The N-current is really a sort of compromise between the L and T-current. Like the T-current, it requires a negative holding potential and is transient, and like the L-current, it requires strong depolarizing steps in order to be observed. From a holding potential of -100 mV, strong depolarizations to -20 mV or more positive elicit N-currents. They are transient and substantially inactivated at -20 mV, half-inactivation being observed at -60 mV. Ba^{2+} carries the current. N-currents are rather sensitive to blockade by Cd^{2+} and are apparently unaltered by dihydropyridines. N-channels have a conductance of 13 psec in 110 mM Ba^{2+}. One particularly fascinating aspect of N-current microphysiology is the existence of "hot-spots" [Fox et al., 1985b]. Thus, in some patches many N-channels (> 100) can be observed, whereas only a few T or L-channels are seen. Why such groups of N-type Ca^{2+} channels should occur is not clear, although such a grouping of Ca^{2+} channels has been suggested to occur around neurotransmitter release sites (vide infra). In addition to DRG cells, N-currents may be found in sympathetic neurones (R. Tsien personal communication) and, in addition, in other neuronal types as well. This will be further discussed below. The existence of three types of Ca^{2+} conductances in sensory neurones (and possibly in other cell types) raises many questions. What is the relative macro- and microdistribution of these channels in the cell, what are their functions, which can be modulated by neurotransmitters and drugs? The answers to most of these questions are as yet unclear. However, as we shall see, the existence of T and L-channels fits in nicely with data previously obtained in a number of central neurones which predicted the existence of two Ca^{2+} conductances with more or less the characteristics observed. Moreover, neurotransmitter release and Ca^{2+} flux data can also be explained by realizing that multiple VSCC exist.

The classification of neuronal VSCC into L, T, and N provides a useful starting point when considering other data from both electrophysiological and other sources. Thus, I shall continue to describe conductances in other cells as being of the "L-type," "T-type," or "N-type." Indeed, as we shall see, there are many good reasons for actually doing so. However, we shall also come across observations that do not fit easily into these categories. Indeed, it seems likely that VSCC other than T, L, and N will be found or at least considerable variations on these themes.

In comparison to sensory neurones, much less is known about Ca^{2+} conductances in other peripheral neurones. Ca^{2+} spikes have been reliably recorded from the cell bodies of sympathetic ganglion cells (particularly the superior cervical ganglion) from rat, rabbit, and bullfrog (Table I), although one older study failed in this respect [Tashiro and Nishi, 1972]. Similar results have also been obtained using cultures of rat superior cervical ganglion cells. In these neurones, the Ca^{2+} conductance is manifest under normal conditions as a "shoulder" on the action potential. In TTX/ TEA media, action potentials solely dependent on the Ca^{2+} conductance can be obtained in all species. These spikes are typically followed by a large AHP which, as discussed above, is a manifestation of the activation of $I_{K(Ca)}$. In Ba^{2+}, action potentials can even be provoked in the axons of rabbit sympathetic neurones in Na^+ free media [Greengard and Straub, 1959]. Soma-recorded Ca^{2+}-dependent spikes and their associated AHPs can be depressed by the activation of α_2-adrenergic, muscarinic, adenosine, and prostaglandin E_1 receptors on sympathetic neurones (see Table IX below). Thus as with DRG cells, such data suggest that I_{Ca}s in sympathetic neurones may be modulated by various neurotransmitters and drugs. Some information is available on the Ca^{2+} currents found in these cells [Freschi, 1983; 1984; Akasu and Koketsu, 1981; Galvan and Adams, 1982; Koketsu and Akasu, 1982; Nerbonne and Gurney, 1985; Belluzzi et al., 1985]. When cells are held around -50 mV, depolarizing steps to -20 mV or more produce a Ca^{2+} current with characteristics very similar to the L-current from sensory neurones. Although data are scanty, certain comparisons can be made. The current in sympathetic neurones activates in approximately the same voltage range, and under the appropriate conditions, it is obviously long-lasting and inactivates slowly, if at all. The sensitivity of this current to various blockers is hard to assess.

However, it is clearly blocked by Cd^{2+} and by D-600 (at least partially), although at the concentrations of D-600 used (5×10^{-5} M), the significance of this block is unclear [Akasu and Koketsu, 1981]. One report has claimed that I_{Ca}s in sympathetic neurones are insensitive to DHPs [Nerbonne and Gurney, 1985]. However, these authors also found no effects of DHPs on sensory neurones. Sympathetic neurone Ca^{2+} currents under voltage clamp are clearly reduced by norepinephrine [Galvan and Adams, 1982; Koketsu and Akasu, 1982]. Interestingly, maximally effective concentrations of norepinephrine (10^{-5} M) only reduced the I_{Ca} by about 50% [Galvan and Adams, 1982]. In addition, Belluzzi et al. [1985] have found that the Ca^{2+} current in sympathetic neurones can be depressed by muscarine. This is different from the classical observation that the major mode of action of muscarinic agonists in these cells is the inhibition of the K^+ current, I_m [Adams et al., 1982]. There is no indication from the published reports as to the existence of a T-type I_{Ca} in sympathetic neurones. Carbone and Lux claim in passing that they could find no evidence for the existence of T-currents in sympathetic neurones, although they clearly observed such currents in DRG cells [Carbone and Lux, 1984a]. As I shall discuss below, other data make it virtually certain that some drug-insensitive VSCC (N or T?) do exist in sympathetic neurones.

While considering sympathetic neurones, it is also appropriate to mention adrenal chromaffin cells and the related pheochromocytoma cell line PC12. Owing to the convenience of culturing chromaffin cells, or PC12 cells in particular, evoked catecholamine release from these cells is often used as a "model" for neurosecretion from sympathetic neurones [Greene and Tischler, 1982]. Actually, adrenal chromaffin cells can also secrete opioid peptides, and PC12 cells can also secrete acetylcholine and neurotensin. Of particular interest is the fact that under the influence of NGF both adrenal chromaffin and PC12 cells undergo morphological differentiation so that they now resemble sympathetic neurones

[Greene and Tischler, 1982; Doupe et al., 1985]. Together with this morphological change from endocrine cells to neurones, several biochemical and physiological changes also occur. The Ca^{2+} conductances in undifferentiated adrenal and PC12 cells have been investigated, although little is known about the differentiated state in each case. Both PC12 cells and adrenal chromaffin cells secrete catecholamines in response to a depolarizing stimulus such as an increase in K^{+}. Under appropriate conditions, adrenal chromaffin cells display Ca^{2+} spikes [Kidokoro and Ritchie, 1980; Brandt et al., 1976]. This is one pathway by which Ca^{2+} enters the cell to trigger exocytosis (the other major one being via nicotinic receptors during cholinergic stimulation of the cell). The Ca^{2+} conductance in bovine adrenal cells has been extensively investigated and appears to be very similar to the DRG L-current [Clapham and Neher, 1984; Fenwick et al., 1982; Hoshi et al., 1984]. This similarity includes general biophysical characteristics, lack of inactivation under appropriate conditions, and significant current run-down. Moreover, Nowycky et al. [1985b] also quote unpublished data showing that the adrenal I$_{Ca}$ is modulated by dihydropyridines, such as BAY K8644, in a manner similar to that of the DRG L-channel. Release of norepinephrine from these cells is also modulated by these same drugs [Cena et al., 1983; Garcia et al., 1984a; Sasakawa et al., 1983, 1984]. T-currents have not been reported in adrenal chromaffin cells. Bossu et al. [1985] mention that they have looked for them but had no success. A particularly interesting feature of the Ca^{2+} currents in chromaffin cells is the existence of facilitation, a phenomenon that is in some ways the opposite of current inactivation [Hoshi et al., 1984]. In this case, the current observed under voltage clamp is larger if it is immediately preceded by a conditioning pulse. The mechanism of this interesting effect and whether it is also found in sympathetic and other neurones is unknown. PC12 cells also fire Ca^{2+} spikes both before and after treatment with NGF [O'Lague and Huttner, 1980; Ogura and Tak-

ahashi, 1984]. In the NGF-treated state, Ca^{2+} spikes can be recorded from the growth cones of growing neurites [O'Lague et al., 1985]. The properties of the Ca^{2+} currents in these cells have only been reported in abstract form. However, there are some very intriguing observations [Scholfield and Weight, 1984; Kunze et al., 1985]. It is clear that PC12 cells treated with NGF (and probably without) have an L-type current. This current appears to be modulated by dihydropyridines as is the current in DRG cells. There are some indications, however, that a second Ca^{2+} conductance might also be present. Thus, Ogura and Takahashi [1984] observed that although evoked release of transmitter from PC12 cells was blocked by the dihydropyridine nicardipine, Ca^{2+} spikes in the same cells were unaltered. The authors, therefore, suggested that two types of VSCC (dihydropyridine-sensitive and insensitive) may be present. Indeed, this idea has much to commend it. Significantly, the authors also found that they had to precondition their cells at -100 mV in order to observe their best Ca^{2+} spikes. In another abstract, Kunze et al. [1985] have reported that the I$_{Ca}$ in PC12 cells was by nitrendipine if evoked from a holding potential of -20 mV, but only a partial block could be obtained if a holding potential of -100 mv was used. This suggests that at hyperpolarized holding potentials, a drug-insensitive current could have been revealed. However, other reasonable explanations for this observation can also be put forward based on well-known characteristics of the dihydropyridine/Ca^{2+} channel interaction [Bean, 1984; Sanguinetti and Kass, 1984a,b]. At any rate, the adrenal/PC12 systems remain to be fully investigated, as they are certainly interesting in terms of their similarities to neurones.

Neuronal clonal cell lines have also been used in the investigation of Ca^{2+} channels. Indeed, as with PC12 cells, such systems have yielded interesting and valuable data. This is particularly true when considering pharmacological aspects of Ca^{2+} channel function. Most of the cells that have been used are in some ways derivatives of C1300, a mouse neuroblastoma clone originally derived from a sympathetic neurone, and so it seems appropriate to consider them at this point [Nirenberg et al., 1983]. Ca^{2+} spikes can be demonstrated in many (but not all) clones of neuroblastomas (Table I). In virtually all cases, the expression of Ca^{2+} conductances is associated with morphological differentiation of the cells produced by cyclic AMP, DMSO, or some other means. Under such conditions, Ca^{2+} currents are associated with growth cones [Anglister et al., 1982] and can also be recorded from the cell soma (Table I). As indicated above, however, even in the undifferentiated state, there is some reported evidence for the presence of VSCC which seem to be predominantly of the T-type [Miyake, 1978; Bodewei et al., 1985]. Interestingly, Ca^{2+} spikes recorded in various neuroblastomas, as in PC12 cells, appear to be very insensitive to blockade by organic VSCC blockers (vide infra). VSCC in neuroblastomas have also been studied by voltage clamp (Table I). Two types of Ca^{2+} conductance have been observed which are extremely similar in their properties to DRG T and L-currents [Fishman and Spector, 1981; Tsunoo et al., 1984, 1985a; Yoshii et al., 1985a,b]. The L-currents appears to be sensitive to dihydropyridines and other VSCC blockers, enhanced by cAMP, and blocked by low concentrations of Cd^{2+}. The T-type current, on the other hand, is not blocked by organic VSCC blockers and is relatively resistant to Cd^{2+}. T-currents in N1E-115 cells have been shown to be blocked by phenytoin [Twombly and Narahashi, 1985], however, which may be a useful observation. (It should be noted that effects of phenytoin on L-type currents have also been reported; vide infra.) Recently, L-currents in these same cells have been shown to be blocked by the neuropeptides enkephalin and somatostatin [Tsunoo et al., 1985b] (vide infra).

Ca^{2+} spikes have been observed in neurones of the enteric ganglia (Table I). In one group of neurones from the myenteric plexus, an AHP is extremely prominent, and so these cells are known as "AH" cells. These neurones produce Ca^{2+} spikes in TTX which can be enhanced by the usual maneuvers such as intracellular injection of Cs^+ [Cherubini and North 1984]. These Ca^{2+} spikes can be suppressed by agonists of GABA-B (but not GABA-A) receptors and by agonists at κ-opiate receptors [Cherubini and North, 1984; 1985]. Norepinephrine can also depress the Ca^{2+} spike, but clonidine is ineffective [Slack, 1985]. The status of the adrenergic control of these Ca^{2+} spikes will be discussed below. Under voltage clamp, AH neurones exhibit an I_{Ca} which appears to have L-like characteristics [Hirst et al., 1985]. Interestingly, even with Ba^{2+} carrying the current, a short inactivating phase can still be observed. However, this is unlikely to be due to a T-current component as it is produced from a relatively depolarized holding potential (-55 mV). The drug sensitivity of this current has not been studied. AH cells have also been observed in the guinea pig submucous plexus [Surprenant, 1984], and these also show Ca^{2+} spikes under appropriate conditions. No voltage clamp datais available on these cells. However, Surprenant observed that the Ca^{2+} action potentials in submucous AH cells were unaffected by 10^- M nifedipine. The AHP was also unaltered. Interestingly, in the same preparation, Ca^{2+} potentials in the adherent smooth muscle cells were completely blocked by nifedipine at 10^{-9}-10^{-7}. This is a most intriguing finding that suggests that the Ca^{2+} conductance underlying the spike in these submucous neurones may be distinct from the dihydropyridine (L-type?) channel.

Central neurones. In spite of the difficulties associated with voltage clamping neurones with complex morphologies, some progress has been made in identifying Ca^{2+} currents in vertebrate central neurones. The development of slice systems has particularly helped in this respect. Voltage clamp data is available from hippocampal pyramidal and granule cells, neurones from the olfactory cortex, and locus coeruleus and spinal motoneurones. Of these, much more data is available in the case of hippocampal pyramidal cells than in any other. In addition, measurements of Ca^{2+} spikes in a variety of other cases has led to considerable insights into underlying Ca^{2+} conductances even when they have not been directly measured. One particularly fascinating aspect of this work is the clear compartmentalization of Ca^{2+} conductances into different portions of the neurone, and the emergence of the dendritic processes as an area in which such VSCC are particularly important [Llinas, 1984; Llinas and Sugimori, 1979]. Where data are available, I shall attempt to compare the properties of central I$_{Ca}$s with those described above for peripheral neurones.

Ca^{2+} spikes have often been reported in pyramidal cells of the hippocampus. These can be demonstrated in hippocampal slice preparations or in primary cultures of hippocampal neurones (Table I). In fact, two types of Ca^{2+}-dependent electrogenesis have been described. One response is the Ca^{2+} spike and the second is a slow depolarizing "envelope," otherwise described as a "burst-firing" response [Brown et al., 1985, 1986, for review]. The importance of the dendrites in these responses can be demonstrated in preparations in which the dendrites of CA1 pyramidal neurones are isolated from their cell bodies by cuts through the proximal stratum radiatum [Masukawa and Prince, 1984; Benardo et al., 1982; Wong et al., 1979]. Intracellular recordings can then be made from the isolated dendrites themselves or from the isolated "soma." The latter portion usually consists of the cell bodies, basal dendrites, and probably the most proximal portions of the apical dendritic tree. Such studies show that the isolated dendrites are capable of generating both Ca^{2+} spikes and the Ca^{2+} dependent slow depolarizing envelope. The isolated somas were also able to generate Ca^{2+} spikes, although it is difficult to say whether the origin of such spikes was in the soma itself or in the dendrites proximal to the cut. Voltage clamp studies have demonstrated an I$_{Ca}$ which again greatly resembles

the L-current from DRG cells [Halliwell, 1983; Brown and Griffiths, 1983b; Halliwell and Scholfield, 1984a,b; Brown et al., 1985, 1986; McClesky et al., 1986b]. Thus, this current is non (or at least very slowly) inactivating, high threshold, enhanced by Ba^{2+}, very sensitive to Cd^{2+} and modulated by dihydropyridines as well as ω-toxin from *Conus geographus* (vide infra). It is thought that this conductance may underlie the slow depolarizing envelope. However, it has been suggested that it is unlikely to underlie pyramidal cell Ca^{2+} spikes [Brown et al., 1985, 1986]. For example, spiking can be inactivated by a depolarizing prepulse which does not alter the slow current. Clearly, a current such as the DRG T-current would be an ideal conductance for production of the spike response. Indeed, such a current has been investigated by Halliwell [1983] who observed a transient I$_{Ca}$ in voltage clamped guinea pig hippocampal neurones if depolarizing jumps were made from hyperpolarized holding potentials. Clearly, this current has a superficial resemblance to the T-current from DRG cells and other sources. Furthermore, Brown and colleagues have also reported the existence of a high threshold transient Ca^{2+} current (N-current?) in pyramidal neurones; however, little data is available on this point as yet [Brown et al., 1985, 1986; Gahwiler and Brown, 1985]. It is also worth noting that Ca^{2+} spikes recorded from CA1 neurones are virtually resistant to organic VSCC blockers [Dingledine, 1983]. This would fit nicely with the idea that a T-type current underlies this response, as such currents seem to be resistant to the effects of these drugs.

Ca^{2+} spikes in hippocampal cells can be modified by various neurotransmitters, as in the case of peripheral neurones. Both GABA and adenosine reduce Ca^{2+} spikes in pyramidal cells [Newberry and Nicoll, 1984; Proctor and Dunwiddie, 1983]. Interestingly, in contradistinction to the observations discussed above, these actions do not appear to be the result of direct modulation of VSCC. Indeed in this case, the effects of GABA and adenosine appear to be the result of enhancement of K^+ currents that would tend to "oppose" inward Ca^{2+} currents [Gahwiler and Brown, 1985; Halliwell and Scholfield, 1984a,b; Newberry and Nicoll, 1984]. In hippocampal granule cells, however, a preliminary report has suggested that an L-like current can be enhanced by adrenergic agonists which presumably act via increases in intracellular cyclic AMP concentrations. This would be analogous to the effects of β-agonists in the heart [Gray and Johnston, 1985a,b].

The concept of multiple types of VSCC that is supported by these studies on hippocampal neurones is also supported by studies on several other types of central neurones. Although voltage clamp data are unavailable in these cases, the experiments conducted so far, particularly by Llinas and his colleagues have provided a great deal of fundamental data concerning neuronal Ca^{2+} conductances [Llinas, 1984]. These studies again illustrate the prevalance of Ca^{2+} conductances in the dendrites, in particular. The situation in cerebellar Purkinje cells appears similar to that discussed for hippocampal pyramidal cells [Llinas and Hess, 1976; Llinas and Sugimori, 1980a,b; Mori-Okamoto et al., 1983]. Intradendritic recordings again reveal the presence of Ca^{2+}-dependent plateau ("envelope") and spike potentials. Unlike hippocampal pyramidal cells, however, Ca^{2+} spikes are not found to originate in the cell bodies of Purkinje cells. Ca^{2+} spikes recorded from the soma appear to have a dendritic origin. Significantly, Ca^{2+} spikes cannot be recorded in the Purkinje cells of immature animals prior to dendritic development [Llinas and Sugimori, 1979]. Furthermore, Crepel et al. [1984] have found that Ca^{2+} spikes were absent from the dendrites of *staggerer* mutant mice, although they could be clearly recorded from control animals. It is not known why this difficiency occurs; however, it may be due to the absence (or mutation) of VSCC.

A slightly different picture is seen in brain slice recordings from thalamic [Jahnsen and Llinas, 1984a,b; Llinas and Jahnsen, 1982;

Deschenes et al., 1982] and inferior olivary neurones [Llinas and Yarom, 1981a,b]. In both these cases, two kinds of Ca^{2+} spikes can be observed under appropriate conditions. One type of spike (low threshold, LTS) can only be evoked if the cell is first conditioned at hyperpolarizing membrane potentials (negative to -70 mV). The conductance underlying this response appears to be inactivated at normal resting potentials. A second feature of this type of spike is that it is followed by a refractory period. The origin of this type of spike appears to be the cell soma or the region close to it. A second type of Ca^{2+} spike can be evoked at higher thresholds without prior hyperpolarization (HTS). This HTS appears to be dendritic in origin and exhibits no refractory period. In keeping with this latter observation in inferior olivary neurones (and probably also in neurones of the red nucleus) [Kubota et al., 1985], Ba^{2+} and TEA could prolong the HTS considerably, although Ba^{2+} was less effective in thalamic neurones. Both LTS and HTS responses have also been recorded from dopaminergic neurones in the pars compacta of the guinea pig substantia nigra. Here again Llinas et al. [1984] concluded that the source of the HTS was the distal dendritic arborization. It was concluded that the LTS was derived from the proximal dendrites close to the soma. There may be several roles for these various Ca^{2+} conductances. However, they are clearly involved in the generation of firing patterns in different portions of the cell. Moreover, the dendritic influx of Ca^{2+} may be involved in the release of transmitters that occur from these processes. Indeed, Ca^{2+} spikes have also been observed in the mitral cells of the turtle olfactory bulb where they are believed to be involved in transmission across reciprocal dendrodendritic synapses with granule cells [Mori et al., 1981].

The similarity of HTS and LTS responses to data on L and T-currents discussed elsewhere will not escape the reader. Indeed, Llinas [Llinas 1984, for review] has proposed that different types of I_{Ca}s underlie the HTS and LTS. The properties of the currents involved are predicted to be similar to an L-current in the former case and a T-current in the latter. It should be noted that although it has been suggested that Ca^{2+} spikes are produced by all thalamic neurones, Crunelli et al. [1985] observed that in the lateral geniculate nucleus (LGN), this was only true for cells in the dorsal portion of the nucleus. Ca^{2+} spikes appeared to be absent from cells in the ventral portion.

Cells from the vertebrate spinal cord exhibit Ca^{2+} spikes either in culture or in slice preparations (Table I). In slices of immature rat spinal cord, Murase and Randic [1983] observed two types of Ca^{2+} spikes that appeared to have properties identical to the HTS and LTS described above. Several studies have also provided data on the existence of I$_{Ca}$s in motoneurones. Barrett and Barrett [1976] first observed Ca^{2+} spikes in frog motoneurones. Other authors suggested the existence of VSCC from observations on the AHP following action potentials in these cells [Krnjevic et al., 1978, 1979]. Schwindt and Crill have studied the ionic currents in cat motoneurones in situ under voltage clamp [Crill and Schwindt, 1983; Schwindt and Crill, 1980a,b,c, 1982]. Depolarization from resting potentials in these cells evokes an inward current designated I$_i$ which is carried by both Ca^{2+} and Ba^{2+}. This current shows only slow inactivation and therefore resembles other L-like currents, at least superficially. Little is known about the modulation of I$_{Ca}$s in spinal neurones. However, it has been reported that Ca^{2+} spikes in cultured spinal cells can be reduced by muscarinic *antagonists* such as atropine [Hedlund et al., 1985]. However, the significance of such an observation is difficult to assess.

The existence of Ca^{2+} currents in neocortical cells is suggested by older observations on the effects of Ba^{2+} and TEA on these cells in situ [Krnjevic et al., 1971]. This has been confirmed in slice and culture preparations [Dichter et al., 1983; Nerbonne et al., 1985]. Under voltage clamp, neurones of the guinea pig olfactory cortex display a persistent inward current similar to that recorded in hippocampal cells [Halliwell and Sholfield, 1984a,b].

In neurones of the rat locus coeruleus, Ca^{2+} currents measured under voltage clamp in slices of the rat pons were found to be transient even when cells were injected with Cs$^+$, and Ba^{2+} was used as the current carrier [Williams and North, 1984; Williams et al., 1984a,b]. Moreover, these transient currents were evoked from holding potentials between -55 and -45 mV. These observations do not seem to fit in precisely with the L/T/N classification used as a model so far. Of course it is possible that the manipulations utilized did not completely eliminate contaminating outward currents. At any rate, the Ca^{2+} currents and Ca^{2+} spikes evoked in these cells can be inhibited by catecholamines [Williams and North, 1984]. However, as previously mentioned in the myenteric plexus, this effect is quite odd as it is not mimicked by clonidine nor is it very sensitive to reversal by phentolamine and is completely resistant to both prazosin and yohimbine. Thus, the type of adrenoreceptor involved is quite unclear (vide infra).

In the hypothalamus, Ca^{2+} components to the action potentials recorded from the cell bodies of magnocellular neurons in situ and in vitro have been recorded (Table I). In some studies, the neurones have also been simultaneously identified using immunohistochemistry (e.g., as containing vasopressin) [Theodosis et al., 1983]. In addition, a Ca^{2+} component to the spike produced by these neurones has also been detected in the neurohypophysis using optical techniques (vide supra) [Obaid et al., 1985; Salzberg et al., 1983, 1985].

Ca^{2+} spikes and currents have been investigated in retinal rods and bipolar cells (Table I). In rod inner segments from the salamander, Ca^{2+} currents have been studied in detail using the whole cell patch clamp technique [Bader et al., 1982; Corey et al., 1984]. From a holding potential of -70 mV, an I$_{Ca}$ could be activated at potentials more positive than about -35 mV. The current was maximal at about 0 mV. When EGTA was included in the internal solution, the Ca^{2+} current did not inactivate.

No evidence for a transient current was found. The Ca^{2+} current did "run-down." However, unlike the other cases discussed, inclusion of ATP and cyclic AMP in the internal medium did not stabilize the situation. Clearly, however, apart from this final observation, the current in salamander rods resembles an L-type current. The lack of effect of ATP/cAMP may be significant. However, the effectiveness of this manipulation clearly depends quite a lot on conditions. Thus, Fedulova et al. [1985] observed that cAMP/ATP did not restore the DRG L-current if it had already completely rundown. Thus, the difference may be more apparent than real (vide infra).

Invertebrate neurones. In comparison to the difficulties associated with recording from vertebrate neurones, performing electrophysiological recordings from many invertebrate neurones is a comparatively easy task. The main reason for this is that some of these neurones are truly gigantic, having diameters of over 500 μm with an approximately spherical cell body. In addition, many of these cells have only a single process. The axon can be removed, and the spherical cell body can be used by itself in various types of recording paradigms [Geletyuk and Veprintsev, 1972; Chen et al., 1971]. Consequently, there is an immense amount of information about ionic currents in these cells, and many hundreds of papers have been published on this subject. How do Ca^{2+} currents in such cells compare to those in vertebrate neurones discussed above? In spite of all the information available, it is still difficult to make absolute comparisons. However, I shall now discuss the most relevant points. As so much information is available, I shall not attempt a comprehensive summary of all the papers in this area. The interested reader should refer to several excellent reviews of this field that have appeared in the last few years [Hagiwara, 1983; Kostyuk, 1981; Eckert and Chad, 1984; Adams et al., 1980].

This subject can, in fact, be traced back to 1959 when Hagiwara and Saito [1959] performed an early voltage clamp study on nerve cell bodies from the mollusc *Onchiduim ver-*

ruculatum, an experiment that was well ahead of its time. In retrospect, evidence for a Ca^{2+} current was obtained in these studies. However, as Hagiwara [1983] discusses in his memoir on the subject, the evidence was ignored at the time, as such things were not known to exist in neurones. However, the existence of a Ca^{2+}/Ba^{2+} spike in these neurones was reported in 1961 by Oomura et al. [1961]. In the next dozen years or so there were several observations demonstrating action potential generation by various molluscan neurones in Na^+- free solutions. Ca^{2+} influx in aequorin-loaded cells was also demonstrated [Stinnakre and Tauc, 1973]. Most studies utilized neurones from snails such as *Helix* [Gerasimov, 1964; Kawa, 1979; Meves, 1966, 1968; Standen, 1975; Wald, 1972; Chamberlain and Kerkut, 1967; Kerkut and Gardner 1967; Gerasimov et al., 1965], or giant neurones or bag cell neurones from *Aplysia* [Junge, 1967; Moreton, 1968; Carpenter and Gunn, 1970; Geduldig and Junge, 1968; Horn and Miller, 1977; Junge and Miller, 1974; Kaczmarek et al., 1980; Strumwasser et al., 1981]. The spikes observed in Na^+- free solutions are now known to be Ca^{2+} spikes by all the usual criteria. Initially, however, some authors considered the possibility that the spikes were due to leftover reservoirs of Na^+ which were not removed in the Na^+-free solutions [Meves, 1966; Moreton, 1968; Chamberlain and Kerkut, 1967; Kerkut and Gardner, 1967]. Further examples of Ca^{2+} spikes in invertebrates include neurones from the crayfish X-organ [Iwasaki and Sato, 1971], crab cardiac ganglion [Tazaki and Cooke, 1979], barnacle visual system [Ross and Stuart, 1978; Stuart and Oertel, 1978], Leech Retzius cells [Kleinhaus, 1976; Kleinhaus and Prichard, 1975, 1977] and N-neurones [Johansen et al., 1985], cockroach motoneurones [Pitman, 1979], and grasshopper neurones [Goodman and Heitler, 1979; Goodman and Spitzer, 1981a,b]. The special case of the squid giant neurone will be considered further below. Of particular interest is a recent observation using the giant motor axon of the jellyfish *Aglantha digitale*. This jellyfish is capable of either fast or slow swimming depending on whether it is dining alone or on the run. Mackie and Meech [1985] showed that the two behaviours were associated with different types of axonal electrical activity. During rapid swimming, fast Na$^+$ spikes were generated. However, during more leisurely behaviour, Ca^{2+} spikes were generated by the same axon.

Studies on the distribution of Na$^+$ and Ca^{2+} conductances in invertebrate neurones have led to the general conclusion that whereas both Na$^+$ and Ca^{2+} currents are found in the cell soma, N$^+$ currents are much more prevalent in the axon [Kado, 1973; Wald, 1972; Junge and Miller, 1974]. It should be noted that Ca^{2+} spikes have been demontrated in the axons of *Aplysia* neurones [Horn, 1977, 1978], squid giant neurones [Watanabe et al., 1967a], and in other cases, as well, under some circumstances [Orchard, 1976; Suzuki, 1976]. In the case of the squid giant axon, however, these spikes are blocked by TTX, indicating that they are due to the entry of Ca^{2+} through voltage-sensitive Na$^+$ channels [Watanabe et al., 1967b], an event that has also been recorded by optical methods [Baker et al., 1973]. However, in the other cases referred to, such as the *Aplysia* neurones, the Ca^{2+} spikes obtained appear to be due to Ca^{2+} entry through VSCC, and their properties resemble other bona fide Ca^{2+} spikes.

Since the early 1970s [Geduldig and Gruener, 1970; Krishtal and Magura, 1970] there have been a large number of studies analyzing I$_{Ca}$s in molluscan neurones. In many of the early studies, however, precise characterization of the I$_{Ca}$ was somewhat compromised due to the presence of contaminating outward currents, most of which were presumably carried by K$^+$ [for references on early studies, see Kostyuk, 1984; Eckert and Chad, 1984; Hagiwara and Byerly, 1981; Adams et al., 1980]. However, the subsequent development of perfusion and patch techniques largely eliminated these problems [Kostyuk, 1981, 1984; Eckert and Chad, 1984; Hagiwara and Byerly, 1981; Adams et al., 1980; Chesnoy-Marchais, 1985; Byerly and Moody, 1984; Chad and Eckert, 1985a,b,c; Brown et al.,

1984b; Byerly et al., 1984, 1985; Lemos et al., 1985]. The complementary use of optical methods has also proved valuable [Ahmed and Connor, 1979; Gorman and Thomas, 1980; Gorman et al., 1982, 1984].

The result of all this activity is a picture of an I$_{Ca}$ that looks suspiciously like an L-current. This is not to say that differences do not exist between various sets of investigators. Indeed, there is no reason to assume a priori that all the VSCC being examined in all the different molluscan neurones are exactly the same. This is certainly borne out by studies of channel pharmacology and modulation (vide infra). However, in many cases, results have several features in common. Certain properties of the type of current that is usually observed in most modern investigations can be seen by using an example. Doroshenko et al. [1984a] recorded I$_{Ca}$s in neurones from *Helix pomatia*. The cells were perfused internally with a K$^+$- free solution. Depending on the strength of the depolarizing steps (from a holding potential of -50 mV), various components of the I$_{Ca}$ can be seen. For weak depolarizations, a very persistent current is observed. For stronger depolarizations, the initial portion of the current exhibits a decay which is then followed by a more sustained phase. At very strong depolarizations, the current is diminished by a very rapid decay which completely obliterates the sustained phase prior to the end of the voltage step. The rapid decay phase appears to be due to the activation on "nonspecific" outward currents activated at strong depolarizations, a phenomenon that is frequently observed [Kostyuk and Krishtal, 1977a]. When this current is blocked by raising the internal pH, the rapid phase of the decay disappears. The slow decay process appears to be due to the blockade of I$_{Ca}$ by rising internal Ca^{2+} concentrations (current-dependent inactivation), as it can be removed by intracellular chelators of divalent cations (EGTA/EDTA) or by using Ba^{2+} which does not appear to inactivate I$_{Ca}$ in the same way. As discussed above, it is now quite well established that most L-type Ca^{2+} currents are subject to current-dependent inactivation, which may be looked upon as a major type of negative feedback regulation of VSCC [Eckert and Chad, 1984]. It may result from the operation of a Ca^{2+}-regulated phosphorylation/dephosphorylation cycle with VSCC as substrate [Chad and Eckert, 1985a,b] (vide infra). This appears to be the major form of Ca^{2+} current inactivation for this type of Ca^{2+} current rather than the classical voltage-dependent inactivation associated with Na^+ channels for example, although other kinds of non-voltage-dependent inactivation (habituation) may also occur [Klein et al., 1980]. There is now a colossal amount of biophysical information concerning this process which has been reviewed in incredible detail [Eckert and Chad, 1984]. In spite of this, some reports persist in claiming that this is not the mechanism of Ca^{2+} channel inactivation in neurones [Lux and Brown, 1984b]. It is of course possible that such discrepancies are due to the fact that different authors are looking at different types of current. One need only compare the difference in properties of the T-, N-, and L-currents in DRG cells to see how this could happen. Thus, inactivation of T- or N-type currents may well have a different mechanism. Actually there is very little convincing evidence that more than one type of VSCC is found in molluscan neurones, and many reports that this is so can be explained more parsimoniously. Indeed, Carbone and Lux [1984a] apparently searched for a T-type current in snail neurones and were unable to find one. However, some recent preliminary reports have provided some evidence for molluscan VSC heterogeneity. The first report has indicated that phorbol esters such as TPA can induce a new (second) type of VSCC activity in *Aplysia* bag cell neurones [Strong et al., 1986; see also Chesnoy-Marchais, 1985] (vide infra). A second report is based on the sensitivity of Ca^{2+}- currents to cyclic AMP [Kostyuk et al., 1985]. Both cyclic AMP-dependent and independent VSCC were indicated. Such observations illustrate the similarities between some slowly inactivating Ca^{2+} currents often recorded in molluscan neurones and the DRG L-type current. Thus, some molluscan I_{Ca}s are

blocked by raising intracellular Ca^{2+} [Eckert and Chad, 1984], some molluscan I_{Ca}s are increased by cAMP [Pellmar, 1981; Hockberger and Connor, 1984], and possibly in some cases by protein kinase C-mediated mechanisms [DeRiemer et al., 1985a,b]. Some molluscan I_{Ca}s wash-out (run down), a process that can be retarded by intracellular perfusion with cAMP/Mg-ATP [Doroshenko et al., 1982, 1984a; Kostyuk et al., 1985] (Table X). Molluscan I_{Ca}s are rather sensitive to blockade by Cd^{2+} Byerly et al., 1985] and in some reports (but not others) by dihydropyridines [Nerbonne and Gurnery, 1985; Walden et al., 1985; Walden et al., 1985] (Table VIII). Molluscan I_{Ca}s can also be modulated by certain neurotransmitters, effects possibly mediated by changes in cell Ca^{2+}, cyclic AMP or IP_3-linked mechanisms (vide infra) [Pellmar, 1981, 1984; Pellmar and Carpenter, 1980; Akopyan et al., 1985; Brezina et al., 1985; Colombaioni et al., 1985; Klein et al., 1980; Paupardin-Tritsch et al., 1985a,b] (Table IX). Thus although it would be reasonable to expect some heterogeneity to emerge with respect to Ca^{2+} currents in invertebrate neurones, it seems as though at least some of these strongly resemble one class of VSCC in vertebrate neurones (L-channels).

A particularly important preparation in research on synaptic transmission and the properties of VSCC has been the squid giant axon and giant synapse in the stellate ganglion. The giant synapse is formed at the junction between the pallialis nerve from the brain and the giant motor axon which innervates the squid mantle. Depolarization-induced uptake of Ca^{2+} into the squid axon demonstrated that Ca^{2+} could enter the axon through voltage-sensitive Na^+ channels [Hodgkin and Keynes, 1957; Baker et al., 1971]. Indeed, under peculiar circumstances, Ca^{2+} entering by this route can produce action potentials in the squid giant axon [Watanabe et al., 1967a,b]. The studies of Baker et al. [1973] using aequorin-filled axons then established that there was an additional pathway of "slow" Ca^{2+} entry that could be blocked by Mn^{2+} but not TTX. These studies were subsequently extended using voltage clamped axons by Rojas and Taylor [1975]. More recently, the VSCC in squid axon has actually been demonstrated electrophysiologically [Di Polo et al., 1983]. The current bears some resemblance to an L-type current. Thus, under the particular experimental conditions examined, it inactivated extremely slowly (half-time for inactivation approximately 45 sec). As in other instances, the density of VSCC seems to be much higher in the presynaptic terminal of the squid giant axon. This terminal is extremely large, and several microelectrodes can be readily inserted into it. Ca^{2+} spikes have been recorded in the presynaptic terminal in several studies [Katz and Miledi, 1969, 1971; Llinas et al., 1976a,b]. As neurotransmitter release can be easily assayed in this preparation by recording simultaneously from postsynaptic cell, the preparation provides a unique opportunity for examining the relationship between presynaptic Ca^{2+} currents and transmitter release. This experiment has been performed on a number of occasions [Augustine and Eckert, 1984; Augustine et al., 1985a,b,c; Charlton et al., 1982; Llinas et al., 1976a, 1981; Smith et al., 1985]. Furthermore, complementary data can be obtained by filling the terminal with aequorin [Llinas and Nicholson, 1975]. The results of these studies are most important with respect to the regulation of neurotransmitter release. From the point of view of the present discussion, however, it seems as though the Ca^{2+} current recorded in these terminals appears similar in properties to that found in the axon, as discussed above.

This latter comment, "appears similar to" has appeared several times in the preceding discussion. Such murky conclusions are unfortunately unavoidable at this point. I have used the model of L-, T-, and N-types of VSCC as a basis for comparison between various systems. In some cases, ther are clearly certain similarities between Ca^{2+} currents in other neurones and the three types of current observed in DRG cells. When purely biophysical data are available, "appears similar to" is about as close as one can go in making such comparisons. Biochemical data (e.g., effects

of cAMP and neurotransmitters) and pharmacological data (e.g., sensitivity to drugs) serve to put such comparisons on much firmer ground. However, variations in experimental conditions are so vast that genuine differences in the effects of even specific drugs may occur from one lab to another. However, as we shall see in subsequent discussions, other nonelectrophysiological data have provided evidence that fits in well with much of the preceding discussion.

BIOCHEMICAL AND MOLECULAR PROPERTIES OF NEURONAL CALCIUM CHANNELS

The preceding discussion has illustrated the large amount of data available on the electrophysiological properties of neuronal VSCC. Biochemical data on this same subject has only become available more recently. These data provide us with a different perspective on the same subject. Happily, many of the conclusions that can be reached from biochemical studies fit in well with conclusions from biophysical/electrophysiological studies.

Clearly, one would like to have as deep an understanding of the molecular properties of neuronal VSCC as one has of Na$^+$ channels or nicotinic receptors. This has not been achieved as yet. However, the situation with VSCC in many ways resembles that with the Na+ channel, for example. Indeed, it cannot be considered a coincidence that most of the detailed biochemical work on VSCC has come from laboratories that were already involved with sophisticated studies of Na+ channels. The key to the biochemical identification of ion channels is possession of a molecule, usually a drug or toxin, that binds to the channel with high affinity and specificity. Such a molecule can be used as a probe for identifying the channel protein in membranes or in the soluble state when it is no longer functional. The analogy of the Na$^+$ channel is a good one. In this case there are several types of toxins that interact with the channel at different sites [Catterall, 1984]. The binding of toxin to a particular site may be voltage-dependent. Moreover, many of the sites interact with one another in an interesting fashion. A similar approach has been taken with VSCC, although the situation in this case is somewhat more complex. In the case of VSCC there are no toxins that have as yet been utilized for biochemical studies in a well-established fashion. There are, however, several good candidates for toxins that may eventually play such a role (vide infra). On the other hand, the pharmacology of VSCC is particularly rich. The therapeutic implications of being able to block VSCC in the cardiovascular system has not been lost on a number of pharmaceutical companies. The result is that a vast number of compounds have been synthesized and tested as potential regulators of VSCC. Several classes of substances have emerged as being effective. These include the dihydropyridines, such as nifedipine, the phenylalkylamines, such as verapamil, and the benzothiazepines, such as diltiazem. As we shall see, all of these have been successfully used as probes for VSCC in neuronal and other tissues. Of the various agents available, the dihydropyridines (DHPs) have been the most useful. There are several reasons for this. To begin with, these drugs interact with VSCC with the highest affinities. This is particularly true in depolarized tissue, an observation that has several important implications. Thus, smooth muscle preparations contracted by depolarizing concentrations of K^+ can be relaxed by some DHPs at subnanomolar concentrations. This high affinity interaction is reflected in biochemical paradigms by the presence of high affinity binding sites for tritiated DHPs in the appropriate tissues. A complicating observation is that in some tissues, functioning VSCC do not appear to be blocked at quite such low DHP concentrations. However, as we shall discuss, adequate explanations are available for this phenomenon. The second useful fact about DHPs is the spectrum effects they produce. Thus, some DHPs act as VSCC blockers (antagonists), whereas some act to enhance the time that channels remain open (agonists). A third important issue concerns stereospecificity.

Often, the pure enantiomers of DHPs prove to have different actions. In a relatively simple case, one isomer may be a potent blocker, and the other isomer less potent or inactive. Thus, the (−)isomers of several DHPs are much more potent antagonists than their (+)isomers [Towar et al., 1982]. In the case of the drugs nicardipine and PN200-110, however, this stereospecificity is reversed [Shibanuma et al., 1980]. Furthermore, pure enantiomers of DHPs may also differ in terms of their overall effects. One isomer may be an agonist and the other an antagonist [Bellemann and Franckowiak, 1985; Franckowiak et al., 1985; Hof et al., 1985; Kongsamut et al., 1985a; J.S. Williams et al., 1985]. Thus (+) −202791 is an antagonist and (−) −202791 is an antagonist. This varied pharmacology raises several points. The first is that it is helpful, where possible, to work with pure isomers of any drug. Secondly, it is clear that there are many potential tools available for probing the specificity of drug binding sites. Verapamil-like and diltiazem-like drugs may also be used to identify VSCC biochemically. The pharmacology of such agents is less sophisticated than that of the DHPs. Moreover, these substances are in general less potent and specific than DHPs. However, some structure-activity data are available, and it is clear that the interactions of such substances with VSCC are stereospecific [e.g., Triggle, 1981]. These interactions may also extend to agonist/antagonist differences as well, although there are as yet only hints of this in the literature [Himori et al., 1975, 1976].

Using radiolabeled derivatives of DHPs (nitrendipine, nimodipine, +/− PN200110, BAY K8644 iodipine), phenylalkylamines (verapamil, desmethoxyverapamil, or D-888), or [^{3}H]D-cis-diltiazem, saturable drug binding sites have been observed in the nervous system and other tissues. Before describing some of the properties of these binding sites in brain, it is important to ask some general questions about how we can be sure these sites are indeed VSCC, particularly in the nervous system [Janis and Triggle, 1984;

Miller and Freedman, 1984; Glossmann et al., 1984, 1985; Janis et al., 1985]. It will be quite clear that as drugs such as DHPs are being used to identify VSCC in the nervous system and elsewhere, such studies only relate to the properties of drug-sensitive (L-type?) channels, and shed no light on the properties of the other non-drug-sensitive channels that are known to exist and for which we have as yet no specific biochemical probes.

The detailed pharmacology of drugs that act upon VSCC has invariably demonstrated that at elevated concentrations they also interact with other molecules [Miller and Freedman, 1984]. Such alternative sites include other kinds of channels, i.e., Na$^+$ [Bustamante, 1985; Galper and Catterall, 1979; Clay and Shrier, 1984; Yatani and Brown, 1985] or K$^+$ channels [Gola and Ducreux, 1985; Hume, 1985; Nerbonne and Gurney, 1985] or neurotransmitter receptors [Triggle, 1981; Atlas and Adler, 1981; Bender and Herz, 1985; De Vries and Beart, 1984; Miller and Freedman, 1984; Canter et al., 1984; McLawhon et al., 1981; Thayer et al., 1985]. Because drug-VSCC interactions are clearly voltage-dependent, they often only block VSCC in functioning tissue that maintains a membrane potential at concentrations slightly below those at which they have other non-VSCC-directed actions [Miller and Freedman, 1984] (Table VIII). It is important, therefore, when comparing specificity and affinity of drugs for binding sites in depolarized tissue fragments with their whole tissue pharmacology, to make comparisons with depolarized tissues. For example, the affinity of drugs for smooth muscle binding sites in a membrane preparation can be appropriately compared with their relaxant effects in K$^+$ contracted tissue. Similarly the effects of drugs on K$^+$-evoked neurotransmitter release can be appropriately compared with their affinities for drug binding sites in neuronal tissue. When this is done, it is usually clear that high affinity drug binding sites and VSCC correspond [Bean, 1984; Bolger et al., 1983]. This is true in neuronal tissue in some cases,

as well. For example, the evoked release of transmitter from DRG cells [Perney et al., 1986] or PC12 cells [Toll, 1982; Ogura and Takahashi, 1984; Takahashi and Ogura, 1983; Kongsamut et al., 1985a] is blocked by very low concentrations of DHPs. It should be pointed out that when DHP binding studies were initiated, an interesting anomaly was observed. Thus, although many high affinity DHP binding sites were observed in the nervous system, several processes, such as evoked neurotransmitter release, seemed insensitive to these agents [see Miller and Freedman, 1984]. This raised the question as to whether such binding sites in the nervous system really represented VSCC. However, electrophysiological (vide supra) and neurochemical (vide infra) studies have now made it abundantly clear that DHP-sensitive VSCC do indeed exist in the nervous system in addition to drug-insensitive VSCC. The question is therefore no longer whether [^{3}H]nitrendipine binding sites in the brain are really VSCC, but rather what are the particular functions of this class of VSCC. Where a particular neuronal Ca^{2+} current or process cannot be blocked by DHPs under appropriate conditions, it is presumably mediated by a non-DHP-sensitive VSCC (e.g., T-like or N-like) and is not represented by a DHP binding site. Clearly, therefore, although we may start out with the assumption that neuronal drug binding sites are VSCC, not all neuronal VSCC will be manifest as drug binding sites.

This heterogeneity of VSCC is certainly a complicating factor. Another concerns the voltage dependence of drug action already referred to. It has been proposed that DHP binding sites in membrane fragments that maintain no membrane potential represent inactivated VSCC [Bean, 1984; Sanguinetti and Kass, 1984a,b]. This assumption is valuable in explaining discrepancies that arise between the affinities of DHPs for their binding sites and the concentrations at which they block VSCC in normal polarized tissue. VSCC can clearly exist in several conformations, and it is not unreasonable that drugs should preferentially bind to particular states. In DHP binding studies, lower-affinity drug binding sites can often be observed [Weiland and Oswald, 1985; Green et al., 1985; Janis et al., 1985; Kenessey et al., 1984; Kunze et al., 1985; Marsh et al., 1983; McBride et al., 1984; Rogart et al., 1986; Shrikande et al., 1985]. What are these low affinity sites? One possibility is that in many cases they are not connected with drug actions at VSCC. Thus, saturable binding sites for DHPs and particularly for less specific drugs such as verapamil have been found in many tissues other than nerve and muscle. These tissues include everything from sperm [Kazazoglou et al., 1985; Trimmer et al., 1985] to zucchini [Andrejaus et al., 1985]. Careful analysis of the pharmacological specificities of such sites usually indicates that they are probably not VSCC. Presumably, they represent neurotransmitter receptors (vide supra), other ion channels (vide supra), transport proteins [Gopalkrishnan and Triggle 1984; Striessnig et al., 1985a,b], or other entities. On the other hand, in some cases low affinity sites may represent other conformations of VSCC (e.g, resting or closed states). It might therefore be supposed that upon depolarization, some of these low affinity sites would be converted to high affinity (inactivated) sites. Interestingly, such an increase in the number of high affinity binding sites for DHPs or an apparent increase in K_D in depolarized intact tissue has been observed in a number of cases [Green et al., 1985; Schwartz et al., 1985; Reuter et al., 1985a,b]. A similar phenomenon can be observed in isolated vesicles from cardiac sarcolemma where binding studies can be carried out at different membrane potentials generated by altering the extra- and intra-vesicular ionic composition [Schilling and Brewe, 1985]. A final complicating issue is important with respect to studies of the nervous system. Recent reports have suggested that VSCC may occur in glial cells as well as neurones [MacVicar, 1984; Newman, 1985; Bender and Herz, 1985; Litzinger and Brenneman, 1985; Walz and MacVicar, 1985; Barres et al., 1985]. Nothing is known as yet of the phar-

macology of such channels. However, it is conceivable that some drug binding observed in neuronal tissue could include binding to glial cells. Indeed, a very recent study using spinal cord cultures has suggested that this is the case [Litzinger and Brenneman, 1985]. It has also been suggested that glial binding sites may be connected with a subclass of benzodiazepine receptor [Canter et al., 1984; Bender and Herz, 1985]. However, the overall importance of such a possibility remains to be determined (vide infra).

The above discussion illustrates some of the questions associated with the use of radiolabeled drugs in the identification of VSCC in tissue, with particular reference to neuronal tissue. Actually, neuronal tissue has not normally been the tissue of choice when performing such experiments. Far higher concentrations of drug binding sites are found in skeletal muscle, T-tubules for example, making it a better tissue source for isolation purposes [Janis and Triggle, 1984; Miller and Freedman, 1984; Glossmann et al., 1984; Janis et al., 1985]. Moreover, because of the uncertainties associated with exactly what neuronal drug-sensitive VSCC "do," comparisons between binding and pharmacology have been easier to make in tissues such as smooth muscle [Bolger et al., 1983]. However, a good deal of information on nerve is available. Much of this information, particularly earlier studies, has been reviewed in considerable detail elsewhere. Consequently, I shall only attempt an overview of the situation.

The distribution of high affinity binding sites for DHPs or phenylalkylamines can best be seen by using autoradiographic techniques [Quirion, 1983; Hanada and Tanaka, 1985; Cortes et al., 1982; Ferry et al., 1984a; Gould et al., 1985; Murphy et al., 1982; Titeler et al., 1985]. As far as can be seen to date, the distribution of such sites is identical, as would be expected. The distribution of binding sites is extremely heterogeneous and is reminiscent of the distribution of some neurotransmitter receptors. This has given rise to the suggestion that an "endogenous ligand" for DHP binding sites may exist. Indeed, there is some preliminary evidence for such a substance [Thayer et al., 1984]. However, the existence of this material is certainly not well established at this point. The heterogeneous binding of DHPs does not appear to be associated with blood vessels and is often associated with areas of the brain where many synaptic connections occur, such as the external plexiform layer of the olfactory bulb and the molecular layer of the dentate gyrus. Table II illustrates the distribution of drug binding sites in rat brain. Measurement of drug binding in tissue homogenates from rat and human brain approximately parallels this distribution [Quirion, 1985; Hanada and Tanaka, 1985; Peroutka and Allen, 1983; Supavilai and Karobath, 1984; Gould et al., 1982; Marangos et al., 1982; Schoemaker et al., 1983]. In addition to the brain, autoradiographic studies have also demonstrated DHP binding sites in the anterior and posterior lobes of the pituitary [Titeler et al., 1985].

The high density of drug binding sites in the hippocampus is interesting and has been studied further. Cortes et al. [1982] produced ablations of hippocampal granule cells by local injection of colchicine. Following such treatment, there was a substantial diminution of drug binding in the molecular layer of the dentate gyrus and in the CA3 subfield, whereas other areas of the hippocampus were unaltered. These studies clearly suggest the presence of DHP binding sites on granule cells of the dentate gyrus [see also Gray and Johnston, 1985a,b].

The density of DHP binding sites in the brain is low at early foetal stages and then increases [Erman et al., 1983; Kazazoglou et al., 1983; Marangos et al., 1984]. The rate of appearance of binding sites varies considerably in different brain areas and between tissues. The density of sites in the cerebellum, for example, continues to rise until about 30 days after birth. Comparison with heart or skeletal muscle shows that postnatally, the density of sites in these tissues rises much more rapidly. Similar "development" of DHP binding sites can also be observed in culture using neuroblastoma cells. For example, morphological differentiation of NbR10-A cells with cyclic nucleotides is accompanied by a large increase in the number of DHP binding sites [Nirenberg et al., 1983]. Such increases in binding correlate well with increases in DHP-sensitive Ca^{2+} fluxes observed in this and other cell lines upon differentiation (vide infra) as well as some electrophysiological studies discussed above.

Binding sites for [^{3}H-]DHPs and other VSCC modulators have been studied in detail in a number of tissues. The properties of such binding sites show small but consistent differences from tissue to tissue (see Table III) [Glossmann et al., 1984, 1985; Gould et al., 1983a]. Thus, irrespective of species, the affinity of brain sites for [^{3}H]nimodipine is about 0.6 nM, whereas it is about 0.25 nM in cardiac membranes and about 1.5 nM in skeletal muscle membranes. Preliminary data available from radiation inactivation studies and other sources suggest that the protein involved in each case may be the same. Differences in affinity and other properties may be due to different factors in the environment of the channel. By analogy it is well known that alterations in membrane lipid composition can alter the affinity of ligands for Na$^+$ channels [Talvenheimo, 1985]. Such differences may be important from the regulatory point of view. However, it is also possible that the differences in affinity observed actually reflect differences in the basic structure of the protein in each case [Chin et al., 1985]. It should be pointed out, however, that in general the properties of binding sites in each tissue show many more similarities than differences. For example, each of the three main classes of organic VSCC modulators binds to the channel in a characteristic manner. The basic picture that emerges is that the channel possesses separate binding sites for DHPs, phenylalkylamines, and benzothiazepines, and these three sites can interact with one another. However, it has also been argued that the

TABLE II. Localizations of Specific [³H]Nitrendipine Binding*

High	Low
Molecular layer of dentate gyrus	Habenula
External plexiform layer of olfactory bulb	Periventricular hypothalamus
Superficial cerebral cortex	Zona incerta
Moderate	Corpus callosum
Thalamus	Hippocampal formation
Ventral thalamic nucleus	Fimbria
Lateral thalamic nucleus	Pyramidal cell layer
Posterior thalamic nucleus	Alveus
Substantia nigra	Medial lemniscus
Zona reticulata	Fornix
Hippocampal formation	Crus cerebri
Stratum lacunosum-moleculate	Optic tract
Stratum radiatum	Olfactory bulb
Subiculum	Olfactory nerve layer
Cortex	Lateral olfactory tract
Layer IV	Midbrain
Olfactory bulb	Pons
Glomerular layer	Medulla oblongata
Granule cell layer	

*From Gould et al., 1985.

TABLE III. Three Types (Represented by Brain, Heart, and Muscle) of Particulate Ca²⁺ Channel Binding, Evaluated with [³H]Nimodipine*

Property	Brain	Heart	Muscle
pH profile	Biphasic	ND	Monophasic
Sulfhydryl reagent sensitivity	+	+	+++
Heparin sensitivity	−	+	+++
K_D of nimodipine (at 37°C)	0.6 nM	0.25 nM	2.0 nM
AQA-39 inhibition	−	+	+++
YS 035 inhibition	−	ND	+++
Diltiazem regulation (at 37°C)	+++	++	−
EDTA sensitivity	+++	++	−

*ND, not determined; −, not sensitive; +, low sensitivity; ++, intermediate sensitivity; +++, high sensitive [from Glossmann et al., 1984].

binding sites for phenylalkylamines and benzothiazepines are actually one and the same [Murphy et al., 1983]. Actually, such arguments are quite hard to resolve using pharmacological data, and presumably the truth of the matter will result from purely biochemical studies now in progress. The concept of several interacting drug binding sites on an ion channel is of course not new. Studies on the nicotinic receptor and Na⁺ channel have produced similar conclusions [Catterall, 1984; Dolly and Barnard, 1984]. Because much of the drug binding data have been derived from tissues other than brain, I shall now give a brief "composite" description. Important differences specific for nervous system binding sites will be mentioned in passing.

Most work has been performed using a variety of DHP ligands (vide supra). The high affinity binding sites labelled by these ligands are destroyed following heat treatment of membranes or by a variety of proteolytic enzymes, indicating the protein nature of the channel [Bolger et al., 1983; Fosset et al., 1983; Janis et al, 1984]. Binding in brain is also decreased by certain glycosidases, indicating the possible glycoprotein nature of the channel [Glossmann et al., 1982], an observation confirmed by channel purification studies utilizing lectin affinity columns [Curtis and Catterall, 1983, 1984; Borsotto et al., 1984, 1985]. Binding of DHPs to their "receptor" is pH-sensitive, although the details of this sensitivity in brain and skeletal muscle differ (Table III).

An intriguing, and probably important, aspect of DHP binding is its sensitivity to divalent cations [Glossmann et al., 1984, 1985; Gould et al., 1982, 1983a]. DHP binding can be greatly reduced by pretreatment of membranes with EDTA. This inhibition can be reversed by divalent cations such as Ca^{2+}, Sr^{2+}, or Ba^{2+}. The ability to reconstitute DHP binding with Ca^{2+}, for example, can be blocked by some inorganic ions which normally act as VSCC blockers, such as La^{3+}. Whether, indeed, the ability to reconstitute or block is really connected in some way with an ion's, normal permeability through the channel or whether this similarity is fortuitous is hard to say at this time. It is thought that cations promote the formation of high affinity DHP binding sites from very low-affinity sites [Glossmann et al., 1984, 1985]. The observation that low affinity DHP binding sites exist in various tissues has been referred to above, as well as the implications of these observations. Indeed, low afinity DHP binding in brain has also been "detected" using kinetic arguments [Weiland and Oswald, 1985]. It was postulated that high and low affinity states may be in equilibrium. The detection of such interconvertible states of differing affinity is clearly interesting in the light of electrophysiological data also indicating different binding affinities of drugs to different states of the channel [Hess et al., 1984; Nowycky et al., 1985b], e.g., high affinity binding to the inactivated state [Bean,

1984; Sanguinetti and Kass, 1984a,b]. It is not clear as yet whether biochemists and electrophysiologists are talking about the same thing when they discuss different states. It would obviously be helpful in neurones as in other cases to examine binding in detail in subcellular preparations (e.g., vesicles or synaptosomes) in which the membrane potential can be regulated. As discussed, such experiments have in fact been performed in some muscle preparations [Schilling and Drewe, 1985; Green et al., 1985; Reuter et al., 1985a,b; Schwartz et al., 1985].

Binding of DHPs to their receptor can be inhibited by a variety of agents [Janis and Triggle, 1984; Miller and Freedman, 1984; Glossmann et al., 1984, 1985; Janis et al., 1985]. Clearly, binding is blocked by other DHPs as would be expected. Interestingly, however, under appropriate conditions DHP binding is enhanced by D-cis-diltiazem. Furthermore, DHP binding is reduced by verapamil-like drugs, but incompletely. Detailed analysis of the situation indicates that diltiazem and verapamil act as positive and negative heterotropic allosteric regulators of the DHP binding site, respectively. The binding sites for diltiazem and verapamil can be labelled separately using the appropriate radioactive ligands [Ferry et al., 1984a; Reynolds et al., 1983, 1985; Wagner et al., 1986]. Interactions of a drug at any one site can influence binding at the other two sites in the manner summarized in Figure 2. The data supporting such interactions have been extensively reviewed and can be found in the original studies [reviewed in Janis and Triggle, 1984; Miller and Freedman, 1984; Glossmann et al., 1984, 1985; Janis et al., 1985]. Of particular note are some reports indicating that DHP agonists, such as BAY K8644, interact differently than DHP antagonists. Various kinds of differences have been discovered [Reuter et al., 1985b]. In particular, it seems clear that DHP agonists do not stimulate [^{3}H]diltiazem binding in the same fashion as DHP antagonists do [Schoemaker and Langer, 1985; Glossmann et al., 1984, 1985]. Whether such differences are actually related

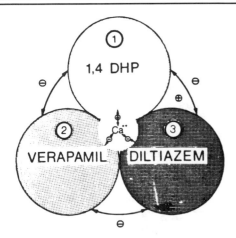

Fig. 2. Interaction of drug binding sites at the calcium channel, as pictured by Glossmann and colleagues [Glossmann et al., 1984].

to the agonist effects of such DHPs is not as yet clear.

A variety of other substances, such as neuroleptics and benzodiazepines, not normally thought of as VSCC modulators can be shown to alter DHP binding [Thorgeirsson and Rudolph, 1984; Gould et al., 1983b, Flaim et al., 1985; Harris et al., 1985b; Mestre et al., 1985; Messing et al., 1985; Quirion et al., 1985; Reynolds et al., 1984]. In some cases, parallel studies have indeed revealed that these agents do possess VSCC blocking actions, and these may help to explain their overall pharmacological effects [Flaim et al., 1985; Mestre et al., 1985; Gould et al., 1983b; Reynolds et al., 1984].

Rather little direct biochemical evidence is available concerning the actual properties of the brain DHP receptor. However, what data there are indicate that the brain receptor is very similar but possibly not identical to the protein in other tissues. Most data have been obtained from skeletal muscle owing to the very high specific activity of binding obtained in purified T-tubular vesicles from this source. The most indirect way of approaching this problem is through the use of radiation inactivation procedures [Janis and Triggle, 1984; Glossmann et al., 1984, 1985; Janis et al., 1985]. Although this kind of technique is fine

for globular proteins in solution, it is frankly exceedingly unreliable for assessing the MW of multisubunit integral membrane proteins. About the best thing that can be said for these studies is that they show that DHP receptors in all tissues are, perhaps not surprisingly, large. Most reports put their size at about 200,000 daltons, which is approximately the same size obtained for virtually every other integral membrane protein assessed by this method. One rather interesting observation, however, has been made by Glossmann and his colleagues [Ferry et al., 1983; Glossmann et al., 1984, 1985]. This group has shown that on preincubation with diltiazem there is apparent loss of mass of about 70,000 daltons from VSCC as assessed by inactivation of [^{3}H-]DHP binding. This of course suggests some conformational change occurs in the channel on binding of diltiazem, probably associated with the dissociation of a diltiazem binding subunit. This is certainly interesting in light of data indicating an interaction between the various binding sites.

Solubilization with the detergents CHAPS or digitonin has provided the most definitive biochemical data on VSCC. The channel can be solubilized from brain or cardiac or skeletal muscle in a state in which [^{3}H-]DHP binding can still be modulated by both verapamil and diltiazem in an appropriate fashion [Curtis and Catterall, 1983, 1984, 1985a,b; Borsotto et al., 1984, 1985; Rengasamy et al., 1985]. In skeletal muscle, at any rate, there is some agreement that the DHP receptor consists of three subunits of MW $130(\alpha)$, $50(\beta)$, and $33(\gamma)$ K_D or 142, 33, and 32 KD, estimates that seem rather close. Recent data have indicated that the structure of the brain receptor may be somewhat different. Specific antisera have been raised against skeletal muscle α-, β-, and γ-subunits [Chin et al., 1985]. Antisera against the β- and γ-subunits cross-reacted with proteins from brain but antisera against the α-subunit did not. Thus on the basis of this immunological evidence, it may be supposed that the α-subunits in brain and skeletal muscle differ structurally in at least some minor fashion. Such differences could be the basis of the somewhat different properties associated with DHP binding observed in tissues (vide supra).

It is unclear as yet which subunits are responsible for binding the various types of ligands. Affinity labelling has been achieved in a preliminary manner with a variety of DHP derivatives. However, it should be pointed out that at this time the use of any of these probes needs to be further substantiated. Affinity labelling has identified binding structures with MWs of 145,000 [Ferry et al., 1984b], 32,000 [Campbell et al., 1984], 42,000 [Venter et al., 1983], and 50,000 [Sarmiento et al., 1985] daltons, depending on the tissue used and the conditions employed. Other indications suggest that a verapamil binding protein can exist, at least in heart, in a form separate from the DHP and diltiazem binding entities [Garcia et al., 1984b]. Thus, it may be that verapamil binds to a separate subunit.

A particularly interesting question relates to the potential modifiability of these channels. Curtis and Catterall [1985a] have demonstrated that, depending on conditions, both the α- and β-subunits of purified skeletal muscle receptors are substrates for cAMP-mediated phosphorylation. In heart, a 42,000-dalton DHP binding protein has also been reported to be a substrate for phosphorylation [Horne et al., 1984].

A further interesting and important group of studies relate to data on reconstitution of VSCC [Curtis and Catterall, 1985b]. Only preliminary reports have as yet emerged on reconstitution of purified (three subunit) DHP receptors. These studies indicate, however, that the purified three-subunit complex from skeletal muscle T-tubules may be identical with functional VSCC—a most important point. VSCC in membrane fractions have also been successfully reconstituted in a functional state. Sources of VSCC for these studies have been skeletal muscle T-tubules [Affolter and Coronado, 1985], cardiac sarcolemmal vesicles [Ehrlich et al., 1985; Rosenberg et al., 1986], or, significantly for the present discussion, brain synaptosomes [Nelson, 1985; Nelson et al., 1984]. In the case of skeletal muscle and heart, the reconstituted channels were shown to be sensitive to both DHP agonists and antagonists. However, in the case of brain, the reconstituted channel is apparently drug-sensitive [Nelson, 1985]. Such an observation fits well with the postulated synaptosomal localization of N-type VSCC (vide infra). Apart from anything else, these studies indicate that VSCC can function in the absence of any endogenous ligand. However, such a substance if it exists could still act normally to modulate their activity. Another set of experiments has also succeeded in obtaining the expression of neuronal VSCC in oocytes following the injection of mRNA from the brain (and other tissues) [Dascal et al., 1985a,b].

In addition to these biochemical studies, other molecular biophysical studies are helping to provide a picture of the way in which Ca^{2+} actually traverses drug-sensitive VSCC. The channel appears to be a large pore with a diameter no less than 6 Å at its narrowest point [McClesky and Almers, 1985; McClesky et al., 1986a]. Selectivity of the channel for Ca^{2+} appears to be the result from high affinity binding of Ca^{2+} to sites within the channel pore. Indeed, in the absence of Ca^{2+}, VSCC are rather nonselective [Hess and Tsien, 1984; McClesky and Almers, 1985; Hess et al., 1986; Lansman et al., 1986; McClesky et al., 1986a]. It will be interesting to see whether the structures of binding sites within VSCC resemble that of other high affinity Ca^{2+} binding proteins, such as calmodulin.

With respect to VSCC biochemistry, another recent set of observations is of note. Nahorski and his colleagues [Kendall and Nahorski, 1985] have demonstrated that depolarization of slices from various brain regions can lead to an increase in IP$_3$ synthesis that can be blocked by nitrendipine and enhanced by BAY K8644. Moreover, studies in skeletal [Veraga et al., 1985] and smooth muscle [Kobayashi et al., 1985b] also indicate that depolarization can lead directly to IP$_3$ production and Ca^{2+} mobilization from intracellular stores. Whether this IP_3 synthesis is the result of Ca^{2+} influx via VSCC resulting in the stimulation of phospholipase C or whether it is the result of the direct modulation of an enzyme-linked coupling mechanism (a voltage-sensitive G-protein?) remains to be seen. However, the fact that a link may exist between mechanisms for Ca^{2+} influx and Ca^{2+} mobilization is extremely interesting.

VOLTAGE-SENSITIVE CALCIUM FLUXES IN NEURONES

The technique of depolarization-induced $^{45}Ca^{2+}$ influx has been widely used in many laboratories to examine neuronal VSCC. In particular, as previously mentioned, such techniques are currently the most direct available for examining the properties of VSCC in nerve terminals which are not amenable to direct recording methods. The use of giant synaptosomal preparations may be a way around this difficulty [Umbach et al., 1984]. Flux experiments have been designed to investigate the properties of neuronal VSCC per se and, in addition, they have often been used to examine the effects of drugs on neuronal VSCC. With respect to the latter, it has frequently been suggested that if the depolarization-induced influx of $^{45}Ca^{2+}$ into synaptosomes is inhibited by a particular drug then this reflects an action of the drug on neuronal VSCC. Naturally, such a conclusion is only valid if $^{45}Ca^{2+}$ influxes really measure Ca^{2+} movement through VSCC. As it turns out, this is only the case under particular conditions which have been realized relatively recently. Thus, although there is a huge amount of literature on $^{45}Ca^{2+}$ fluxes in neuronal tissue and their modulation by drugs, very little of it can be interpreted unequivocally with respect to actions at VSCC.

It is probably best to approach these studies by describing the situation as it is presently understood. This will enable us to place both older and newer studies in their proper perspectives. When performing Ca^{2+} influx studies, most workers have examined the influx of $^{45}Ca^{2+}$ into synaptosomal preparations or neuronal cell lines. Interestingly, the picture that emerges from these two systems is strikingly different. However, it can be nicely integrated into the scenario discussed above on multiple types of neuronal VSCC. In addition to $^{45}Ca^{2+}$ fluxes, some studies have also utilized optical methods [Ashley et al., 1984; Heinonen et al., 1985]. Indeed, several such studies have already been mentioned above.

There are certain problems associated with the interpretation of $^{45}Ca^{2+}$ influx data using synaptosomes (vide supra). In particular, the heterogeneity of the preparation means that the results obtained are necessarily an overall average picture, and individual neuronal differences, which may be of great importance, are likely to be missed. A general consensus now appears to have been reached about the basic pattern of polarization-induced $^{45}Ca^{2+}$ fluxes seen in synaptosomes. The important conclusions reached from these studies make a great deal of sense in the light of the electrophysiological studies discussed above. Much of this work is the result of a long series of studies conducted by Blaustein and his colleagues. Initially, Blaustein demonstrated that the rate of $^{45}Ca^{2+}$ influx into synaptosomes was greatly increased upon depolarization [Blaustein, 1975; reviewed in McGraw et al., 1982]. These influxes could be blocked by inorganic VSCC blockers, and so it was suggested that they represented the movement of Ca^{2+} through VSCC. This has ultimately proved to be only partly true. Using methods with increased time resolution, Nachshen and Blaustein observed that depolarization-induced $^{45}Ca^{2+}$ influx seemed to occur in two phases. The initial "fast phase" appeared to be complete within a second or two, whereas the second "slow phase" occurred over many seconds or minutes [Nachshen, 1984, 1985; Drapeau and Nachshen, 1984; Nachshen and Blaustein, 1980, 1982]. It was also observed that the properties of these two phases differed profoundly in several ways. For example, the rapid phase was considerably more sensitive to blockade by inorganic VSCC blockers than the slow phase [Nachshen, 1984, 1985; Drapeau and Nachshen, 1984; Nachshen and Blaustein, 1980, 1982]. Moreover, it was also demonstrated that the rapid phase underwent rapid inactivation that appeared to be voltage-dependent rather than current-dependent [Nachshen, 1984, 1985; Drapeau and Blaustein, 1983; Nachshen and Blaustein, 1980]. It was therefore suggested that the observations were consistent with the existence of two types of VSCC in synaptosomes that mediated the fast and slow phases of ^{45}Ca^{2+} uptake, respectively. Such fast and slow phases of depolarization-induced ^{45}Ca^{2+} uptake have been reproduced in several laboratories [Harris, 1984; Harris and Bruno, 1985; Hoss and Formaniak, 1984; Harris et al., 1985b; Leslie et al., 1983a,b]. The relative contributions of the two phases differ in different brain areas [Leslie et al., 1983a]. An important advance, however, was subsequently made by Turner and Goldin [1985a]. These workers found that the slow phase could be abolished by substituting all the external Na$^+$ by choline. They concluded that the slow phase actually represented a reversal of the electrogenic Na$^+$/Ca^{2+} exchange that is known to exist in synaptosomes. These observations are certainly consistent with all the previous data. Thus, it appears that only the rapid phase of ^{45}Ca^{2+} uptake truly reflects flux via VSCC. These observations allowed previous studies to be put into proper perspective. When experiments with synaptosomes have utilized fluxes in the range of < 1 sec to about 2 sec, they represent VSCC. Several studies conducted over several seconds, say 3–15, really represent fluxes mediated by a combination of VSCC and Na$^+$/Ca^{2+} exchange. Studies carried out over long periods of time, however, probably only reflect Na$^+$/Ca^{2+} exchange, as the relatively small fluxes via the rapidly inactivating VSCC are effectively masked. If such a model is accepted, a great deal of sense can be made out of the reported observations. If the rapid phase of uptake reflects VSCC function, can

the properties of these VSCC be compared with those described electrophysiologically in vertebrate neurones? Let us consider the properties of the rapid flux. The VSCC mediating this flux are permeable to Ca^{2+}, Sr^{2+}, and Ba^{2+} [Nachshen and Blaustein, 1982] and also Mn^{2+} [Drapeau and Nachshen, 1984]. Secondly, the VSCC undergo a rapid voltage-dependent inactivation [Nachshen, 1985; Drapeau and Blaustein, 1983; Leslie et al., 1985; Nachshen and Blaustein, 1980, 1982]. Thirdly, the rapid phase VSCC are very sensitive to blockade by inorganic VSCC blockers. Of particular interest are their great sensitivity to Cd^{2+} and also La^{3+} [Nachshen, 1984]. Furthermore, it appears that these VSCC may be blocked by the ω-toxin from Conus geographus (vide infra) [Kerr and Yoshikami, 1984; Hirning and Miller, unpublished observations]. Comparison of such data with the electrophysiological observations discussed previously shows that the N-channel described by Nowycky et al. [1985a], has properties suspiciously like the VSCC mediating the rapid flux. The rapid flux has been shown to be responsible for the influx of Ca^{2+} that triggers the release of neurotransmitter in several cases [Drapeau and Blaustein, 1983; Drapeau and Nachshen, 1984; Leslie et al., 1985]. Thus, it might be postulated that an N-type VSCC-mediated Ca^{2+} influx is responsible for stimulus-secretion coupling from nerve terminals in many cases. Further evidence on this point will be discussed below. One further feature of N-type channels is that they are insensitive to modulation by DHPs [Nowycky et al., 1985a]. It is therefore instructive to ask whether this is also true of rapid phase fluxes. Here we run into something of a discrepancy, although most of the data are still consistent with the above hypothesis. The effects of organic VSCC blockers on fluxes into synaptosomes have been examined in several cases (Table IV) [Nachshen, 1985; Akerman and Nicholls, 1981; Aronstam and Hoss, 1985; Turner and Goldin, 1985a; Nachshen and Blaustein, 1980, 1979b; Norris and Bradford, 1985; Taft and DeLorenzo,

TABLE IV. Some Observations on the Modulation of Voltage-Sensitive Calcium Fluxes in Neurones*

Organic VSCC modulators

D-600 blocks F and S with similarly low potency [Nachshen and Blaustein, 1980]

F only blocked by Nit > 10^{-5} M [Daniell et al., 1983]

VP (mM) blocks S [Akerman and Nicholls, 1981]

VP (μM or less) blocks S [Norris and Bradford, 1985]

VP Cn, Flu block F/S 40%, 1–10 μM [Wibo et al., 1983]

D-600 > 10^{-5} M blocks F/Z (?) in neurohypophysis [Dreifuss et al., 1973]

VP, D-600 > 10^{-5} M partly blocks F/S mixture. Nif no effect [Nachshen and Blaustein, 1979b]

F is partly but potently blocked by DHPs, D-600, and DZ [Turner and Goldin, 1985a]

BAY K8644 no effect on F/S [Rampe et al., 1984]

BAY K8644 increases F [Turner and Goldin, 1985b]

DHPs do not block F/S even with predepolarization [Harris et al., 1985a]

BAY K8644 small increase in S [Woodward and Leslie, 1985]

Nim $IC_{50} \simeq 10^{-6}$ inhibits F/S mixture [Nordstrom et al., 1986]

Nit and BAY K8644 potently alter fluxes in cultures of cerebellar granule cells [Carboni and Wojcik, 1985]

Depolarization-induced increase in quin-2 signal in some diencephalic neurones blocked by nitrendipine [Connor, 1985]

Predepolarization increases effect of VP in F [Nachshen, 1985]

Benzodiazepines

Diazepam enhances evoked Ca fluxes, and

this is reversed by DHPs [Mendelson et al., 1984]

S is blocked by benzodtazepines and DHPs at mM concentrations [Taft and DeLorenzo, 1984]

Narcotics

S is blocked by morphine [Kamikubo et al., 1983; End et al., 1981]

Morphine has no effect on F/S [Leslie et al., 1982]

Adenosine

Adenosine blocks F/S [Wu et al., 1982; Ribeiro et al., 1979]

Adenosine has no effect [Barr et al., 1985]

Other agents

ETOH blocks F. Extent depends on brain region [Leslie et al., 1983b]

Phenothiazines (10^{-6}–10^{-3}) block F/S [Hoss and Formaniak, 1984]

Melatonin blocks S 10^{-8}–10^{-6} [Vacus et al., 1984]

Colchicine (10^{-2} M) blocks S $\simeq$ 58% [O'Leary and Suszkiw, 1983]

4-AP (10^{-4} M) enhances evoked Ca^{2+} influx. Mostly F. [Agoston et al., 1983]

Tricyclic antidepressants (10^{-6}–10^{-3}) block F/S [Aronstam and Hoss, 1985]

Phenytoin blocks F. $IC_{50} \simeq 10^{-4}$ M [Harris et al., 1985b; Sohn and Ferrendelli, 1973]

F blocked by phenytoin, pentobarbital, ETOH. IC_{50} = 1 mM, 1 mM and 1,000 nM [Harris and Bruno, 1985]

F blocked by ETOH $IC_{50} \simeq$ 400 nM [Harris, 1984]

Ca flux blocked by phenytoin [Sohn and Ferrendelli, 1976; Pincus and Hsaio, 1981; Ferrendelli and Daniels-McQueen, 1982]

*F, Fast phase Ca^{2+} flux; S, slow phase Ca^{2+} flux; F/S, mixed flux; VP, verapamil; Nim, nimodipine; Nit, nitrendipine; Cn, cinnarizine; Flu, flunirazine.

1984; Daniell et al., 1983; Dreifuss et al., 1973; Harris et al., 1985b; Rampe et al., 1984; Wibo et al., 1983]. In most cases, DHPs even at high concentrations appear rather ineffective in blocking rapid fluxes, and indeed, they are also usually ineffective in blocking neurotransmitter release (vide infra). However, this does have its limits. For example, it can be shown that synaptosomal $^{45}Ca^{2+}$ fluxes can be blocked by DHPs at concentrations approaching 1 mM [Taft and De-

Lorenzo, 1984]. Effects of various VSCC blockers have indeed been observed at elevated concentrations. However, in virtually every case, these effects are clearly exerted on the slow rather than the fast phase of evoked $^{45}Ca^{2+}$ influx (Table IV). Thus, these observations only further illustrate that many of these agents are nonspecific when used at higher concentrations and will readily inhibit Na^+/Ca^{2+} exchange, among other things. If we accept the fact that the rapid phase is basically resistant to DHPs, its properties resemble an N-type channel even more closely. However, there are observations that do not quite fit in with this picture. As discussed above, DHP-sensitive VSCC do appear to exist in the nervous system by biochemical and electrophysiological criteria. Why is it then that they have not in general been observed in rapid flux measurements in synaptosomes? One possibility is that N-type channels are selectively localized in nerve terminals and mediate transmitter release, whereas DHP-sensitive VSCC are found in other regions of the neurone such as the soma and subserve other functions. Alternatively, DHP-sensitive VSCC may occur in nerve terminals but may only be activated under certain conditions which are not usually achieved during flux experiments. Another possibility is that DHP-sensitive VSCC are found in terminals and normally mediate transmitter release but only do so in a minority of cases and are, therefore, not seen in a highly heterogeneous synaptosomal preparation. As we shall see, there is evidence that all of these possibilities may be important. It is interesting to note in passing a recent observation using cultures of neocortical neurones which contain a variety of neuronal types. Connor [1985] observed that many neurones exhibited an increased Ca^{2+} influx upon depolarization as assessed by an increase in quin-2 fluorescence. However, only in a minority of cases was this blocked by DHPs. This indicates that only some neurones may contain DHP-sensitive VSCC. For example, DHP-sensitive VSCC appear to be present as assessed by fluxes in cultures of cerebellar granule cells [Carboni and Wojcik, 1985]. At any rate, we might speculate from the evidence discussed so far that in most, but not all, cases, it is a N-type channel that mediates stimulus-secretion coupling in nerve terminals.

Recently, however, Turner and Goldin [1985a,b] have reported that when synaptosomal rapid phase fluxes are very carefully examined, effects of organic VSCC modulators can be observed. In contrast to previous studies, they observed that a portion of the rapid phase could be blocked by a group of drugs including DHPs at low concentrations [Turner and Goldin, 1985a]. This portion approached 50% of the flux in some cases. Furthermore, these authors also found that a similar portion of evoked transmitter release could also be blocked. In addition, they have recently observed that rapid phase flux could be enhanced by BAY K8644 [Turner and Goldin, 1985a]. A further complication concerns observations recently reported by Nachshen [1985] that predepolarization could enhance the blocking effects of both inorganic VSCC blockers and verapamil on the rapid phase of influx. This indicates that the effects of drugs observed may depend quite critically on the way in which the experiment is carried out. However, it should be noted that predepolarization has been reported to not enhance the effects of DHPs on rapid phase fluxes in another study [Harris et al., 1985b]. Having said this, however, there is nothing particularly obvious in the method of Turner and Goldin that would explain why they have observed the effects that they have. One possibility is that these authors have more effectively excluded slow phase Na$^+$/Ca^{2+} exchange contamination than other groups. Clearly these studies need to be confirmed [as possibly in Carboni and Wojcik, 1985; Woodward and Leslie, 1985] and extended, as they have interesting implications. In summary, therefore, it is clear that the majority of rapid phase fluxes into synaptosomes and, moreover, the majority of cases of evoked neurotransmitter release (vide infra) seem to utilize a DHP-insensitive N-type VSCC. The contribution of DHP-sensitive VSCC to these processes appears unclear. Some evidence suggests that such VSCC contribute to synaptosomal VSCC fluxes but many do not. I shall attempt to further integrate these VSCC into an overall model following the subsequent discussion of neurotransmitter release mechanisms.

In addition to organic VSCC blockers, there are many other reports on the effects of drugs on depolarization-induced influxes of $^{45}Ca^{2+}$ into synaptosomes (Table IV). These include benzodiazepines [Taft and DeLorenzo, 1984; Leslie et al., 1980a; Mendelson et al., 1984b], ethanol [Harris, 1984; Harris and Hood, 1980; Leslie et al., 1983b], phenytoin and barbiturates [Harris, 1984; Blaustein and Ector, 1975; Ferrendelli and Daniels-McQueen, 1982; Harris and Bruno, 1985; Elrod and Leslie, 1980; Sohn and Ferrendelli, 1973, 1976; Pincus and Hsaio, 1981; Harris et al., 1985b; Leslie et al., 1980b], melatonin [Vacas et al., 1984], opiates [Hoss and Formaniak, 1983; End et al., 1981; Kamikubo et al., 1983; Leslie et al., 1982; West et al., 1982; Yamamoto et al., 1981], tricyclic antidepressants [Aronstam and Hoss, 1985], colchicine [O'Leary and Suszkiw, 1983], neuroleptics [Hoss and Formaniak, 1984; Leslie et al., 1979], 4-aminopyridine [Agoston et al., 1983], and adenosine analogues [Barr et al., 1985; Ribeiro et al., 1979; Wu et al., 1982]. As with studies on VSCC blockers, many of these studies have only served to show that certain drugs can alter slow phase Na^+/Ca^{2+} exchange rather than anything else (Table IV). However, in other cases, a genuine effect on fast phase VSCC is apparent. In most instances, however, the effects observed are not particularly potent but may be of therapeutic importance in some cases. Of particular interest are two reports of enhancement of voltage-dependent uptake by 4-aminopyridine [Agoston et al., 1983] and diazepam [Mendelson et al., 1984b], rather than inhibition. Similar enhancing effects of 4-AP have also been observed electrophysiologically [Rogawski and Barker, 1983]. The report that diazepam enhances evoked $^{45}Ca^{2+}$ influx is interesting as it was reported to be blocked by DHPs. However, other workers have reported that benzodiazepines produce the opposite effects [Taft and DeLorenzo, 1984]. Moreover, as both the reports on benzodiazepines examined synaptosomal fluxes after several minutes and were, therefore, presumably examining Na^+/Ca^{2+} exchange, it is hard to know exactly what to make of them.

Voltage-sensitive $^{45}Ca^{2+}$ uptake or increases in quin-2 fluorescence has also been examined in a variety of clonal neuronal cell lines (Table V). Such cell lines appear to contain a variety of VSCC, just as authentic neurones (vide supra). Indeed, DHP-sensitive VSCC in neuronal cells were first observed in neuronal cell lines using flux techniques [Freedman et al., 1984]. Both T-type and L-type channels have been reported in a number of cases [Fishman and Spector, 1981; Tsunoo et al., 1984, 1985a]. Interestingly, $^{45}Ca^{2+}$ fluxes in these cells have revealed only L-type channels which appear relatively uncontaminated by Na^+/Ca^{2+} exchange or other problems [Freedman et al., 1984]. Thus upon depolarization, an increased uptake of $^{45}Ca^{2+}$ is observed which can be shown to be entirely due to flux via VSCC even if incubations are continued for several minutes. In all cases where the pharmacology of these fluxes has been examined, the VSCC involved are very sensitive to DHPs and other organic VSCC modulators [Freedman and Miller, 1984; Freedman et al., 1984a,b; Kongsamut et al., 1985a; Nirenberg et al., 1983]. Moreover, if cells are depolarized by raising K^+, the resulting fluxes can be blocked by VSCC blockers at concentrations comparable to their effects in smooth muscle depolarized the same way. It is interesting to note that in some cell lines the expression of DHP sensitive fluxes is associated with morphological differentiation of the cells [Freedman et al., 1984a; Nirenberg et al., 1983]. If cell lines such as NG108-15, N4TG1, or NBr10a are differentiated with cyclic nucleotides or other appropriate substances, there is a substantial increase in DHP-sensitive $^{45}Ca^{2+}$ uptake and also a similar increase in high affinity [^3H]-DHP binding. It is not clear why these cell lines show predominantly DHP-sensitive fluxes, whereas those in synaptosomal preparations are predominantly sensitive. One possibility is that it is due to the fact that most of the lines that have been investigated are related to the original C1300 line. It is possible, therefore, that this particular phenotype was characteristic of the original tumor. In a survey including other unrelated cell lines, one might turn up a cell type exhibiting predominantly DHP-insensitive synaptosomal type (N-type?) fluxes. A further possibility is that as fluxes are performed on cultures of whole cells, they may predominantly reflect fluxes into the cell soma. If DHP-sensitive VSCC were predominantly localized in this portion of the cell, then they would dominate fluxes measured in whole cells rather than in synaptosomes. At any rate, those lines so far examined are excellent models for investigating neuronal phenomena mediated by L-type VSCC. This includes DHP-sensitive neurotransmitter release (vide infra). It should also be noted that Ca^{2+} fluxes in adrenal medullary cells appear to be blocked quite effectively by DHPs [Sasakawa et al., 1984]. These cells also contain [^{3}H]DHP binding sites [Garcia et al., 1984a; Sasakawa et al., 1984]. This is also true of PC12 pheochromocytoma cells [Toll, 1982; Takahashi and Ogura, 1983; Harris et al., 1985a; Greenberg et al., 1984; Meldolesi et al., 1984]. Release of catecholamines from both cell types is also sensitive to these same drugs, at least when nondifferentiating culture conditions are utilized (vide infra) [Takahashi and Ogura, 1983; Albus et al., 1984; Garcia et al., 1984a; Harris et al., 1985a; Kongsamut et al., 1985a,b; Shalaby et al., 1984; Sasakawa et al., 1984].

CALCIUM CHANNELS AND NEUROTRANSMITTER RELEASE

A further valuable way in which to ascertain the properties of VSCC in neurones is to examine the consequences of their activation. Clearly, Ca^{2+} entering a neurone may trigger many events depending on the type of neurone and the position in the neurone where the VSCC are located. For example, as discussed above, Ca^{2+} ions are clearly concerned in the regulation of a number of types of ion channels. Thus, spike AHPs which are usually due to the activation of I$_{K(Ca)}$ can often be used to obtain information about the

influx of Ca^{2+} that triggers them. Moreover, incoming Ca^{2+} may be associated with phenomena such as increased protein phosphorylation [Zurgil and Zisapel, 1983] or increases in cGMP concentrations [Study et al., 1978], the significance of which is not completely clear at this time. However, by far, the best-characterized function of VSCC in neurones is mediation of the entry of Ca^{2+} for the release of neurotransmitters following depolarization of the nerve terminal (stimulus-secretion coupling). It is established without question that during the depolarization-induced release of transmitter-containing vesicles, influx of Ca^{2+} from the cell exterior is required. Evidence for this scheme was obtained in now classical studies utilizing the frog neuromuscular junction and squid giant synapse preparations [reviewed in Llinas and Walton, 1980]. Thus, it has often been shown that the evoked release of transmitter can be blocked in Ca^{2+}-free medium or by inorganic cations that block all types of VSCC. Although all this is clear, further information may be obtained by asking the question, What types of VSCC are concerned in the stimulus-secretion coupling process? This is particularly relevant from the point of view of the present discussion. Thus, if [^{3}H]DHP binding sites in neurones represent functional VSCC, we might expect to find examples in which transmitter release was modulated by organic VSCC modulating agents. Indeed, in many ways the same considerations apply to the study of drug effects on transmitter release as apply to the investigations on ^{45}Ca^{2+} fluxes discussed above. It should also be noted that modulation of transmitter release by drugs may have direct practical implications for potential drug therapy. Thus, the use of VSCC modulators as neuroactive agents may represent an entirely novel approach to therapy in a number of cases.

The clearest case of modulation of transmitter release by DHPs is found with PC12 cells. As already discussed, voltage-sensitive ^{45}Ca^{2+} fluxes in these cells are potently blocked by DHPs such as nitrendipine and enhanced by VSCC agonists such as BAY K8644. The evoked release of catecholamines from these cells parallels the Ca^{2+} flux data precisely (Tables V and VI). Low concentrations of DHPs are effective. An analogy can be drawn here to the effects of DHPs on smooth muscle, as already mentioned. Thus, it is clear that when smooth muscle is contracted by K^+ polarization, it can be relaxed by low concentrations of DHPs that clearly correspond to the actions of these agents at high affinity binding sites. This fits in well with ideas correlating such high affinity sites with inactivated channels (vide supra). Similarly, if DHP-sensitive (L-type) channels are involved in stimulus-secretion coupling, transmitter release should be blocked by low concentrations of DHPs if high K^+ is used as a stimulus. This is true, at any rate, if the drug-sensitive VSCC in neurones and smooth muscle are basically similar, which seems to be the case. In the case of the PC12 cell, the VSCC mediating transmitter release are indeed blocked by low drug concentrations.

TABLE V. Some Observations on Neurotransmitter Release and Calcium Fluxes in Clonal Cell Lines and Adrenal Chromaffin Cells*

Neuroblastomas
  NG108-15, NCB-20, and N4TG1 cells. Fluxes potently blocked by DHPs. Fluxes modulated by cyclic nucleotides in culture [Freedman et al., 1984a]
  NBr10A, NBr20A exhibit [^{3}H]nitrendipine binding and DHP-sensitive fluxes when cultured with cyclic nucleotides [Nirenberg et al., 1983; Rotter et al., 1979]
  NG108-15 fluxes modulated by (+) and (−)−202791 [Kongsamut et al., 1985a]
  NG108-15, N1E-115, NH15CA2. Fluxes blocked by veratridine and batrachotoxin [Kongsamut et al., 1985b]
  NG108-15 fluxes enhanced by BAY K8644 and CGP 28392 [Freedman and Miller, 1984]
  NG108-15 fluxes enhanced by maitotoxin [Freedman et al., 1984b]
  DHP-sensitive Ca fluxes in single NG108-15 cells using quin-2 method [Perney et al., 1984]
  DHP-sensitive fluxes in NG108-15 cells [Carboni and Wojcik, 1985]
  VP blocks Ca flux in SH-SY5Y cells [Scott et al., 1985]
  DHP block substance P release from F11 cells (Perney et al., 1986]
PC12 cells
  BAY K8644 blocks [^{3}H]DHP binding to PC12 cells and enhances Ca fluxes [Greenberg et al., 1984, 1985]
  DHPs modulate PC12 NE release [Shalaby et al., 1984]
  Kinetics of Ca fluxes in PC12 cells [Stallcup, 1979]

[^{3}H]HP binding to PC12 cells. Ca fluxes are modulated by DHPs [Toll, 1982]
PC12 Ca fluxes blocked by nicardipine [Takahashi and Ogura, 1983; Ogura and Takahashi, 1984]
PC12 Ca fluxes are blocked by TPA (phorbol esters) [Harris et al., 1985a]
PC12 NE release is modulated by (+) and (−)−202791 [Kongsamut et al., 1985a]
[^{3}H]DHP binding to PC12. DHPs modulate NE release [Albus et al., 1984]
PC12 Ca flux blocked by VP [Meldolesi et al., 1984]
NGF regulates DHP sensitivity of PC12 NE release but not Ca flux [Kongsamut and Miller, 1986]
NGF regulates DHP sensitivity of PC12 NE release [Takahashi et al., 1985]
PC12 Fluxes blocked by phenytoin [Messing et al., 1985]
Adrenal chromaffin cells
  DHPs modulate Ca flux and catecholamine release from adrenal cells [Sasakawa et al., 1984]
  BAY K8644 enhances catecholamine release from adrenals. [^{3}H]DHP binding to adrenal [Garcia et al., 1984a; Montiel et al., 1984]
  CGP 28392 and BAY K8644 enhance adrenal catecholamine release [Holden and Knight, 1984]
  VP blocks adrenal Ca flux and catecholamine release [Sasakawa et al., 1983]
  D-600 blocks adrenal Ca flux and catecholamine release [Corcoran and Kirschner, 1983]
  NGF regulates adrenal NE release [Takahashi et al., 1985]

*VP, verapamil; DHP, dihydropyridine.

TABLE VI. Some Effects of Organic Calcium Channel Modulators on Neurotransmitter Release*

Frog neuromuscular junction
  No effect of VP or Pren $< 3 \times 10^{-4}$ M [Van der Kloot and Kita, 1975]
  VP 5×10^{-5} M. No effect on miniature end plate potentials [Nachshen and Blaustein, 1979b]
  VP and D-600. No effect except and high concentrations where they block. Action potential propagation [Gotgil'f and Magazanik, 1977]
Guinea pig ileum
  VP 10^{-6} M. No effect on ACh release [Rezvani et al., 1983]
  D-600, Nic, DZ 10^{-5} M. No effect on ACh release [Kaplita and Triggle, 1983]
Heart
  Nif $> 10^{-6}$ M reduces evoked NE release [Starke and Schumann, 1973]
  VP $> 10^{-5}$ M reduces evoked NE release [Haeusler, 1972]
  VP, D-600, Pren $> 10^{-5}$ M reduces evoked NE release [Gothert et al., 1979]
  DZ 10^{-5} M reduces evoked NE release [Zelis et al., 1982]
Arteries, veins, etc.
  VP, Nif 2×10^{-5} M. No effect. Rabbit ear artery [Steinsland et al., 1985]
  Nif 3×10^{-6} M. No effect. Rabbit basilar and facial arteries [Hogestatt et al., 1982]
  Flun, DZ 10^{-4} M. No effect [Kajiwara and Casteels, 1983]
  VP, Bep 10^{-5} M. Small effect on excitatory junction potential. Guinea pig mesenteric arteries [Zelcer and Sperelakis, 1981]
  VP IC$_{50}$ = 10^{-4} M, DZ IC$_{50}$ = 6×10^{-5} M, Nic IC$_{50}$ = 6×10^{-5} M. Inhibition of NE release from canine saphenous vein [Takata and Kato, 1985]
  Nim 3×10^{-5} M reduces ACh and 5-HT release from cerebral arteries [Porter et al., 1985]
  VP 2×10^{-4} M. Small inhibition of NE release from rabbit aorta [Karaki et al., 1984]
  VP 10^{-10-4} M. "Enhanced" NE release evoked from the tail artery [Zsoter et al., 1984]
Vas deferens
  BAY K8644 enhances evoked NE release from rat vas deferens [Cena et al., 1985]
  BAY K8644 does not enhance evoked NE release from rat vas deferens [Docherty et al., 1984]
  DHPs have no effect up to 10^{-4} M. VP blocks at concentration where it also blocks nerve conduction. Guinea pig vas deferens [Beattie et al., 1985]
Other isolated preps
  3×10^{-6} Nif. No effect. DZ 5×10^{-5} M small inhibition. VP 10^{-6} M enhanced NE release from rabbit urethra [Larsson et al., 1984]
  Nit 2×10^{-5} M. No effect on NE release from rat phrenic nerve [Fairhurst et al., 1983]

DZ $> 10^{-5}$ M. Inhibits transmission in superior cervical ganglion but is no more potent than propanolol [Ito and Nishi, 1982]
D-600 = IC$_{50}$ 10^{-5} M. Inhibits evoked oxytocin release from neurohypophysis [Dreifuss et al., 1973]
Cultured neurones
  Nic blocked (partially) evoked release of GABA from chick retinal cells with IC$_{50}$ = 10^{-8} M [Takahashi and Ogura, 1983]
  Nit, BAY K8644 10^{-5} M. No effect on evoked DA release from cultured rat nigro striatal neurones [Shalaby et al., 1984]
  Various DHPs potently (10^{-9}–10^{-6} M) block evoked substance P release from cultured rat DRG cells but not NE release from sympathetic neurones [Perney et al., 1986]
Brain slices and synaptosomes
  D-600 and DZ blocked evoked NE release from cortical vesicular prep IC$_{50}$ 2×10^{-5} and 2.5×10^{-5} M. 5×10^{-5} Nif. No effect [Ebstein and Daly, 1982]
  VP, DZ, and ryosidine had little effect on evoked ACh or DA release from rabbit caudate slices except at very high concentrations [Starke et al., 1984]
  D-600 10^{-5} M. Inhibited evoked NE or GABA release from synaptosomes about 60% [Haylock et al., 1978]
  VP IC$_{50}$ = 5×10^{-7} M. Blocks evoked glutamate release from cortical synaptosomes [Norris and Bradford, 1983; Norris et al., 1983]
  DHPs potently block about 40% of the evoked release of NE from cortical synaptosomes. BAY K8644 has no effect [Turner and Goldin, 1985a,b]
  Nim and other DHPs had no effect on evoked DA release from striatal synaptosomes. BAY K8644 caused a small enhancement of release that could be reversed by Nim [Daniell et al., 1983; Woodward and Leslie, 1985]
  5-HT release from cortical slices, ACh from hippocampus, NE from hypothalamus. Not blocked by DHPs. BAY K8644 produces some enhancement of evoked release that can be reversed by DHP blockers [Middlemiss, 1985; Middlemiss and Spedding, 1985; Spedding and Middlemiss, 1985]
  D-600 IC$_{50}$ = 10^{-4} M. Blocks evoked NE or GABA release from synaptosomes [Vargas et al., 1977]
  VP IC$_{50}$ = 4×10^{-5} M. Blocks evoked GABA release from synaptosomes [Sihra et al., 1984]
  VP IC$_{50}$ = 2.5×10^{-5} M, Nim 5×10^{-6} M. Block evoked glutamate release from cortical synaptosomes [White and Bradford, 1985]
  Nim IC$_{50}$ = 10^{-6} M. Inhibited evoked ACh release from striatal or cortical slices, and evoked DA

TABLE VI. Continued

VP, Pren 3×10^{-4} M. No effect on crayfish neuromuscular transmission [Van der Kloot and Kita, 1975]	release was enhanced [Nordstrom et al., 1986]

*VP, verapamil; Pren, prenylamine; Nif, nifedipine; DZ, diltiazem; Flun, flunrzrizine; Bep, bepridil; Nic, nicardipine; Nit, nitrendipine; Nim, nimodipine.

What is the relevance of the observations made with PC12 cells? Actually under normal growth conditions, PC12 cells probably resemble adrenal chromaffin cells more than sympathetic neurones. It is quite clear that VSCC and amine release in authentic chromaffin cells show similar drug sensitivities to the PC12 cell line (Table V). Indeed, release from other excitable endocrine cells is similarly drug-sensitive [Enyeart et al., 1985]. Thus, the results with PC12 cells are probably more relevant to endocrine cells than to neurones per se. However, these results do illustrate a situation that might be expected to exist in neurones as well.

A large amount of data does exist concerning the effects of drugs and other agents on neurotransmitter release. Clearly, most of it is not relevant to the present discussion. It will be obvious that agents may interfere with the release of transmitters at numerous sites, of which VSCC are only one. Thus, the observation that a drug blocks release does not give us any information about VSCC except under particular circumstances. We might, however, consider the effects of organic VSCC modulators in particular. The actions of these agents might be expected to reveal important information about the types of VSCC involved in the release process. However, even this approach may be problematic. Thus, it is quite clear that at concentrations above a few μM, VSCC blockers are no longer specific. At such concentrations, these drugs can interact with virtually every biological process known to man [Triggle, 1981; Miller and Freedman, 1984]. This is particularly true with drugs such as verapamil and diltiazem. It is less true with some DHPs which may maintain their relative VSCC specificity even at quite high concentrations.

At any rate, the "window" between the concentrations at which many DHPs produce specific and nonspecific effects is rather large compared to other VSCC blockers. It is essential to recognize, therefore, that when a particular study demonstrates that 5×10^{-5} M verapamil, say, blocks transmitter release, this tells us nothing at all about VSCC. It is probably more likely that the drug is interacting with another element of the release system rather than VSCC. However, drug studies can be terribly revealing if certain important rules are recognized. The first rule I would suggest derives from the well-known observation that it is usually much easier to "kill" an enzyme, channel, or receptor by some nonspecific treatment than to get it to work better! Thus, although it may be difficult to interpret data using organic VSCC blockers and neurotransmitter release, use of VSCC agonists is likely to be less problematic. Thus, actual enhancement of evoked transmitter release by BAY K8644 constitutes really good evidence for the involvement of DHP-sensitive VSCC and is really more meaningful than a blocking experiment. In addition, consideration of the arguments used above with PC12 cells indicates that if DHP-sensitive VSCC are involved, a block should be obtained with low concentrations of drugs if K^+ depolarization is used to elicit the release process. It may not be necessary to block all transmitter release in this way, as conceivably a situation could arise in which both drug-sensitive and -insensitive VSCC were involved. However, some portion of release evoked by K^+ should be blocked by DHPs in the nM to low μM range.

With these caveats in mind, I shall now discuss what data are available concerning the effect of drugs on evoked neurotransmitter release. Data are available on the effects of drugs on peripheral noradrenergic and cholinergic neurones and from central neuronal preparations such as brain slices, synaptosomes, or cultured cells (Tables V and VI). Virtually all of these data demonstrate that drug-sensitive VSCC are not involved in the release process. Actually many studies do demonstrate some blocking effect of drugs at elevated concentrations. However, as discussed, most of this data clearly illustrates the *insensitivity* of the channels involved. These observations fit in well with the above discussion on voltage-sensitive ^{45}Ca^{2+} fluxes in neurones. It seems, therefore, that in most cases so far investigated, the VSCC mediating fluxes and transmitter release are drug-insensitive. However, there are also examples of evoked transmitter release processes that are clearly drug-sensitive by all reasonable criteria and are therefore presumably mediated by VSCC of the type that mediate release in PC12 cells or many endocrine cells (L-type?).

One might start by considering the case of catecholamine release from sympathetic neurones. The effects of drugs on this release process have been widely studied. In general, the results clearly show that organic VSCC blockers will inhibit evoked [^{3}H]norepinephrine release, but only at colossal concentrations (Table VI). The basis of this inhibition is presumably, therefore, nonspecific and probably has nothing to do with VSCC. One might, therefore, conclude that VSCC providing Ca^{2+} for release in these neurones are DHP-insensitive, perhaps an N-type channel. Indeed, experiments with PC12 cells reflect this situation. Thus, when such cells are treated with NGF and change from an adrenal-like to a neuronal-like morphology, the evoked release of catecholamine also becomes predominantly DHP-insensitive, whereas under nondifferentiating conditions, release is highly drug-sensitive (vide supra) [Kongsamut and Miller, 1986; Takahashi et al., 1985]. Some experiments on sympathetic neurones using BAY K8644 have come to a rather different conclusion. Thus, Cena et al. [1985] reported that the release of transmitter

from nerves innervating the rat vas deferens was enhanced by BAY K8644 at reasonable concentrations, although Docherty et al. [1984] did not. Similar results have recently been obtained by Perney et al. [1986] who observed that the evoked release of [^{3}H]norepinephrine from cultured sympathetic neurones was not blocked by nimodipine but could be enhanced by BAY K8644. Moreover, they also found that cultured sympathetic neurones possessed high affinity [^{3}H]-DHP binding sites.

Experiments examining transmitter release from central neurones have generally utilized synaptosomal or brain slice preparations. Again most studies have indicated that the evoked release of transmitters is drug-insensitive, indicating a role for drug-insensitive VSCC (Table VI). This fits in well with the above discussion illustrating that most voltage sensitive ^{45}Ca^{2+} uptake in synaptosomes is similarly drug-insensitive. However, recently, some reports have indicated that drug-sensitive release processes may occur centrally as well. One group has claimed that as with sympathetic neurones, K$^+$-evoked release of 5-HT from the cortex, norepinephrine from the hypothalamus, and acetylcholine from the hippocampus, is resistant to blockade by antagonist DHPs but can be enhanced by BAY K8644 [Middlemiss, 1985; Middlemiss and Spedding, 1985; Spedding and Middlemiss, 1985]. Moreover, the BAY K8644-induced enhancement could be reversed by nitrendipine. Thus, this pattern of effects has been observed in several cases. Preliminary data also indicate that the release of dopamine from striatal synaptosomes may also be modulated in this way [Woodward and Leslie, 1985], although not all studies have demonstrated drug effects on dopamine release [Shalaby et al., 1984]. In contrast, the studies of Turner and Goldin have demonstrated that the evoked release of norepinephrine from cortical synaptosomes could be partially blocked by DHPs [Turner and Goldin, 1985a] but could not be enhanced by BAY K8644 [Turner and Goldin, 1985b]. On the other hand, K$^+$-evoked ^{45}Ca^{2+} uptake into such synaptosomes was sensitive to both DHP agonists and antagonists [Turner and Goldin, 1985a,b]. Thus, one is left with the general impression that, as with sympathetic neurones, central transmitter release processes are generally drug-insensitive and utilize drug-insensitive VSCC, but that drug-sensitive VSCC may sometimes be persuaded to play a role in the process if BAY K8644 is used. Perhaps the clearest case of drug-sensitive transmitter release occurs with sensory neurones. This is obviously a good place to look for such a phenomenon, as DHP-sensitive L-type VSCC have been clearly identified in such neurones [Nowycky et al., 1985a,b]. Perney et al. [1986] have demonstrated that the evoked release of substance P from cultures of 2-day-old rat dorsal root ganglion cells is very DHP-sensitive. Thus, release is blocked by low concentrations of DHPs such as nimodipine and enhanced by agonists such as BAY K8644. Moreover, the (+) and (−) isomers of the DHP 202-791 produce agonist and antagonist effects, respectively.

How can all these diverse observations be explained? One possibility is suggested by the aforementioned recent experiments on PC12 cells [Kongsamut and Miller, 1986; Takahashi et al., 1985]. These cells go from a DHP-sensitive to a DHP-insensitive state upon morphological differentiation by NGF. Interestingly, however, voltage-dependent $^{45}Ca^{2+}$ uptake into the cells is equally DHP-sensitive in both growth states [Kongsamut and Miller, 1986]. Under the conditions used, such flux experiments easily monitor fluxes through large noninactivating L-type channels but not through rapidly inactivating N- or T-type channels. Thus, such channels even if present would not make an appreciable contribution to the overall flux observed. It is known that in neurones, release of transmitter takes place primarily from terminal varicosities, although some release from the cell soma may occur [Chow and Poo, 1985; Suetake et al., 1981]. It is possible that in nerve terminals, VSCC cluster around transmitter release sites ("active zones"), as suggested from morphological [Pumplin et al., 1981] and biophysical [Simon and Llinas, 1985] evidence. Moreover, as discussed above, clusters of N-type VSCC have been observed electrophysiologically [Fox et al., 1985b]. If this is the case, then these channels may have an overriding influence on transmitter release because they are positioned in exactly the correct place, i.e., right next to the area of vesicle exocytosis. Such a scheme can potentially explain why transmitter release may be predominantly insensitive to DHP blockers (as in sympathetic neurones or differentiated PC12 cells) but still possess high affinity [^{3}H]DHP binding sites or DHP-sensitive, voltage-sensitive $^{45}Ca^{2+}$ fluxes. Consider, for example, the several instances in which it has been reported that evoked transmitter release was not blocked by DHP antagonists but was enhanced by DHP agonists such as BAY K8644. It may be supposed that, as suggested, sites for transmitter release are surrounded by DHP-insensitive VSCC, whereas DHP-sensitive VSCC are not organized in this way. They may even be in quite different parts of the cell. Normally when the cell is depolarized with K^+-rich solutions, Ca^{2+} enters the neurone via all VSCC types. However, the area around the transmitter release zones is primarily influenced by DHP-insensitive VSCC. Thus, release is not blocked by DHP antagonists. In the presence of BAY K8644, however, influx of Ca^{2+} through DHP-sensitive VSCC is greatly enhanced. So much Ca^{2+} may now enter via this pathway that there is a "spill-over" effect, and this Ca^{2+} begins to contribute to exocytosis. Thus, we might actually expect a pattern in which evoked release was not blocked by DHP antagonists, but was enhanced by DHP agonists. If, indeed, the DHP-sensitive VSCC were usually localized outside the nerve terminal then this would also explain why fluxes measured in synaptosomes are DHP-insensitive, as synaptosomes represent the terminal varicosities of neurones. Indeed, it has recently been demonstrated that there is a different nerve terminal of single molluscan neurones [Graubard and Ross, 1985]. An alternative scenario would not involve selective localization of VSCC but selective VSCC in-activation. Thus, one could suppose that both DHP-sensitive and insensitive VSCC oc-curred at the nerve terminal, but that the DHP-sensitive channels were selectively in-activated. For example, it has been observed that L-type VSCC in PC12 cells or DRG cells can be inactivated by the phorbol ester TPA [Rane and Dunlap, 1985a,b; Werz and MacDonald, 1985c; Harris et al., 1985a]. Thus, in certain cases, it is possible that local (synaptosomal) levels of some intracellular feedback modulator of L-channels, such as diacylglycerol, are particularly high, and so L-channels no longer influence the release process except presumably under special con-ditions. However, although such schemes seem to adequately explain the situation in the majority of cases, there are obviously certain cases (e.g., DRG cells) in which they do not apply, and where predominantly DHP-sensi-tive transmitter release does not occur. It is not clear why this is, but it may be due to an unusually large complement of L-type chan-nels in such cells, a selective clustering of L- rather than N-type VSCC, or else a large amount of release from nonterminal sites. These explanations obviously represent "ide-alized" cases. However, they do seem to fit much of the available data. There may be in reality many situations which represent vari-ations on these themes. Clearly, however, by using different combinations of DHP-sensi-tive and insensitive channels and variations in their microdistribution, different neurones could tailor transmitter release to exactly suit their particular requirements.

MODULATION OF CALCIUM CHANNELS

Toxins

At this point, naturally occurring toxins have not played the key role in VSCC re-search that they have in research on nicotinic receptors or sodium channels. In the case of VSCC, this key role has been taken by drugs such as DHPs rather than toxins. Indeed, there is not even one really well-established exam-ple of a toxin that interacts with VSCC. How-

ever, there are some promising leads as well as some "blind alleys" [Miller, 1984b] (Table VII).

Most of the fuss and publicity in this area has centered on a marine toxin known as maitotoxin. This toxin is isolated from the dinoflagellate *Gambierdiscus toxicus*, which is found in tropical and subtropical seas and is responsible for a syndrome known as "cig-uatera" poisoning. The structure of the toxin is unknown, but it does not appear to be a polypeptide. Many studies on the effects of the toxin have been published (Table VII). All these papers have highly descriptive titles in-cluding phrases describing maitotoxin (MTX) as "the most lethal," "most potent," "most nauseating" (sic) substance known to man. At any rate, it is certainly quite clear that if MTX is added to cells that possess VSCC, Ca^{2+} uptake through these channels is observed [Freedman et al., 1984b; Schettini et al., 1984; Takahashi et al., 1982, 1983], as well as subsequent muscle contraction [Ohizumi and Yasumoto, 1983; Legrand and Bagnis, 1984; Kobayashi et al., 1985a]; and hormone [Login et al., 1985; Schettini et al., 1984] or neurotransmitter release [Kim et al., 1985; Takahashi et al., 1982, 1983]. Such observa-tions are obviously consistent with the pro-posal that MTX directly activates VSCC. Indeed, this has been proposed as its mecha-nism of action. Several reports have, indeed, now assumed that this is the case. Unfortu-nately, however, this is probably not how the toxin works. Electrophysiological data on the action of MTX are very scanty. However, the data available do not unequivocally support the proposal that MTX directly activates VSCC, although some of it are consistent with this idea [Miyamoto et al., 1984; Ogura et al., 1984; Yoshii et al., 1986]. Some un-published data, however, are much clearer in this respect. MTX has no effect on slow Ca^{2+} action potentials in guinea pig papillary mus-cle (T. Kamp and M. Sanguinetti, personal communication) nor does it alter Ca^{2+} cur-rents under voltage clamp in N1E-115 neuro-blastoma cells (M. Lazdunski, personal communication). It is probable, therefore, that

TABLE VII. Toxins That May Act Upon Calcium Channels

Veratradine and batrachotoxin
  Romey and Lazdunski, 1982; Bolger et al., 1983; Kongsamut et al., 1985b; Yoshii et al., 1985b
ω-Conus geographus toxin
  Kerr and Yoshikami, 1984; Feldman and Yoshikami, 1985; McClesky et al., 1986b; Olivera et al., 1984
Leptinotarsin-Dor H/Leptinotoxin
  Crosland et al., 1984; Koenig et al., 1985; Madeddu et al., 1985a,b,c; McClure et al., 1980; Yoshino et al., 1980
Atrotoxin
  Hamilton et al., 1985
Talaromycin
  Griffiths et al., 1985; Lynn et al., 1982
Maitotoxin
  Neuronal: Freedman et al., 1984b; Ogura et al., 1984; Takahashi et al., 1982, 1983; Yoshii et al., 1984, 1986
  Other: Legrand and Bagnis, 1984; Ohizumi and Yasumoto, 1983; Kim et al., 1985; Kobayashi et al., 1985a; Login et al., 1985; Miyamoto et al., 1984; Ohizumi et al., 1983; Schettini et al., 1984

MTX somehow depolarizes cells leading to the opening of VSCC. It does not appear to do so by causing an increase in Na^+ permeability, although its action is partially dependent on the presence of external Na^+ [Freedman et al., 1984b; Takahashi et al., 1982, 1983]. Thus, its mechanism of action is unknown. This is a most interesting substance. Research on its mechanism of action would be greatly aided by the elucidation of its structure.

A second toxin about which there is a certain amount of controversy is a polypeptide derived from the haemolymph of the Colorado potatoe beetle and variously known as leptinotarsin-d (orh) [Crosland et al., 1984; Koenig et al., 1985; McClure et al., 1980; Yoshino et al., 1980] or leptinotoxin (LTX) [Madeddu et al., 1985a,b,c]. It was originally reported that this toxin was able to stimulate the release of several neurotransmitters (Ach, norepinephrine, GABA) from synaptosomes in a Ca^{2+}-dependent fashion. This release could be blocked by Cd^{2+}. Moreover, LTX depolarized synaptosomes, also in a Ca^{2+}-dependent fashion. Subsequent work has

shown that its effects are specific for mammalian synaptosomes, as it does not act on PC12 cells, molluscan neurones, paramecium, or squid optic lobe neurones [Koenig et al., 1985]. LTX was also found to increase the fura-2 (Ca^{2+}) signal in a subclass of brain diencephalic neurones in culture [Koenig et al., 1985]. Interestingly, the effects of LTX on synaptosomal transmitter release were unaffected by DHPs, whereas those on fura-2 signals were inhibited. These effects suggest that LTX may be an activator of some type of mammalian neuronal VSCC. Unfortunately, however, data from another group are at odds with this proposal. Thus, Meldolesi and his colleagues [Madeddu et al., 1985a,b,c] have suggested that LTX may act as an ionophore in a similar fashion to black widow spider venom (α-latrotoxin) (α-Lx), albeit at a different receptor. These authors have demonstrated that LTX does not interact with the same binding site as α-Lx. However, both toxins increased $^{45}Ca^{2+}$ uptake, depolarization, and, in contrast to the above, norepinephrine release from PC12 cells. Significantly, these actions were not blocked by verapamil, which, as discussed above, does block the VSCC in nondifferentiated PC12 cells. These latter data suggest some ionophore-like action for the toxin. Clearly, therefore, the mechanism of action of the toxin is as yet unresolved.

A really promising candidate for a VSCC-specific toxin, however, is the polypeptide (27 amino acids) known as ω-toxin isolated from the venom of the marine snail *Conus geographus* [Olivera et al., 1984]. This amazing animal has an interesting venom apparatus that contains little harpoons filled with a wide variety of toxins. The snail can fire these harpoons at anything swimming in its vicinity. This is usually a fish but on rare occasions may be a tourist. Having paralyzed its prey, the snail now proceeds to gobble it up in a single gulp. The Kraken waketh! ω-CTx has been shown to reduce the evoked release of transmitter at the neuromuscular junction without reducing the ability of the spike to invade the nerve terminal [Kerr and Yoshikami, 1984]. In addition, it was also initially observed that the toxin would abolish the Ca^{2+} component of combined Ca^{2+}/Na^{+} spikes in DRG cells in culture. These actions suggest that the toxin might be able to block VSCC. Subsequently, electrophysiological studies have revealed that this is indeed the case [Feldman and Yoshikami, 1985; Mc-Clesky et al., 1986b]. In studies using cultured DRG cells, ω-CTx blocked both N- and L-channels but not T-channels. The toxin also blocked a component of the Ca^{2+} current in hippocampal pyramidal cells but not in *Aplysia* bag cells or in cardiac or skeletal muscle. This is most interesting as it could suggest some structural similarity between DRG L- and N-type channels. Moreover, it could also suggest a structural diversity between the L-type channels found in different tissues. Clearly, however, other explanations are also possible. Thus, the toxin may bind to a specific receptor which is not actually a VSCC and then subsequently influence channel function. Clearly CTx is a promising compound and may be of great use to research in this area.

The second major hope for a VSCC-specific toxin is a second polypeptide named atrotoxin, partially purified from the venom of the rattlesnake *Crotalus atrox* [Hamilton et al., 1985]. This material increases Ca^{2+} currents under voltage clamp in the heart and, therefore, seems to have VSCC agonist effects. Even more interestingly, the toxin was found to inhibit the binding of [^{3}H]nitrendipine to cardiac muscle membranes in an allosteric fashion. Reuter et al. [1985b] have observed that DHP agonists reduce the binding of DHP antagonists in an allosteric fashion. Thus, it is possible that the toxin interacts with VSCC in the same fashion as a DHP agonist. There are no reports as yet as to the effects of atrotoxin on neurones.

In addition to these various candidates, there are also other scattered reports of non-peptidergic toxins that interact with VSCC. Romey and Lazdunski [1982] reported that veratradine and batrachotoxin, which are best known as activators of Na^{+} channels, were able to block Ca^{2+} current in voltage clamped N1E-115 neuroblastoma cells. The protocol employed would suggest that they were observing a T-type current. Indeed, they reported that the current was not blocked by verapamil. Further reports have indicated that these toxins may also interact with DHP-specific sites on VSCC and even possibly with some K^{+} channels [Bolger et al., 1983; Kongsamut et al., 1985b; Yoshii et al., 1985b]. Finally, a fungal toxin known as talaromycin may also be a candidate for a blocker of VSCC [Griffiths et al., 1985; Lynn et al., 1982].

It can be seen from the above discussion that most of the candidate toxins seem to interact with L-type channels. There is clearly a great need for agents that specifically interact with all VSCC, particularly T-type channels.

Effects of Drugs

Clearly, examining the sensitivity of neuronal Ca^{2+} currents to various drugs is important for many reasons. In particular, in the absence of well-established toxin probes, drugs are very useful aids in trying to classify neuronal VSCC. In the discussion so far, we have shown that the nervous system possesses a large number of high affinity binding sites for DHPs and other organic VSCC blockers. Some indications have been given that these do in fact represent a class of VSCC. Thus, DHP effects on Ca^{2+} fluxes and neurotransmitter release have been alluded to. I shall now discuss data on the effects of such drugs on neuronal Ca^{2+} conductances as assessed electrophysiologically. One may start out with the proposal that VSCC are either drug-sensitive (L-type) or insensitive (N- or T-type). However, in reality this may be quite an oversimplification. Thus, there may be several subtypes of VSCC which actually vary somewhat in their drug sensitivities. Indeed, I have already pointed out several preliminary indications of differences in L-type VSCC based on differences in biochemical properties (e.g., affinity, Table III) and preliminary data on antibody crossreactivity [Chin et al., 1985]

TABLE VIII. Effects of Organic Calcium Channel Modulating Drugs on Neuronal Calcium Conductances

Sensory neurones

   Rabbit. Nodose Ca spike 10^{-5} M DZ, VP and Nif block 76, 84 and 87% [Ito et al., 1984]

   Rabbit. Nodose Ca spike 10^{-5} M. DZ, VP block nearly completely [Ito, 1982]

   Mouse. DRG Ca spike partially inhibited by Nit [Pun and Litzinger, 1984]

   Rat DRG. I_{Ca} (L) blocked > 80% by 100 μg/ml VP [Kostyuk et al., 1981b]

   Rat DRG. 10^{-4} M VP blocks (L) but not (T) [Fedulova et al., 1985]

   Frog sensory neurons. I_{Ca} (L) blocked by VP, DZ, D-600 (10^{-6} M). Drugs also effective from inside [Ishizuka et al., 1984]

   Rat DRG. I_{Ca} (L) blocked by VP [Fedulova et al., 1981]

   Chick DRG. I_{Ca} (L) blocked completely by VP > 2×10^{-5} M. Nif increases and BAY K8644 decreases I_{Ca} (L) [Boll and Lux, 1985]

   Chick DRG. BAY K8644 enhances I_{Ca} (L) [Fox et al., 1985a; Nowycky et al., 1985b]

   Chick DRG. BAY K8644 enhances I_{Ca} (L) but not (T) or (N) [Nowycky et al., 1985a]

   Mouse DRG. Partial block of Ca spike by nitrendipine 10^{-9}–10^{-5} M [Litzinger et al., 1985]

   Mouse DRG. BAY K8644 enhances I_{Ca} (L) [Jia and Litzinger, 1985]

   Mouse DRG. DHPs have no effect on I_{Ca} (L) [Nerbonne and Gurney, 1985]

   Mouse DRG. Barbiturates (50–2,000 μM) inhibit Ca spike, AHP and I_{Ca} (L) [Werz and MacDonald, 1985b]

Other peripheral neurones

   Bullfrog sympathetic neurone. I_{Ca} blocked 50–70% by 5×10^{-5} M D-600 [Akasu and Koketsu, 1981]

   Guinea pig submucous plexus neurone. Ca spike unaffected by 10^{-5} M Nif [Surprenant, 1984]

   Superior cervical and ciliary ganglia neuronal I_{Ca} unaffected by DHPs [Nerbonne and Gurney, 1985]

Central neurones

   Inferior olivary neurone. High threshold Ca spike blocked by D-600 [Llinas and Yarom, 1981a]

   Cerebellar Purkinje cells. Ca spike blocked by D-600 10^{-5} g/ml) [Llinas and Sugimori, 1980a,b]

   Cortical neurons. Ca spike blocked by VP at 10^{-4} M [Dichter et al., 1983]

   Locus coeruleus. I_{Ca} unaffected by 10^{-5} M nitrendipine [Williams et al., 1984]

   Olfactory cortex. Ca spikes unaffected by Nif

or D-600 [Kuan et al., 1985]

   Hippocampal pyramidal cells. VP and D-600 (3×10^{-3} M) reduce Ca spike [Dingledine, 1983]

   Hippocampal pyramidal cells. D-890 (10^{-5} M) reduce Ca spike [Deisz and Prince, 1985]

   Hippocampal pyramidal cells. VP (10^{-4} M) blocks I_{Ca} (L) [Brown and Griffiths, 1983b]

   Hippocampal pyramidal cells. Nim blocks. BAY K8644 enhances I_{Ca} (L) at modest concentrations [Brown et al., 1985, 1986]

   Spinal neurones. Ca spike unaffected by > 2.5×10^{-5} M D-600 or Nif [Bixby and Spitzer, 1984b]

   Spinal neurones. I_{Ca} blocked by atropine [Hedlund et al., 1985]

   Motoneurones. VP had no effect in vivo [Krnjevic et al., 1979]

   Rods. Ca spike blocked by D-600, 10^{-4} M [Fain et al., 1980]

   Muscle spindle. Ca spike blocked reversibly by 50 μg/ml VP [Ito et al., 1982b]

Neuroblastomas and PC12 cells

   NG108-15. I_{Ca} (L) blocked by nimodipine, enhanced by BAY K8644 [Docherty and Miller, 1985]

   NG108-15. Ca spike blocked by high concentrations of D-600 and DHPs [Reiser et al., 1977]

   NG108-15. Ca spike blocked by D-600. IC_{50} = 10^{-4} M [Atlas and Adler, 1981]

   Neuroblastoma. I_{Ca} (L) enhanced by BAY K8644 [Fox et al., 1984]

   N1E-115. I_{Ca} (T) unaffected by VP or D-600 [Moolenaar and Spector, 1979b]

   N1E-115. I_{Ca} (T) unaffected by VP or D-600 below 10^{-4} M [Romey and Lazdunski, 1982]

   N1E-115. I_{Ca} (L) blocked by VP or veratridine. No effect on I_{Ca} (T) [Twombly and Narahashi, 1985; Tsunoo et al., 1984, 1985]. I_{Ca} (T) blocked by phenytoin or tetramethrin. No effect on I_{Ca} (L) [Yoshii et al., 1985a,b]

   NG108-15. Ca spike. 100% block by VP 3×10^{-6} M [Furuya et al., 1983]

   PC12. Ca spike unaffected by nicardipine [Ogura and Takahashi, 1984]

   PC12. Nit enhances Ca spike [Brown et al., 1984a]

   PC12. Nit blocks I_{Ca} completely evoked from depolarized (−30) but not hyperpolarized (−100 mV) holding paths [Kunze et al., 1985]

   Adrenal I_{Ca} (L) blocked by trifluoperazine IC_{50} = 10^{-5} M [Clapham and Neher, 1984]

— Continued

Intervertebrate neurons

Helix neurones. I$_{Ca}$ blocked by VP (2 × 10^{-4} M) [Doroshenko et al., 1984a]

Helix neurones. I$_{Ca}$ blocked by D-600 and Nif IC$_{50}$ = 2.6 × 10^{-5} and 2.3 × 10^{-5} M. Less effective by intracellular route [Kostyuk, 1983]

Helix neurones. I$_{Ca}$ blocked by VP 7.5 × 10^{-5} M. Similar IC$_{50}$ for I$_K$ [Kostyuk et al., 1975]

Helix neurones. I$_{Ca}$ blocked by VP and DZ both IC$_{50}$ = 5 × 10^{-5} M [Akaike et al., 1981b]

Helix neurones. I$_{Ca}$ blocked by propanolol IC$_{50}$ = 5 × 10^{-5} M [Akaike et al., 1981a]

Helix neurones. I$_{Ca}$ blocked by Nif 5 × 10^{-6} M. Spec of block ratio I$_{Ca}$/I$_K$. 1.25: 16.6: 2.5: 22.72 for Nif, DZ, VP, and propanolol [Nishi et al., 1983]

Helix neurones. I$_{Ca}$ blocked by D-600 and Nif, IC$_{50}$ = 2.6 × 10^{-5} and 2.3 × 10^{-5} M [Kostyuk and Shuba, 1982]

Helix neurones. I$_{Ca}$ partially blocked by D-600 at 10^{-2} M [Eckert and Lux, 1976]

Helix neurones. I$_{Ca}$ blocked by D-600 and Nif IC$_{50}$ = 3.4 × 10^{-5} M [Kostyuk and Krishtal, 1977a,b; Kostyuk et al., 1983]

Helix neurones. D-600 blocked I$_{Ca}$, IC$_{50}$ = 1.3 × 10^{-4} M. Blocked I$_{K(Ca)}$ IC$_{50}$ = 1.7 × 10^{-5} M. Nif > 10^{-4} M did not block I$_{Ca}$ [Gola and Ducreux, 1985]

Helix neurones. I$_{Ca}$ increased by BAY K8644. Reduced by Nif [Walden et al., 1985]

Aplysia neurones. Ca spike blocked by D-600 10^{-4}–10^{-3} [Klee et al., 1973]

Aplysia bag cell I$_{Ca}$ blocked by Nif IC$_{50}$ = 1.7 × 10^{-6} M. I$_k$ blocked by Nif IC$_{50}$ 3 × 10^{-6} M [Nerbonne and Gurney, 1985]

Snail neurones. ZN^{2+} blocked by VP 10^{-4} gm/ml [Kawa, 1979]

Lymnea neurons. I$_{Ca}$ blocked 30% by 10^{-4} M Nif [Byerly et al., 1985]

Aglantha digitale. Ca spike in giant axon partially reduced by 10^{-4} M Nif [Mackie and Meech, 1985]

Squid axon aequorin signal blocked by D-600 and VP 100 μg/ml [Baker et al., 1973]

Leech neurones. Ca spike blocked by diazepam. IC$_{50}$ = 10^{-4} M [Johansen et al., 1985]

Helix U-neurones. D-600 blocked I$_{Ca}$, IC$_{50}$ = 1.3 × 10^{-4} M. Blocked I$_{K(Ca)}$ IC$_{50}$ = 1.7 × 10^{-5} M. Nif > 10^{-4} M did not block I$_{Ca}$ [Gola and Ducreux, 1985]

and sensitivity to toxins [McClesky et al., 1986b]. These details will presumably become clearer as time goes on. However, at the moment it is useful to at least attempt to categorize VSCC according to "drug-sensitive" and "drug-insensitive" criteria. Table VIII lists the various observations in the literature on the effects of drugs on neuronal Ca^{2+} spikes or currents. Of particular interest are observations that clearly indicate drug sensitivity or lack of it according to the criteria discussed above. From this point of view, it is clear that many of the observations listed in Table VIII are uninterpretable. Data from experiments employing 50–100 μM D-600 or diltiazem, for example, that yield a partial inhibition of a current or spike are impossible to assess. This is because of the uncertainties associated with using such high drug concentrations. Thus, such observations may or may not indicate a specific interaction with

VSCC—it is just impossible to tell. However, it is rather likely that such effects are quite nonspecific. Having discounted these studies, one may now ask what remains. There are several observations which clearly indicate that some conductances are very drug-sensitive or, in other cases, completely insensitive. There is also a murky area in between where "partial" effects of drugs are seen at "moderate" concentrations. Clearly, observations based on the use of DHPs are in general much easier to interpret than those based on the use of verapamil-like or diltiazem-like drugs.

In vertebrate neurones, there are several reports showing a total lack of effect of DHPs on some Ca^{2+} conductances, even at elevated concentrations. Thus, high concentrations of DHPs fail to block Ca^{2+} spikes or currents in neurones of the guinea pig submucous plexus [Surprenant, 1984], locus coeruleus [Williams et al., 1984], olfactory cortex [Kuan et al., 1985], or in embryonic frog spinal neurones [Bixby and Spitzer, 1984b]. Interestingly, in the former case, nifedipine completely blocked Ca^{2+} spikes in adjoining smooth muscle cells at nM concentrations, even though the neuronal spikes were resistant [Surprenant, 1984]. The best example of drug-sensitive VSCC in vertebrate neurones is in the DRG cell. It is quite clear from the most complete studies that the L-type conductance in these cells is modulated by DHPs in an appropriate fashion [Fox et al., 1985a; Nowycky et al., 1985a,b]. Some preliminary reports differ slightly in the details of the DHP modulation, but sensitivity is still observed [Boll and Lux, 1985; Jia and Litzinger, 1985; Pun and Litzinger, 1984]. Only one report failed to observe DHP sensitivity of VSCC in such cells [Nerbonne and Gurney, 1985]. Even when nonDHP blockers are used, they are clearly very effective in DRG cells, producing large inhibitions of L-type currents or Ca^{2+} spikes at moderate concentrations in several reports [Ito, 1982; Boll and Lux, 1985; Fedulova et al., 1985; Ishizuka et al., 1984; Ito et al., 1984]. It is just as clear that T-type (and N-type) VSCC in these cells are drug-insensitive, although data on this point are less extensive.

No other neuronal Ca^{2+} conductance has been as well studied as the DRG L-channel with respect to its DHP sensitivity. However, there is good evidence that a VSCC found in hippocampal pyramidal cells may be similar. These cells also clearly possess at least two separate types of VSCC which appear comparable to DRG T- and L-channels [Halliwell, 1983]. Indeed, the hippocampal L-type conductance also appears to be blocked by DHP antagonists and enhanced by DHP agonists [Brown et al., 1985, 1986]. It should be stressed that DHP antagonists can actually be shown to produce small agonist effects in various tissues, including neurones, under certain conditions [Boll and Lux, 1985; Sanguinetti and Kass, 1984b; Brown et al., 1984a; Hess et al., 1984]. Thus, the precise effects observed on a DHP-sensitive Ca^{2+} current

may depend on the conditions used in the experiment. However, what is not yet clear is whether these mixed effects are due to intrinsic "partial agonist" properties of pure substances or due to the mixed effects of racemic mixtures whose isomers exhibit the opposite actions (vide supra).

Data from clonal cell lines are also interesting. In a number of cases, it has been reported that Ca^{2+} spikes in neuroblastomas [Atlas and Adler, 1981; Reiser et al., 1977] or PC12 cells [Ogura and Takahashi, 1984] are resistant to organic VSCC blockers except at very high concentrations. This differs from conclusions reached using $^{45}Ca^{2+}$ fluxes (vide supra). However, the data can be explained from observations that such cells contain [Fishman and Spector, 1981; Twombly and Narahashi, 1985; Tsunoo et al., 1984, 1985a; Yoshii et al., 1985a,b] or probably contain [Kongsamut and Miller, 1986; Ogura and Takahashi, 1984; Kunze et al., 1985] both L- and T-type VSCC. The neuroblastoma T-type current is predictably rather resistant to verapamil and D-600, at any rate [Moolenaar and Spector, 1979b; Romey and Lazdunski, 1982]. On the other hand, the L-type channel is predictably drug-sensitive [Docherty and Miller, 1985; Fox et al., 1984; Tsunoo et al., 1985a; Yoshii et al., 1985a].

Clearly, it would be interesting to find agents that specifically interacted with T- rather than L-channels. There are some indications that the drug tetramethrin may do this [Tsunoo et al., 1985a; Yoshii et al., 1985b]. The antiepileptic drug phenytoin may also fall into this category [Twombly and Narahashi, 1985; see also Selzer, 1979; McLean and MacDonald, 1983; Ribares and Miller, 1985; Tuttle and Richelson, 1979; Messing et al., 1985], as may the drug menthol [Swandulla et al., 1985]. There are reports that veratradine and batrachotoxin block T-channels in neuroblastomas [Romey and Lazdunski, 1982]; however, other reports indicate that these substances interact with L-type channels [Kongsamut, 1985b; Bolger et al., 1983; Yoshii et al., 1985b]. Other agents which have been shown to block L-type currents include barbiturates [Werz and MacDonald, 1985b], trifluoperazine [Clapham and Neher, 1984], and possibly atropine [Hedlund et al., 1985].

There are also several reports on the effects of drugs on invertebrate neuronal VSCC. It is certainly more difficult to put this data in perspective, particularly as there are no [^{3}H]DHP binding data and little transmitter release data with which to relate it. On purely biophysical grounds, there certainly appear to be invertebrate Ca^{2+} currents that are similar to vertebrate L-type currents (vide supra). However, exactly how similar they are is impossible to tell. Drug data are potentially helpful in making such comparisons.

The most detailed study has examined the effects of DHP on Ca^{2+} currents in *Aplysia* bag cell neurones [Nerbonne and Gurney, 1985]. These currents were clearly inhibited by DHPs at reasonable concentrations (IC$_{50}$ for nifedipine ~ 1.7×10^{-6} M). BAY K8644 had little effect on its own, but "antagonized" the effects of nifedipine. Interestingly, DHPs were also found to be quite effective blockers of K$^+$ currents in these cells, with IC$_{50}$s $\simeq 5 \times 10^{-6}$ M. One should remember that even in the vertebrate heart, DHPs do also have appreciable effects on K$^+$ currents [Hume, 1985]. Nifedipine also blocked Ca^{2+} currents in *Helix* neurones at a reasonable concentration (IC$_{50} = 5 \times 10^{-6}$ M) [Nishi et al., 1983], and *Helix* neuronal currents are enhanced by BAY K8644 [Walden et al., 1985]. Verapamil and diltiazem were both about an order of magnitude less effective, as was propanolol, which is not usually thought of as a VSCC blocker [Akaike et al., 1981a]. It is also clear that DHPs are not effective in blocking all invertebrate neuronal Ca^{2+} currents. Thus, nifedipine blocked Ca^{2+} currents in some *Helix* neurones less potently (IC$_{50} = 2.3 \times 10^{-5}$ M) [Kostyuk, 1983; Kostyuk and Krishtal, 1977a,b; Kostyuk and Shuba, 1982; Kostyuk et al., 1983], and 10^{-4} M nifedipine had hardly any effect on Ca^{2+} currents in neurones from *Limnea stagnalis* [Byerly et al., 1985] or in U neurones from *Helix* [Gola

and Ducreux, 1985], although such currents were potently blocked by Cd^{2+}. Furthermore, $> 10^{-4}$ M nifedipine did not completely block the Ca^{2+} spike in the axons of the giant neurones of the jellyfish *Aglantha digitale* [Mackie and Meech, 1985]. Several other reports demonstrate the blocking effects of verapamil on invertebrate Ca^{2+} currents, and these are associated with the usual uncertainties. In addition, it has been reported that mM concentrations of benzodiazepines, active at "peripheral"-type benzodiazepine receptors, block the Ca^{2+} spike in leech neurones (Table VIII).

At this point, it is still quite unclear exactly how closely VSCC in invertebrate neurones resemble those in vertebrate neurones. However, the observations that some are really quite DHP-sensitive, together with certain biophysical characteristics and their sensitivity to phosphorylating conditions (vide infra), seem to indicate considerable similarities, at least in some cases.

Effects of Neurotransmitters

One of the most interesting and important aspects of research in this area concerns the possible regulation of VSCC by neurotransmitters. Such effects are obviously of great fundamental importance in any consideration of the regulation of interneuronal communication. It is by such mechanisms that neurotransmitters may modify both their own release and the release of other substances and generally modify neuronal excitability directly. Similar considerations, of course, apply to the now well documented neurotransmitter-induced modulation of neuronal K$^+$ conductances. Indeed, in many of the cases reported, substances that modulate neuronal VSCC have also been shown in other cases to modulate neuronal K$^+$ channels, often with the same end result. Sometimes these two possibilities are not easy to distinguish. Thus, an agonist may reduce neurotransmitter release by either directly inhibiting Ca^{2+} influx or by reducing it subsequent to the enhancement of a repolarizing K$^+$ flux.

Modulation of neurotransmitter release due to K^+ channel modification has been extensively studied in a number of invertebrate systems, particularly in *Aplysia* [Klein et al., 1980]. From the point of view of the present discussion, however, I shall only consider examples in which there is good reason to believe that VSCC are the locus of neurotransmitter action (Table IX). In the following section, I shall consider some possibilities for the molecular mechanisms underlying these observations.

The classic example of direct VSCC modulation actually occurs not in neurones but in the heart. The positive inotropic effects of catecholamines are clearly the result of a cAMP-mediated phosphorylation of VSCC or some closely associated entity. The details of this system have been investigated rather thoroughly at the molecular level [Reuter, 1983; Bean et al., 1984]. Although both T- and L-type VSCC are known to exist in the heart, cAMP-mediated modulation is directed toward the latter species, resulting in an increase in the probability of channel opening and also, in some species, an increase in the number of VSCC available for opening [Bean, 1985; Nilius et al., 1985]. In vertebrate neurones, however, there is only one report of this type of mechanism, and that is preliminary in nature. Thus, it appears that in hippocampal granule cells, β-adrenergic stimulation may increase a Ca^{2+} current in a fashion analogous to that reported for the heart [Gray and Johnston, 1985a,b]. In all other reports on vertebrate neurones, neurotransmitters seem only to depress Ca^{2+} currents and neurotransmitter release (Table IX). As with studies on VSCC, most reports are derived from observations on peripheral neurones, particularly DRG cells. A particularly good example is provided by examining the effects of opiates and their endogenous counterparts, the opioid peptides [Miller, 1984a]. These substances reduce neurotransmitter release from DRG neurones and in many other cases as well. These effects are associated with a decrease in the size of the action potential measured in the cell soma. Further investigation, however, reveals an interesting

complexity. Thus, whereas opiates acting on μ-, δ-, and κ-opiate receptors, all reduce the size of the spike in DRG cells [Werz and MacDonald, 1984a,b, 1985a; MacDonald and Werz, 1985; Mudge et al., 1979], only those acting on κ-receptors (e.g., dynorphin) reduce the pure Ca^{2+} spike [Werz and MacDonald, 1984a,b, 1985a] or Ca^{2+} currents [MacDonald and Werz, 1985; Werz and MacDonald, 1984b], as measured by voltage clamp techniques. Inspection of the data appears to show that the locus of these κ-opiate effects is the DRG L-channel. A maximally effective concentration of dynorphin blocked about 50% of the Ca^{2+} current. In contrast to the effects of κ-opiates, μ- and δ-specific agents appear to reduce Ca^{2+} influx by enhancing a K^+ current ($I_{K(Ca)}$) [reviewed in Miller, 1984a]. Here then is an excellent example of closely related agents producing the same net result by different neuromodulatory mechanisms. One wonders whether these mechanisms only operate in cultured young DRG neurones (which are in many respects atypical) or whether they operate generally. However, virtually identical results even with respect to μ-, δ-, and κ-specificity have been reported for neurones in the adult guinea pig myenteric plexus, thus encouraging the view that opiates may generally operate in this fashion [Cherubini and North, 1985]. However, it should be pointed out that other data do not quite fit with this elegant story. Thus, in N1E-115 neuroblastoma cells, it appears that an L-type Ca^{2+} current measured under voltage clamp can be inhibited by δ-specific opiates [Tsunoo et al., 1985b]. The peptide somatostatin was also an effective blocker in this system. In addition, pure Ca^{2+} spikes have been reported to be inhibited by δ-opiate agonists in Rohon-Beard neurones [Bixby and Spitzer, 1983a,b] and even in DRG cells [Mudge et al., 1979]. Thus, one may conclude at this point that VSCC seem to be modulated by opioids, but the exact pharmacological specificity of this effect remains to be clearly defined.

Another agent which appears to have clear effects on neuronal VSCC is GABA. Traditionally, of course, GABA was thought to

TABLE IX. Modulation of Neuronal Calcium Conductances by Neurotransmitters

Sympathetic neurones
  I_{Ca} reduced by muscarine [Belluzzi et al., 1985]
  I_{Ca} reduced by adrenaline 10^{-4} M by 75% [Koketsu and Akasu, 1982]
  Ca spike and AHP reduced by adrenaline (3×10^{-5}–10^{-3} M). No effect of isoproterenol. No effect on Ca spike in spinal ganglion neurones [Minota and Koketsu, 1977]
  Ca spike reduced by adenosine (L-PIA and 2-CADO). Also AHP reduced [Henon and McAfee, 1980]
  Ca spike reduced by catecholamines. Also AHP. $> 10^{-6}$ M. Blocked by phentolamine [Horn and McAfee, 1980]
  Ca spike and AHP reduced by PGE$_1$ (10–500 nM) [Mo et al., 1985]
  I_{Ca} reduced by 50% by norepinephrine 5×10^{-5} M [Galvan and Adams, 1982]
Enteric neurones
  Ca spike reduced by GABA-B agonists in myenteric neurones [Cherubini and North, 1984]
  Ca spike reduced by κ-opiates but not μ- or δ-opiates in myenteric neurones [Cherubini and North, 1985]
  Ca spike reduced by Met-enk in cultured by myenteric neurones [Willard and Nishi, 1985]
  Ca spike reduced by norepinephrine but clonidine had no effect. α_2 blockers reversed NE effect [Slack, 1985]
Sensory neurones
  Ca spike and I_{Ca} (L) reduced by GABA-B agonists [Schlichter et al., 1984]
  GABA-B agonists 10^{-5}–10^{-4} M reduce I_{Ca} (L) 46% and I_{Ca} (T) 22% [Deisz and Lux, 1985]
  Ca spike and I_{Ca} reduced by NE, GABA and 5-HT. NE 10^{-4} M reduced I_{Ca} by 30% [Dunlap and Fischbach, 1981]
  Ca spike reduced by GABA-B agonists [Desarmenien et al., 1984]
  Ca spike reduced by GABA-B agonists [Dunlap, 1981]
  Ca spike reduced by GABA, 5-HT, and NE [Dunlap and Fischbach, 1978]
  Ca spike reduced by DA, NE, and 5-HT all IC$_{50}$ = 10^{-6} M. Nonadditive. No effect of clonidine. Not a typical α_2 receptor [Canfield and Dunlap, 1984]

NE reduces I_{Ca} (L) [Forscher and Oxford, 1985a]
NE reduces I_{Ca} (L) and I_{Ca} (T) effect is bigger on I_{Ca} (T) [Forscher and Oxford, 1985b]
Ca spike and I_{Ca} (L) reduced by adenosine [MacDonald et al., 1985a]
I_{Ca} (L) reduced by adenosine 50–90% [Dolphin et al., 1985]
I_{Ca} (L) reduced by dynorphin but not Leu-enk [MacDonald and Werz, 1985; Werz and MacDonald, 1984b]
Ca spike reduced by enkephalin [Mudge et al., 1979]
Ca spike blocked by dynorphin. Also AHP reduced [Werz and MacDonald, 1984a, 1985a]
Ca spike in *Xenopus* DRG reduced by enkephalin [Bixby and Spitzer, 1983a]
Central neurones
  Ca spike in hippocampal pyramidal cell reduced by adenosine [Proctor and Dunwiddie, 1983]
  I_{Ca} in hippocampal pyramidal cells unaffected by adenosine [Halliwell and Scholfield, 1984a,b]
  I_{Ca} in hippocampal granule cells increased by β-adrenergic agonists [Gray and Johnston, 1985a,b]
  Ca spike in Rohan-Beard cells reduced by enkephalin [Bixby and Spitzer, 1983a]
Neuroblastomas
  N1E-115 I_{Ca} (l) reduced by enkephalin and SRIF [Tsunoo et al., 1985b]
Invertebrate neurones
  Helix neurones. Ca spike and I_{Ca} reduced by DA [Paupardin-Tritsch et al., 1985a]
  Helix neurones. Ca spike and I_{Ca} reduced by FMRF-NH$_2$ [Colombaioni et al., 1985]
  Aplysia neurones. I_{Ca} reduced by FMRF-NH$_2$ [Brezina et al., 1985]
  Limnea neurones. I_{Ca} reduced by DA, A, and 5-HT [Akopyan et al., 1985]
  Aplysia neurones. I_{Ca} increased by 5-HT [Pellmar, 1984; Pellmar and Carpenter, 1980]
  Helix neurones. I_{Ca} increased by 5-HT [Paupardin-Tritsch et al., 1985b]

produce its effects by opening a Cl− channel. This action is known to be enhanced by benzodiazepines, mimicked by muscimol, and blocked competitively by bucuculline and noncompetitively by picrotoxin. However, more recently it has become clear that a second type of GABA receptor exists. This is known as a GABA-B receptor to distinguish it from the traditional GABA-A receptor. Activation of GABA-B receptors has been shown to lead to both inhibition of Ca^{2+} conductances [Dunlap, 1981; Cherubini and North, 1984; Deisz and Lux, 1985; Dunlap and Fischbach, 1978, 1981; Desarmenien et al., 1984; Schlichter et al., 1984] and also enhancement of K^+ currents [Gahwiler and Brown, 1985; Newberry and Nicoll, 1984], although in this case, as yet not in the same neuronal type. Thus, effects on Ca^{2+} conductances have been reported in myenteric [Cherubini and North, 1984] and DRG neurones [Dunlap, 1981; Deisz and Lux, 1985; Dunlap and Fischbach, 1978, 1981], whereas those on K^+ conductances were observed in hippocampal pyramidal cells [Gahwiler and Brown, 1985; Newberry and Nicoll, 1984]. One report has gone so far as to analyze the relative GABA-B effects of DRG T- and L-currents [Diesz and Lux, 1985]. These authors found that the effect was predominantly exerted on the L-conductance, although an appreciable inhibition of the T-current was also observed.

Effects similar to those reported for GABA-B agonists have been reported for adenosine receptor agonists, although the pharmacology of these effects is less clear. Adenosine and associated agonists (e.g., 2-Cl-adenosine) reduce Ca^{2+} spikes in sympathetic neurones [Henon and McAfee, 1983], DRG cells [MacDonald et al., 1985a,b], and possibly in hippocampal pyramidal cells. Voltage clamp data indicate that in DRG neurones at any rate, this is due to an inhibition of a Ca^{2+} current generally resembling the L-current [Dolphin et al., 1985; MacDonald et al., 1985a]. However, the specificity of these effects do not fit very clearly into either of the A_1 or A_2 categories for purinergic receptors [MacDonald et al., 1985]. Moreover, in hippocampal pyramidal cells and olfactory neurones, voltage clamp studies revealed no effect of adenosine analogues on Ca^{2+} currents [Halliwell and Scholfield, 1984].

The most widely studied modulator of vertebrate Ca^{2+} currents is norepinephrine. Apart from the effects referred to in hippocampal granule cells, all these effects are inhibitory and "α_2-adrenergic" in nature. Norepinephrine inhibits Ca^{2+} spikes in sympathetic [Horn and McAfee, 1980; Minota and Koketsu, 1977], myenteric [Slack, 1985; Nishi and North, 1973a,b] and DRG neurones [Canfield and Dunlap, 1984; Dunlap and Fischbach, 1978, 1981], and also in the locus coeruleus [Williams and North, 1985]. Quite extensive voltage clamp studies have demonstrated corresponding norepinephrine inhibition of Ca^{2+} currents in locus coeruleus [Williams and North, 1985] and sympathetic neurones [Galvan and Adams, 1982; Koketsu and Akasu, 1982] and DRG cells [Dunlap and Fischbach, 1981; Forscher and Oxford, 1985a,b]. As with the other neurotransmitters discussed above, α_2-adrenergic stimulation also activates a K^+ conductance in a number of instances [Slack, 1985; North and Surprenant, 1985; Sah et al., 1985; Williams et al., 1984, 1985]. Although it is not entirely clear what type of VSCC is being modulated by norepinephrine, in most cases it appears to have the characteristics of an L-type conductance [Dunlap and Fischbach, 1981; Forscher and Oxford, 1985a; Galvan and Adams, 1982]. However, one preliminary report has indicated that T-type VSCC may also be modulated and that the effect of norepinephrine may be even greater on this conductance [Forscher and Oxford, 1985b]. These are, however, some extremely curious features associated with reported effects of norepinephrine on Ca^{2+} currents. Although there are indications that the effect is α_2-adrenergic in nature, there are other observations that do not fit in with this idea. Among these are data showing that in certain cases clonidine [Slack, 1985; Canfield and Dunlap, 1984; Williams and North, 1985] is not an effective agonist, that yohimbine (or even prazosin) was not an effective blocker [Williams and North 1985], or that dopamine and 5-HT were as effective as norepinephrine [Canfield and Dunlap, 1984]. All such data indicate that the receptor mediating these effects is not an α_2-receptor. On the other hand, the receptor mediating the norepinephrine actions on K^+ conductances fits easily into a traditional α_2-category [Slack, 1985; Williams and North, 1985]. One must be left with some doubts, therefore, as to the physiological significance of the observations with norepinephrine. There is no doubt that such effects occur when catecholamines are squirted onto cells. However, the possibility must be considered that they represent nonspecific interactions of catecholamines with VSCC. Other substances that have been shown to inhibit vertebrate neuronal Ca^{2+} conductances include PGE$_1$ [Mo et al., 1985] and muscarine [Belluzzi et al., 1985]. Again, in the latter case, muscarinic effects are more often associated with actions on a K$^+$ conductance (I$_m$) [Adams et al., 1982].

Several clear-cut examples of the effects of neurotransmitters on Ca^{2+} currents in invertebrate neurones also exist (Table IX). Dopamine (and other biogenic amines) inhibit Ca^{2+} currents in neurones from the snails *Helix* [Paupardin-Tritsch et al., 1985a] and *Limnea* [Akopyan et al., 1985]. The peptide FMRF-NH$_2$ produces similar effects again in *Helix* [Colombaioni et al., 1985] and also in *Aplysia* [Brezina et al., 1985]. The studies in *Helix* are particularly interesting as both DA and FMRF-NH$_2$ can also decrease a K$^+$ conductance in some neurones of this snail. Effects on Ca^{2+} and K$^+$ conductances are often observed in different cells but sometimes in the same cell. Clearly, these effects would have potentially opposite actions on the duration of the action potential in such a neurone. However, when these effects are both observed in the same neurone, the action on Ca^{2+} currents prevails, and the size of the spike is reduced [Colombaioni et al., 1985; Paupardin-Tritsch et al., 1985a]. 5-HT has been shown to increase a Ca^{2+} current in neurones from *Aplysia* [Pellmar, 1984; Pellmar and Carpenter, 1980] and *Helix* [Paupardin-Tritsch et al., 1985b]. Such actions are clearly different from the better publicized effects of 5-HT on the S-type K$^+$ current also reported in *Aplysia* [Siegelbaum et al., 1982].

Effects of Intracellular Mediators

The effects of the various neurotransmitters described above raise questions as to how these actions are mediated. There are clearly two major possibilities. The first is that the receptor involved directly "gates" the VSCC in a manner similar to the action of acetylcholine at the nicotinic receptor. The second possibility is that intracellular second messengers mediate the effects of receptor stimulation on VSCC. This would be analogous to the β-adrenergic effects on VSCC in cardiac muscle. As I shall now discuss, there is considerable evidence that neuronal Ca^{2+} currents can be directly modulated by various second messengers including Ca^{2+}, cyclic nucleotide, and diacylglycerol (DAG)-mediated events (Table X). As many of the neurotransmitters discussed have been shown to exert their actions in other instances through the mediation of second messengers, one's initial bias would be that they must also do so when producing effects on VSCC. However, this may not necessarily be the case. For example, a preliminary report suggests that in patch experiments with DRG cells, norepinephrine is only effective when placed inside the patch pipette and is ineffective when placed outside [Forscher and Oxford, 1985b]. This is a classic paradigm for examining the involvement of a second messenger system and would suggest direct gating of VSCC by a norepinephrine receptor. However, in this case, one should remember the caveats discussed above associated with interpreting the effects observed with catecholamines.

One of the clearest indications of the effects of intracellular mediators on Ca^{2+} currents derives from studies of Ca^{2+} current "rundown" or "wash-out," a phenomenon referred to several times already. Such observations suggest, of course, that some intracellular components are required to keep VSCC working in the normal fashion. A clue as to what such mechanisms may involve comes from studies on a related phenomenon, Ca^{2+}-mediated VSCC inactivation [Eckert and Chad, 1984]. Eckert and colleagues have examined the phenomenon of Ca^{2+} current wash-out in invertebrate neurones [Armstrong and Eckert, 1985; Chad and Eckert, 1985a,b,c; Kalman and Eckert, 1985]. They postulate that two processes may be involved. One process is an irreversible loss of VSCC,

TABLE X. Effects of Intracellular Second Messengers on Neuronal Calcium Conductances

Vertebrate neurones

cAMP/Mg-ATP slows run-down of I_{Ca} in perfused rat DRG neurone [Fedulova et al., 1981, 1985; Kostyuk et al., 1981b]

Mg-ATP/ATP plus regenerating system stabilized I_{Ca} in DRG neurone. EGTA, cAMP, and cGMP had no effect [Forscher and Oxford, 1985a,b]

Run-down of I_{Ca} in petrose or nodose neurones is increased by raising $[Ca^{2+}]_i$ to 10^{-7} M [Bossu et al., 1985]

I_{Ca} (L) in N1E-115 neuroblastoma is increased by cAMP [Tsunoo et al., 1984]

I_{Ca} in rods is unaffected by cAMP [Corey et al., 1984]

Inhibitory effect of Ca^{2+} in I_{Ca} [Eckert and Chad, 1984]

TPA and analogues block I_{Ca} (L) in DRG neurones [Werz and MacDonald, 1985c; Rane et al., 1985a,b]

Effects of GABA and NE on I_{Ca} are blocked by pertussis toxin. [Holz et al., 1985]

Invertebrate neurones

cAMP, cGMP no effect of I_{Ca} in *Helix* neurones. EGTA removes inactivation [Paupardin-Tritsch et al., 1985a]

Run-down in perfused *Helix* neurones slowed by cAMP/MG-ATP or F^-. Increased by raising $[Ca^{2+}]_i$ [Doroshenko et al., 1982]

Invertebrate neurones (continued)

Run-down in perfused *Helix* neurones slowed by protein kinase and Mg-ATP [Doroshenko et al., 1984b]

Two phases of inactivation. Phase (A) irreversible is slowed by leupeptin, inhibitor of Ca-activated protease. Phase (b) reversible, enhanced or mimicked by raising $[Ca^{2+}]_i$ or by calcineurin, a Ca-activated phosphatase. Slowed by protein kinase or ATPγS [Armstrong and Eckert, 1985; Chad and Eckert, 1985a,b,c; Eckert and Chad, 1984; Kalman and Eckert, 1985]

cAMP induces an I_{Ca} in *Aplysia* neurones [Pellmar, 1981]

EGTA and cAMP do not alter I_{Ca} in *limnea* neurones [Akopyan et al., 1985]

cAMP induced an I_{Ca} in slug neurones [Hockberger and Connor, 1984]

cGMP (but not cAMP) or TPA induced an I_{Ca} in *Helix* neurones [Paupardin-Tritsch et al., 1985b]

TPA induces an increase in I_{Ca} and Ca spike in *Aplysia* bag cell neurones. This is due to the increased activity of a large VSCC [DeRiemer et al., 1985a,b; Strong et al., 1986]

Hermissenda I_{Ca} enhanced by TPA [Fisher et al., 1985]

and the second process is reversible. The irreversible process is mediated by a Ca^{2+}-activated protease and can be prevented by the protease inhibitor leupeptin. The second process can be mimicked by a Ca^{2+}-activated phosphatase, calcineurin, and enhanced by raising intracellular Ca^{2+} concentrations. This latter observation indicates the following possibility. It may be supposed that normally VSCC must be phosphorylated in order to respond normally. When Ca^{2+} enters the cell through VSCC, it activates a phosphatase that dephosphorylates the VSCC and thus "inactivates" it. This then would be the mechanism underlying the phenomenon known as Ca^{2+}-dependent VSCC inactivation. In addition, in perfused cells or whole cell patch systems, an irreversible protease-mediated degradation of VSCC seems to occur. The "physiological" significance of this latter mechanism is less clear. There are several pieces of evidence which support the idea that a phosphoryla-

tion-dephosphorylation cycle may be important for VSCC function in many cases. It should also be noted that the VSCC involved here appear generally to be in the L-type class. Experimental manipulations which are designed to raise $[Ca^{2+}]_i$ usually increase the rate of inactivation, whereas those designed to decrease $[Ca^{2+}]_i$ usually decrease it [Eckert and Chad, 1984]. Hence, it is easy to explain the effects of EGTA or Ba^{2+} on Ca^{2+} current inactivation. Interestingly, in cultured sensory neurones, increasing $[Ca^{2+}]_i$ specifically inactivates L-like channels leaving T-like channels unaltered [Bossu et al., 1985]. Indeed, T-like channels have been shown not to "run down" in a number of cases [Armstrong and Matteson, 1985; Bossu et al., 1985; Fedulova et al., 1985]. If the proposed scheme is true, it should be possible to reverse Ca^{2+}-mediated "inactivation" or "run-down" utilizing conditions that enhance phosphorylation. It will also be apparent that whether we describe the phenomenon as Ca^{2+} current "inactivation" or reversible "run-down" merely depends on the experimental paradigm which is employed. There are several observations that indicate that cAMP-mediated phosphorylation mechanisms may be responsible for keeping neuronal VSCC in a functional phosphorylated state. For example, Kostyuk and colleagues have demonstrated that in perfused *Helix* neurones cAMP/Mg-ATP, F$^-$, or the purified catalytic subunit from cAMP-dependent protein kinase can at least partially restore run-down of Ca^{2+} currents and reverse the increased rate of run-down induced by raising [Ca^{2+}]$_i$ [Doroshenko et al., 1982, 1984b]. Similar mechanisms also appear to occur in DRG neurones. Here again run-down is reversed by cAMP/Mg-ATP [Fedulova et al., 1981, 1985; Kostyuk et al., 1981b], although one study found no requirement for cAMP [Forscher and Oxford, 1985a]. Interestingly, the effects of such conditions were only exerted on L-type currents [Fedulova et al., 1985]. In some instances, effects of such phosphorylating conditions on Ca^{2+} current wash-out have not been noted [Corey et al., 1984]. However, in such instances the appropriate conditions may not have been employed, or else they may represent special cases. Evidence similar to that provided by Kostyuk's group has also been provided by Eckert's group [Armstrong and Eckert, 1985; Chad and Eckert, 1985a,b,c; Eckert and Chad, 1984; Kalman and Eckert, 1985]. An alternative view of all these results, however, is provided by Byerly and Yazejian [1985]. Using neurones from the snail *Limnea*, it was shown that Ca^{2+} current wash-out could be prevented by Mg-ATP, but that when good Ca^{2+} buffering was provided, cAMP or a kinase was not required. Thus, these authors postulate that the main effect of cAMP is to increase the Ca^{2+} differing capability of some cellular organelle rather than to enhance VSCC phosphorylation per se. This is obviously an interesting idea.

The idea that intracellular Ca^{2+} can decrease and intracellular cAMP can increase the "functionality" of VSCC in neurones by promoting phosphatase or kinase activity, respectively, provides an obvious mechanism for the effects of neurotransmitters. Thus in certain cases, cAMP or cGMP have been shown to induce a Ca^{2+} current in invertebrate neurones [Pellmar, 1981, 1984; Hockberger and Connor, 1984; Carpenter and Gunn, 1970; Paupardin-Tritsch et al., 1985b; Carpenter, 1980], thus mimicking the action of a neurotransmitter such as 5-HT. However, it is not possible to tell whether such effects involve mechanisms analogous to those already discussed or possibly the induction of a new channel type. In contrast, we have already discussed several observations in which neurotransmitters were found to inhibit neuronal Ca^{2+} currents. It would seem possible that several of these agents could exert their effects by raising [Ca^{2+}]$_i$ or by reducing intracellular concentrations of cAMP. Indeed, if a neurotransmitter were able to increase [Ca^{2+}]$_i$, one might expect to observe both a decrease in Ca^{2+} currents for the reasons discussed above and also an increase in a K$^+$ conductance of the I$_{K(Ca)}$ variety; these may occur in different portions of the same neurone. Clearly such effects often do go hand in hand (vide supra). It is also quite obvious that many of the agents that reduce neuronal Ca^{2+} currents have also been shown to be inhibitory regulators of adenylate cyclase, e.g., α_2 [Limbird et al., 1983], GABA-B [Hill, 1985], opiates [Miller, 1984a]. Thus, one can make an equally good theoretical case for supposing that inhibitory effects on neuronal Ca^{2+} currents are mediated by decreases in cellular cAMP concentrations.

At this point one should also note the possibilities provided by the third major second messenger system, that is, the pathway linked to the generation of diacylglycerol/IP$_3$ and subsequent activation of protein kinase C. Of course it is likely that this system is not actually completely independent of the Ca^{2+} and cyclic nucleotide systems already referred to. There are now important indications of direct effects of protein kinase C on neuronal VSCC. In *Aplysia* bag cell neurones, the phorbol ester TPA (which mimics the effects of endogenous DAG) stimulates a Ca^{2+} current and increases the size of the cell Ca^{2+} spike [DeRiemer et al., 1985a,b]. Further investigations have revealed that the major effect of TPA is actually to increase the activity of a large conductance VSCC which is normally virtually inert. A second type of VSCC with lower conductance is present both before and after TPA treatment [Strong et al., 1986]. This observation is extremely interesting. However, it is not yet known whether the large conductance VSCC that appear are modified versions of the low conductance channel or a totally different species. TPA also appears to have similar effects in some neurones in *Helix* [Paupardin-Tritsch et al., 1985b]. Quite different effects of phorbol esters have been reported in vertebrate neurones. Two groups have demonstrated that in DRG cells, TPA inhibits a Ca^{2+} current [Werz and MacDonald, 1985c; Rane and Dunlap, 1985a,b]. This is probably an L-type current. Moreover, in PC12 cells, TPA clearly inhibits voltage-sensitive $^{45}Ca^{2+}$ influx via L-type channels [Harris et al., 1985a]. This mechanism provides another method by which various neurotransmitters could inhibit neuronal Ca^{2+} currents. Moreover, it is also conceivable that activation of protein kinase C by incoming Ca^{2+} could contribute to the phenomen of CA^{2+}- current inactivation already discussed [Harris et al., 1985a].

Clearly, therefore, there are numerous ways in which neurotransmitters might produce their effects on neuronal Ca^{2+}- channels. It is also equally evident that we have so far only seen the tip of the iceberg, and no general rules have yet emerged. Similar conclusions can be applied to the study of the various types of neuronal K^+- channels [Levitan, 1985].

CONCLUSIONS

It will be clear from the above discussion that the state of our knowledge concerning the nature and functions of neuronal VSCC is growing at a tremendous rate. Because of the enormous importance of Ca^{2+} not only as a charge carrier, but also as a second messenger, its roles in neuronal function are clearly considerably more diverse than those of Na^+ or K^+. Moreover, many of the tools that enable us to study Ca^{2+} at the cellular level (e.g., dihydropyridines, quin-2, etc.) have only recently been developed.

At the beginning of this article, I described the issues of the heterogeneity, modifiability, and distribution of VSCC as been of particular interest at this time. Clearly, many questions relating to these subjects remain to be answered. It is important to realize, however, that until the last few years, neuronal VSCC remained solely biophysical entities. Thus, no biochemical or pharmacological "aid" was available to play a role similar to that of tetrodotoxin in the study of sodium channels. The use of radiolabelled dihydropyridines and other drugs has rapidly changed the situation, however. Indeed, it is these types of data that have probably had the greatest recent impact on the way we now view neuronal VSCC. Thus, one type of neuronal VSCC can now be clearly identified from both the biophysical and biochemical points of view. Because we can now approach the study of these entities from so many directions, information concerning their nature and function will inevitably be rapidly forthcoming. Indeed, it has already been observed that several manipulations can alter the properties of neuronal "dihydropyridine receptors." These include various drug treatments such as administration of narcotics [Ramkumar and El-Fakahany, 1984], PCP [Bolger et al., 1985a], reserpine [Powers and Colucci, 1985], ethanol [Lucchi et al., 1985], and chlorpromazine [Ramkumar and El-Fakahany, 1985]. Moreover, changes in these binding sites have also been associated with hypertension [Lee et al., 1985; Ishii et al., 1983], cardiomyopathy [Wagner et al., 1986], and aging [Govoni et al., 1985]. Thus, we are already obtaining information about the plasticity of this type of VSCC even before we are entirely clear about what it does.

Finally, the realization that dihydropyridine-sensitive VSCC exit in neurones has had several important implications. One of these is that administration of such drugs to the whole organism should lead to behavioural modifications. Indeed, there are now several reports concerning the behavioural effects of dihydropyridines [Bolger et al., 1985a; Draski et al., 1985; Grebb et al., 1985; Hoffmeister et al., 1982; Mendelson et al., 1984a,b; Shelton et al., 1985]. It is not difficult to predict that the studies discussed in this article will usher in an entirely new approach to neuropharmacology.

ACKNOWLEDGMENTS

This work was supported by PHS grants DA-02121 and MH40165-01A1. Grants were also received from Miles Pharmaceutical Ltd. and the Brain Research Foundation of the University of Chicago. The author is indebted to many colleagues for providing him with prepublication manuscripts. These include David Brown, Steve Nahorski, Solomon Snyder, Ron Janis, Mike Sanguinetti, Irwin Levitan, Bill Caterall, and W. Glossmann. I am also indebted to Della Akres for typing the manuscript and to my students and colleagues at the University for critical advice.

REFERENCES

Adams DJ, Smith SJ, Thompson SH (1980): Ionic currents in molluscan soma. Ann Rev Neurosci 3:141–167.

Adams PR, Brown DA, Constanti A (1982): Pharmacological inhibition of the M-current. J Physiol 332:223–262.

Adams WB (1985): Slow depolarizing and hyperpolarizing currents which mediate bursting in Aplysia neurone R15. J Physiol 360:51–68.

Adams WB, Levitan IB (1985): Voltage and ion dependences of the slow currents which mediate bursting in Aplysia neurone R15. J Physiol 360:69–93.

Affolter H, Coronado R (1985): Agonists BAY K8644 and CGP 28392 open calcium channels reconstituted from skeletal muscle transverse tubules. Biophys J 48:341–347.

Agoston D, Hargittai P, Nagy A (1983): Effects on a 4-aminopyridine on calcium movements and changes of membrane potential in pinched off nerve terminals from rat cerebral cortex. J Neurochem 41:745–751.

Ahmed Z, Connor JA (1979): Measurement of calcium influx under voltage clamp in molluscan neurones using the metallochromatic dye Arsenazo III. J Physiol 286:61–82.

Akaike N, Nishi K, Oyama Y (1981a): Inhibitory effects of propanolol on the calcium current of Helix neurones. Br J Pharmacol 73:431–434.

Akaike N, Brown AM, Nishi K, Tsuda Y (1981b): Actions of verapamil, diltiazem and divalent cations on the calcium current of Helix neurones. Br J Pharmacol 74:87–95.

Akasu T, Koketsu K (1981): Voltage clamp studies of a slow inward current in bullfrog sympathetic ganglion cells. Neurosci Lett 26:259–262.

Akasu T, Hirai K, Koketsu K (1983a): Modulatory actions of ATP on membrane potentials of bullfrog sympathetic ganglion cells. Brain Res 258:313–317.

Akasu T, Nishimura T, Koketsu K (1983b): Substance P inhibits the action potentials in bullfrog sympathetic ganglion cells. Neurosci Lett 41:161–166.

Akerman KEO, Nicholls DG (1981): Ca^{2+} transport by intact synaptosomes: The voltage dependence Ca^{2+} channel and re-evaluation of the role of Na$^+$/Ca^{2+} exchange. Eur J Biochem 117:491–497.

Akerman KEO, Nicholls DG (1983): Ca^{2+} transport and regulation of transmitter release in isolated nerve endings. Trends in Biochem Sci 8:63–64.

Akopyan AR, Chemeris NK, Iljin VI (1985): Neurotransmitter induced modulation of neuronal Ca^{2+}-currents is modulated by intracellular Ca^{2+} or cAMP. Brain Res 326:145–148.

Albus U, Habermann E, Ferry DR, Glossmann H (1984): Novel 1,4-dihydropyridine (BAY K8644) facilitates calcium dependent ^{3}H-noradrenaline release from PC12 cells. J Neurochem 42:1186–1189.

Almers W, McClesky EW, Palade PT (1984): A nonselective cation conductance in frog muscle membrane blocked by micromolar external calcium ions. J Physiol 353:565–583.

Alvarez-Leefmans FJ, Miledi R (1980): Voltage sensitive calcium entry in frog motoneurones. J Physiol 308:241–257.

Andrejaus E, Hertel R, Marme D (1985): Specific binding of the calcium antagonist [^{3}H]-verapamil to membrane fractions from plants. J Biol Chem 260:5411–5414.

Anglister L, Farber IC, Shahar A, Grinvald A (1982): Localization of voltage sensitive calcium channels along developing neurites: Their possible role in regulating neurite elongation. Devel Biol 94:351–365.

Armstrong CM, Matteson DR (1985): Two distinct populations of Ca^{2+}-channels in a clonal pituitary cell line. Science 227:65–67.

Armstrong D, Eckert R (1985): Phosphorylating agents prevent washout of unitary calcium currents in excised membrane patches. J Gen Physiol 86:25a.

Aronstam RS, Hoss W (1985): Tricyclic antidepressant

inhibition of depolarization induced uptake of calcium by synaptosomes from rat brain. Biochem Pharmacol 34:902–904.

Ashley RH, Brammer MJ, Marchbanks R (1984): Measurement of intrasynaptosomal free calcium by using the fluorescent indicator quin-2. Biochem J 219: 149–158.

Atlas D, Adler M (1981): Alpha-adrenergic antagonists as possible Ca^{2+} channel inhibitors. Proc Natl Acad Sci USA 78:1237–1241.

Augustine GJ, Eckert R (1984): Divalent cations differentially support transmitter release at the squid giant synapse. J Physiol 348:257–271.

Augustine GJ, Charlton MP, Smith SJ (1985a): Calcium entry into voltage clamped presynaptic terminals of squid. J Physiol 367:143–162.

Augustine GJ, Charlton MP, Smith SJ (1985b): Calcium entry and transmitter release at voltage clamped nerve terminals of squid. J Physiol 367:163–181.

Augustine GJ, Charlton MP, Smith SJ (1985c): Neurotransmitter release from voltage clamped nerve terminals of squid. J Physiol (in press).

Baccaglini PI (1978): Action potentials of embryonic dorsal root ganglion neurones in xenopus tadpoles. J Physiol 283:585–603.

Baccaglini PI, Cooper E (1982): Electrophysiological studies of newborn rat nodose neurones in cell culture. J Physiol 324:429–439.

Baccaglini PI, Spitzer NC (1977): Developmental changes in the inward current of the action potential of Rohon-Beard neurones. J Physiol 271:93–117.

Bader CR, Bertrand D, Schwartz EA (1982): Voltage activated and calcium activated currents studied in solitary rod inner segments from salamander retina. J Physiol 331:253–284.

Bader CR, Bertrand D, Dupin E, Kato AC (1983): Development of electrical membrane properties in cultured avian neural crest. Nature 305:808–810.

Baker PF, Hodgkin AL, Ridgway EB (1971): Depolarization and calcium entry in squid giant axons. J Physiol 218:709–755.

Baker PF, Meves H, Ridgway EB (1973): Effects of manganese and other agents on the calcium uptake that follows depolarization of squid axons. J Physiol 231:511–526.

Baraban JM, Snyder SH, Alger BE (1985): Protein kinase C regulates ionic conductance in hippocampal pyramidal neurones: Electrophysiological effects of phorbol esters. Proc Natl Acad Sci USA 82:2538–2542.

Barr E, Daniell LC, Leslie SW (1985): Synaptosomal calcium uptake unaltered by adenosine and 2-chloroadenosine. Biochem Pharmacol 34:713–715.

Barres BA, Chun LLY, Corey DP (1985): Voltage dependent ion channels in glial cells. Soc Neurosci Abstr 11:147.

Barrett EF, Barrett JN (1976): Separation of two voltage

sensitive potassium currents and demonstration of a tetrodotoxin resistant calcium current in frog motoneurones. J Physiol 255:737–774.

Barros F, Katz GM, Kaczorowski GJ, Vandlen RL, Reuben JP (1985): Calcium currents in GH_3 cultured pituitary cells under whole cell voltage clamp. Inhibition by voltage dependent potassium currents. Proc Natl Acad Sci USA 82:1108–1112.

Bean BP (1984): Nitrendipine blocks cardiac calcium channels: High affinity binding to the inactivated state. Proc Natl Acad Sci USA 81:6388–6392.

Bean BP (1985): Two types of calcium channel in canine atrial cells. Differences in kinetics, selectivity and pharmacology. J Gen Physiol 86:1–30.

Bean BP, Nowycky MC, Tsien RW (1984): Beta-adrenergic modulation of calcium channels in frog ventricular heart cells. Nature 307:371–372.

Beattie DT, Cunnane TC, Muir TC (1985): The effects of Ca^{2+} entry blockers on spontaneous and electrically evoked release of transmitter from guinea-pig vas deferens. Br J Pharmacol 84:29p.

Bellemann P, Franckowiak G (1985): Different receptor affinities of the enantiomers of BAY K8644, a dihydropyridine Ca channel activator. Eur J Pharmacol 118:187–188.

Bellemann P, Schade A, Towart R (1983): Dihydropyridine receptor in rat brain labelled with ^{3}H-nimodipine. Proc Natl Acad Sci USA 80:2356–2360.

Belluzzi G, Sacchi O, Wanke E (1985): Identification of delayed potassium and calcium currents in rat sympathetic neurone under voltage clamp. J Physiol 358:107–129.

Benardo LS, Masukawa LM, Prince DA (1982): Electrophysiology of isolated hippocampal pyramidal dendrites. J Neurosci 2:1614–1622.

Bender AS, Herz L (1985): Pharmacological evidence that the non-neuronal diazepam binding site in primary cultures of glial cells is associated with a Ca^{2+}-channel. Eur J Pharmacol 110:287–288.

Berridge MJ, Irvine RF (1984): Inositol triphosphate, a novel second messenger in cellular signal transduction. Nature 312:315–321.

Biales B, Dichter M, Tischler A (1976): Electrical excitability of cultured adrenal chromaffin cells. J Physiol 262:743–753.

Bixby JL, Spitzer NC (1983a): Enkephalin reduces calcium action potentials in Rohon-Beard neurones in vivo. J Neurosci 3:1014–1018.

Bixby JL, Spitzer NC (1983b): Enkephalin reduces quantal content at the frog neuromuscular junction. Nature, 301:431–432.

Bixby JL, Spitzer NC (1984a): The appearance and development of neurotransmitter sensitivity in Xenopus embryonic spinal neurons in vitro. J Physiol 353:143–155.

Bixby JL, Spitzer NC (1984b): Early differentiation of vertebrate spinal neurones in the absence of voltage dependent Ca^{2+} and Na$^+$ influx. Devel Biol 106: 89–96.

Blaustein MP (1975): Effects of potassium, veratridine and scorpion venom on calcium accumulation and transmitter release by nerve terminals in vitro. J Physiol 247:617–655.

Blaustein MP, Ector AC (1975): Barbiturate inhibition of calcium uptake by depolarized nerve terminals in vitro. Molec Pharmacol 11:369–378.

Bodewei R, Herring S, Schubert B, Wollenberger A (1985): Sodium and calcium currents in neuroblastoma x glioma hybrid cells before and after morphological differentiation by dibutyryl cyclic AMP. Gen Physiol Biophys 4:113–117.

Bolger GT, Gengo P, Klockowski R, Luchowski E, Siegel H, Janis RA, Triggle AM, Triggle DJ (1983): Characterization of binding of the Ca^{2+} channel antagonist nitrendipine to guinea-pig ileal smooth muscle. J Pharmacol Exp Ther 225:291–309.

Bolger GT, Rafftery MF, Skolnick P (1985a): Phencyclidine increases the affinity of dihydropyridine calcium channel antagonist binding in rat brain. Naunyn-Schmiederberg's Arch Pharmacol 330:227–234.

Bolger GT, Weissman BA, Skolnick P (1985b): The behavioural effects of the calcium agonist BAY K8644 in the mouse: Antagonism by the calcium antagonist nifedipine. Naunyn-Schmiedeberg's Arch Pharmacol 328:373–377.

Boll W, Lux HD (1985): Action of organic antagonists on neuronal calcium currents. Neurosci Lett 56: 335–339.

Bolton TB (1979): Mechanisms of action of transmitters and other substances on smooth muscle. Physiol Rev 59:606–718.

Borsotto M, Barhanin J, Norman RI, Lazdunski M (1984): Purification of the dihydropyridine receptor of the voltage dependent Ca^{2+} channel from skeletal muscle transverse tubules using (+)-^{3}H-PN 200110. Biochem Biophys Res Commun 122:1357–1366.

Borsotto M, Barhanin J, Fosset M, Lazdunski M (1985): The 1,4-dihydropyridine receptor associated with skeletal muscle voltage dependent Ca^{2+}-channel. J Biol Chem 260:14255–14263.

Bossu J-L, Feltz A (1984): Patch clamp study of the tetrodotoxin resistant sodium current in group C sensory neurones. Neurosci Lett 51:241–246.

Bossu J-L, Feltz A, Thomann JM (1985): Depolarization elicits two distinct calcium currents in vertebrate sensory neurones. Pflug Arch 403:360–368.

Bourque CW, Renaud CP (1985): Calcium dependent action potentials in rat supraoptic neurosecretory neurones recorded in vitro. J Physiol 363:419–428.

Brandt BL, Hagiwara S, Kidohoro Y, Miyazaki S (1976): Action potentials in the rat chromaffin cell and effects of acetylcholine. J Physiol 263:417–439.

Brezina V, Erxleben C, Eckert R (1985): FMRF-amide suppresses calcium current in Aplysia neurones. Biophys J 47:435a.

Briggs CA, Brown TH, McAfee DA (1985a). Neuropharmacology and pharmacology of long term potentiation in the rat sympathetic ganglion. J Physiol 359:503–521.

Briggs CA, McAfee DA, McCaman RE (1985b): Long term potentiation of synaptic acetylcholine release in the superior cervical ganglion of the rat. J Physiol 363:181–190.

Brown AM, Camerer H, Kunze DL, Lux HD (1982): Similarity of unitary Ca^{2+} channels in three different species. Nature 299:156–158.

Brown AM, Kunze DL, Yatani A (1984a): Agonist effect of a dihydropyridine Ca channel blocker on guinea pig and rat ventricular myocytes. J Physiol 357:59.

Brown AM, Lux HD, Wilson DL (1984b): Activation and inactivation of single calcium channels in snail neurones. J Gen Physiol 83:751–769.

Brown AM, Wilson DL, Lux HD (1984c): Activation of calcium channels. Biophys J 45:125–127.

Brown DA, Griffiths WH (1983a): Calcium activated outward current in voltage clamped hippocampal neurones of the guinea-pig. J Physiol 337:287–301

Brown DA, Griffiths WH (1983b): Persistent slow inward calcium current in voltage clamped hippocampal neurones of the guinea-pig. J Physiol 337:303–320.

Brown DA, Constanti A, Docherty RJ, Galvan M, Gahwiler B, Halliwell JVC (1985): Pharmacology of calcium currents in mammalian central neurones. Proc IX IUPHAR Symposium 2:343–348.

Brown DA, Docherty RJ, Gahwiler BH, Halliwell JC (1986): Calcium currents in mammalian central neurones. *XI Bayer Symposium*. Cardiovascular effects of dihydropyridine type Ca antagonists and agonists. (in press).

Brown TH, McAfee DA (1982): Long term synaptic potentiation in the superior cervical ganglion. Science 215:1411–1413.

Bustamante JO (1985): Block of Na$^+$-currents by the Ca^{2+}-antagonist D-600 in human heart cell segments. Pflug Arch 403:225–227.

Byerly L, Moody WJ (1984): Intracellular calcium ions and calcium currents in perfused neurones of the snail *Lymnea stagnalis*. J Physiol 352:637–652.

Byerly L, Yazejian B (1985): Intracellular factors for the maintenance of calcium currents in perfused neurones of the snail *Lymnea stagnalis*. J Physiol (in press).

Byerly L, Chase PB, Stimers JR (1984): Calcium current activation kinetics in neurones of the snail Lymnea stagnalis. J Physiol 348:187–207.

Byerly L, Chase PB, Stimers JR (1985): Permeation and interaction of divalent cations in calcium channels in snail neurones. J Gen Physiol 85:491–518.

Cahalan M (1980): Molecular properties of sodium channels in excitable membranes. In Cotman CW, Poste G, Nicolson GL, (eds): "The Cell Surface and Neuronal Function." Elsevier/North Holland pp 1–37.

Campbell KP, Lipshutz GM, Denny GH (1984): Direct photoaffinity labeling of the high affinity nitrendipine binding site in subcellular membrane fractions isolated from canine myocardium. J Biol Chem 259: 1–4.

Canfield DR, Dunlap K (1984): Pharmacological characterization of amine receptors on embryonic chick sensory neurones. Br J Pharmacol 82:557–563.

Canter EH, Kenessey A, Semenuk G, Spector S (1984): Interaction of Ca channel blockers with non-neuronal benzodiazepine binding sites. Proc Natl Acad Sci USA 81:1549–1552.

Carbone E, Lux HD (1984a): A low voltage activated fully inactivating Ca^{2+} channel in vertebrate sensory neurones. Nature 310:501–502.

Carbone E, Lux HD (1984b): A low voltage activated calcium conductance in embryonic chick sensory neurones. Biophys J 46:413–418.

Carbone E, Lux HD (1985): Isolation of low threshold Ca currents invertebrate sensory neurons. Pflug Arch 405(S2):R39.

Carboni E, Wojcik WJ (1985): ^{3}H-Nitrendipine binding sites correlate with dihydropyridine sensitive uptake in cultures of cerebellar granule cells and NG108-15 hybrid cells. Soc Neurosci Abstr 11:793.

Carpenter D, Gunn R (1970): The dependence of pacemaker discharge of Aplysia neurones upon Na^+ and Ca^{2+}. J Cell Physiol 75:121–127.

Catterall WA (1984): The molecular basis of neuronal excitability. Science 223:653–661.

Cena U, Nicolas GP, Sanchez-Garcia P, Kirpekar SM, Garcia AG (1983): Pharmacological dissection of receptor associated and voltage sensitive ionic channels involved in catecholamine release. Neuroscience 10:1455–1462.

Cena U, Garcia AG, Khoyi MA, Salaices M, Sanchez-Garcia P (1985): Effect of the dihydropyridine BAY K8644 on the release of ^{3}H-noradrenaline from the rat isolated vas deferens. Br J Pharmacol 85:691–696.

Chad J, Eckert R (1985a): Leupeptin, an inhibitor of Ca^{2+} dependent proteases, retards the kinase irreversible, Ca^{2+}-dependent loss of Ca^{2+}-current in perfused snail neurones. Biophys J 47:266a.

Chad J, Eckert R (1985b): Calcineurin, a calcium dependent phosphatase, enhances Ca-mediated inactivation of Ca current in perfused snail neurones. Biophys J 47:266a.

Chad JE, Eckert R (1985c): Ca current inactivation is slowed in dialyzed snail neurones by the substitution of ATPγS for internal ATP. J Gen Physiol 86: 27a.

Chamberlain SG, Kerkut GA (1967): Voltage clamp studies on snail (Helix aspersa) neurones. Nature 216:89.

Charlton MP, Smith SJ, Zucker RS (1982): Role of presynaptic calcium ions and channels in synaptic facilitation and depression at the squid giant synapse. J Physiol 323:173–193.

Chen CF, von Baumgarten R, Takeda R (1971): Pacemaker properties of completely isolated neurones in Aplysia californica. Nature New Biol 233:27–29.

Cherubini E, North RA (1984): Inhibition of Ca spikes and transmitter release by γ-aminobutyric acid in guinea-pig myenteric plexus. Br J Pharmacol 82: 101–105.

Cherubini E, North RA (1985): μ and κ opiate opioids inhibit transmitter release by different mechanisms. Proc Natl Acad Sci USA 82:1860–1863.

Chesnoy-Marchais D (1985): Kinetic properties and selectivity of calcium permeable single channels in Aplysia neurones. J Physiol 367:457–488.

Chin H, Krueger K, Beeler T, Nirenberg M (1985): Polyclonal antibodies with specificity for voltage sensitive calcium channel proteins. Soc Neurosci Abstr 11:516.

Chow I, Poo MM (1985): Release of acetylcholine from embryonic neurons upon contact with muscle cells. J Neurosci 5:1076–1082.

Clapham DE, Neher E (1984): Trifluoperazine reduces inward ionic currents and secretion by separate mechanisms in bovine chromaffin cells. J Physiol 353:541–564.

Clay JR, Shrier A (1984): Effects of D-600 on sodium current in squid axons. J Memb Biol 79:211–214.

Clusin WT, Bennett MVL (1977): Calcium activated conductance in skate electroreceptors. J Gen Physiol 69:121–143.

Cognard C, Lazdunski M, Romey G (1985): Different types of Ca^{2+} channels in mammalian skeletal muscle cells in culture. Proc Natl Acad Sci USA (in press).

Colombaioni L, Paupardin-Tritsch D, Vidal P, Gerschenfeld HM (1985): The neuropeptide FMRF-amide decreases both the Ca^{2+} conductance and a cyclic 3'5'-adenosine monophosphate dependent K^+-conductance in identified molluscan neurons. J Neurosci 5:2533–2538.

Colquhoun D, Neher E, Reuter H, Stevens CF (1981): Inward current channels activated by intracellular Ca in cultured cardiac cells. Nature 294:752–754.

Connor JA (1985): Ca^{2+} measurements using the fluorescent indicators quin-2 and fura-2 combined with digital imaging in mammalian CNS cells. Soc Neurosci Abstr 11:176.

Connors BW, Gutnick MT, Prince DA (1982): Electrophysiological properties of neocortical neurons in vitro. J Neurophysiol 48:1308–1320.

Corcoran JJ, Kirschner NC (1983): Inhibition of calcium uptake, sodium uptake and catecholamine secretion by methoxyverapamil (D-600) in primary cultures of adrenal medulla cells. J Neurochem 40: 1106–1109.

Corey DP, Dubinsky JM, Schwartz EA (1984): The calcium current in inner segments of rods from the salamander (Ambystoma triginum) retina. J Physiol 354:557–575.

Cortes R, Supavilai P, Karobath M, Palacios JM (1982): The effects of lesions in the rat hippocampus suggest the association of calcium channel blocker binding sites with a specific neuronal population. Neurosci Lett 42:249–254.

Crepel F, Dupont J-L, Gardette R (1984): Selective absence of calcium spikes in Purkinje cells of staggerer mutant mice in cerebellar slices maintained in vitro. J Physiol 346:111–125.

Crill WE, Schwindt P (1983): Active currents in mammalian central neurones. Trends Neurosci 6:236–240.

Crosland RD, Hsaio TH, McClure WO (1984): Purification and characterization of β-leptinotarsin-h, an activator of presynaptic Ca channels. Biochemistry 23:734–741.

Crunelli V, Leresche N, Pirchio M (1985): Lack of calcium potentials in principal neurones of the rat ventral LGN. J Physiol 365:39p.

Curtis BM, Catterall WA (1983): Solubilization of the calcium antagonist receptor from rat brain. J Biol Chem 258:7280–7283.

Curtis BM, Catterall WA (1984): Purification of the calcium channel antagonist receptor of the voltage sensitive calcium channel from skeletal muscle transverse tubule. Biochemistry 23:2113–2118.

Curtis BM, Catterall WA (1985a): Phosphorylation of the calcium antagonist receptor of the voltage sensitive calcium channel by cAMP dependent protein kinase. Proc Natl Acad Sci USA 82:2528–2532.

Curtis BM, Catterall WA (1985b): Molecular properties of voltage sensitive calcium channels. J Gen Physiol 86:6a.

Daniell, LC, Barr EM, Leslie SW (1983): ^{45}Ca^{2+} uptake into rat whole brain synaptosomes unaltered dihydropyridine Ca^{2+} antagonist. J Neurochem 41: 1455–1459.

Dascal N, Snutch TP, Lubbert H, Davidson NR, Lester HA (1985a): Voltage dependent calcium channels in Xenopus oocytes injected with exogenous mRNA. Soc Neurosci Abstr 11:793.

Dascal N, Snutch TP, Lubbert H, Davidson NR, Lester HA (1985b): Voltage dependent calcium channels in Xenopus oocytes injected with exogenous mRNA. J Gen Physiol 86:24a.

Deisz RA, Lux HD (1985): γ-Aminobutyric acid induced depression of calcium currents of chick sensory neurones. Neurosci Lett 56:205–210.

Deisz RA, Prince DA (1985): D890: A novel intracellular calcium antagonist in pyramidal cells of the guinea pig neocortex. Soc Neurosci Abstr 11:517.

DeRiemer SA, Strong JA, Albert KA, Greengard P, Kaczmarek LK (1985a): Enhancement of calcium current in Aplysia neurones by phorbol ester and protein kinase C. Nature 313:313–316.

DeRiemer SA, Schweitzer B, Kaczmarek CK (1985b): Inhibitors of calcium dependent enzymes prevent the onset of an afterdischarge in the peptidergic bag cell neurones of Aplysia. Brain Res 340:175–180.

Desarmenien M, Feltz P, Occhipinti G, Santangelo F, Schlichter M (1984): Coexistence of GABA-A and GABA-B receptors on A δ and C-primary afferents. Br J Pharmacol 81:327–333.

Deschenes M, Roy JP, Steriade M (1982): Thalamic bursting mechanism: An inward slow current revealed by membrane hyperpolarization. Brain Res 239:289–293.

DeVries DJ, Beart PM (1984): Competitive inhibition of ^{3}H-spiperone binding to D-2 dopamine receptors in striatal homogenates by organic calcium channel antagonists and polyvalent cations. Eur J Pharmacol 106:133–139.

Dichter M, Fischbach GD (1977): The action potential of chick dorsal root ganglion neurones maintained in cell culture. J Physiol 267:281–298.

Dichter MA, Lisak J, Biales B (1983): Action potential mechanism of mammalian cortical neurones in cell culture. Brain Res 289:99–107.

Dingledine R (1983): N-methyl-aspartate activates voltage dependent calcium conductance in rat hippocampal pyramidal cells. J Physiol 343:385–405.

Di Polo R, Caputo C, Bezanilla F (1983): Voltage dependent calcium channel in the squid axon. Proc Natl Acad Sci USA 80:1743–1745.

Docherty JR, Hyland L, Warnock P (1984): Pre and postsynaptic actions of BAY K8644 in the rat vas deferens. Br J Pharmacol 82:213p.

Docherty RJ, Miller RJ (1985): Actions of 1,4-dihydropyridines on voltage sensitive calcium current in neuroblastoma x glioma hybrid NG108-15 cells. J Physiol (in press).

Dolly JO, Barnard EA (1984): Nicotinic acetylcholine receptors: An overview. Biochem Pharmacol 33: 841–858.

Dolly JO, Halliwell JU, Black JD, Williams RS, Pelchen-Matthews, Breeze AL, Mehraban F, Othman IB, Black AR (1984): Botulinum neurotoxin and dendrotoxin as probes for studies on transmitter release. J Physiol (Paris) 79:280–303.

Dolphin AC, Forda SR, Scott RH (1985): The adenosine analogue 2-chloroadenosine inhibits Ba^{2+} currents in rat dorsal root ganglion neurones in culture. J Physiol (in press).

Doroshenko PA, Kostyuk PG, Martynyuk AE (1982): Intracellular metabolism of adenosine 3'5' cyclic monophosphate and calcium inward current in perfused neurones of Helix pomatia. Neuroscience 7: 2125–2134.

Doroshenko PA, Kostyuk PG, Martynyuk AE (1984a): Inactivation of the calcium current in the somatic membrane of snail neurones. Gen Physiol Biophys 3:1–17.

Doroshenko PA, Kostyuk PG, Martynyuk AE, Kursky MD, Vorobetz ZD (1984b). Intracellular protein kinase and calcium inward currents in perfused neurones of the snail Helix pomatia. Neuroscience 11: 263–267.

Doupe AJ, Landis SC, Patterson PH (1985): Environmental influences in the development of neural crest derivatives: Glucocorticoids, growth factors and chromaffin cell plasticity. J Neurosci 5:2119–2142.

Drapeau P, Blaustein MP (1983): Initial release of ^{3}H-dopamine from rat striatal synaptosomes: Correlation with Ca^{2+}-entry. J Neurosci 3:703–713.

Drapeau P, Nachshen DA (1984): Manganese fluxes and manganese dependent neurotransmitter release in presynaptic nerve endings isolated from rat brain. J Physiol 348:493–510.

Draski LJ, Johnston JE, Isaacson RL (1985): Nimodipines interactions with other drugs. II. Diazepam. Life Sci 37:2123–2128.

Dreifuss JJ, Crau JD, Nordmann JJ (1973): Effects on the isolated neurohypophysis of agents which affect the membrane permeability to calcium. J Physiol 231:96–98p.

Dunlap K (1981): Two types of γ-aminobutyric acid receptor on embryonic sensory neurones. Br J Pharmacol 74:579–585.

Dunlap K (1985): Forskolin prolongs action potential duration and blocks potassium current in embryonic chick sensory neurones. Pflug Arch 403:170–174.

Dunlap K, Fischbach GD (1978): Neurotransmitters decrease the calcium component of sensory neurone action potentials. Nature 276:837–839.

Dunlap K, Fischbach GD (1981): Neurotransmitters decrease the calcium conductance activated by depolarization of embryonic chick sensory neurones. J Physiol 317:519–535.

Ebstein RP, Daly JW (1982): Release of norepinephrine and dopamine from brain vesicular preparations effects of calcium antagonists. Cell Mol Neurobiol 2: 205–213.

Eckert R, Chad JE (1984): Inactivation of channels. Prog Biophys Mol Biol 44:215–267.

Eckert R, Lux HD (1976): A voltage sensitive persistent calcium conductance in neuronal somata of Helix. J Physiol 254:129–151.

Ehrlich E, Schen CR, Garcia TL, Kaczorowski GJ (1985): Cardiac calcium channels incorporated into planar lipid bilayers: Stereoselective blockade by

isomers of D-600. J Gen Physiol 86:21a.

Elrod SU, Leslie SW (1980): Acute and chronic effects of barbiturates on depolarization-induced calcium influx into synaptosomes from rat brain regions. J Pharmacol Exp Ther 212:131–142.

End DW, Carchman RA, Dewey WL (1981): Interaction of narcotics with synaptosomal calcium transport. Biochem Pharmacol 30:674–676.

Enyeart JJ, Aizawa T, Hinkle PM (1985): Dihydropyridine Ca^{2+} antagonists: Potent inhibitors of secretion from normal and transformed pituitary cells. Am J Physiol 248:C510–C519.

Erman RD, Yamamura HI, Roseke WR (1983): The ontogeny of specific binding sites for the calcium channel antagonist, nitrendipine, in mouse heart and brain. Brain Res 278:327–331.

Ewald D, Williams SA, Levitan IB (1985): Modulation of single Ca^{2+}-dependent K^+ channel activity by protein phosphorylation. Nature 315:503–506.

Fain GL, Gerschenfeld HM, Quandt FN (1980): Calcium spikes in toad rods. J Physiol 303:495–513.

Fairhurst AS, Thayer SA, Colker JE, Beatty DA (1983): A calcium antagonist drug binding site in skeletal muscle sarcoplasmic reticulum: Evidence for a calcium channel. Life Sci 32:1331–1339.

Fedulova SA, Kostyuk PG, Veselovsky NS (1981): Calcium channels in the somatic membrane of the rat dorsal root ganglion neurons: Effect of cAMP. Brain Res 214:210–214.

Fedulova SA, Kostyuk PG, Veselovsky NS (1985): Two types of calcium channels in the somatic membrane of newborn rat dorsal root ganglion neurones. J Physiol 359:431–446.

Feldman DH, Yoshikami D (1985): A peptide toxin from Conus geographus blocks voltage gated calcium channels. Soc Neurosci Abstr 11:517.

Fenwick EM, Marty A, Neher E (1982): Sodium and calcium channels in bovine chromaffin cells. J Physiol 311:599–635.

Ferrendelli JA, Daniels-McQueen S (1982): Comparative actions of phenytoin and other anticonvulsant drugs on potassium and vratradine-stimulated calcium uptake in synaptosomes. J Pharmacol Exp Ther 220:29–34.

Ferry DR, Goll A, Glossmann H (1983): Calcium channels: Evidence for oligomeric nature by target size analysis. EMBO J 2:1729–1732.

Ferry DR, Goll A, Gadow C, Glossmann H (1984a): $(-)-^3$H-Desmethoxyverapamil labelling of putative calcium channels in brain: Autoradiographic distribution and allosteric coupling to 1,4-dihydropyridine and diltiazem binding sites. Naunyn-Schmiedeberg's Arch Pharmacol 327:183–187.

Ferry DR, Rombusch M, Goll A, Glossmann H (1984b): Photoaffinity labelling of Ca^{2+} channels with ^{3}H-azidopine. FEBS Lett 169:112–118.

Fishman MC, Spector I (1981): Potassium current

suppression by quinidine reveals additional calcium currents in neuroblastoma cells. Proc Natl Acad Sci USA 78:5245–5249.

Fisher D, Auerbach S, Farley J (1985): Protein kinase C reduces K$^+$-currents and enhances a Ca^{2+}-current in *Hemissenda* type B cells. Soc Neurosci Abstr 11: 788.

Flaim SF, Brannan MD, Swigart SC, Gleason MM, Muschek LD (1985): Neuroleptic drugs attenuate Ca^{2+} influx and tension development in rabbit thoracic aorta: Effects of pimozide, penfluoridol, chorpromazine and haloperidol. Proc Natl Acad Sci USA 82:1237–1241.

Forscher P, Oxford GS (1985a): Norepinephrine affects Ca^{2+} channel currents through tight receptor channel coupling in DRG cells. Biophys J 47:515a.

Forscher P, Oxford GS (1985b): Modulation of calcium channels by norepinephrine in internally dialyzed avian sensory neurones. J Gen Physiol 85:743–763.

Fosset M, Jaimovich E, Delmont E, Lazdunski M (1983): ^{3}H-nitrendipine receptors in skeletal muscle. J Biol Chem 258:6086–6092.

Fox AP, Hess P, Lansman JB, Nowycky M, Tsien RW (1984): Slow variations in the gating properties of single calcium channels in guinea-pig heart cells, chick neurones and neuroblastoma cells. J Physiol 313:75p.

Fox AP, Hess P, Lansman JB, Nilius B, Nowycky MC, Tsien RW (1985a): Shifts between modes of calcium channel gating as a basis for pharmacological modulation of calcium influx in cardiac, neuronal and smooth muscle derived cells. In Poste G, Crooke ST (eds): "New Insights Into Cell and Membrane Transport Processes." (in press).

Fox AP, Nowycky M, Tsien RW (1985b): Kinetic and pharmacological properties distinguish N-type calcium channels from other types of calcium channel in chick sensory neurons. Soc Neurosci Abstr 11: 792.

Franckowiak G, Bechem M, Schramm M, Thomas G (1985): The optical isomers of the 1,4-dihydropyridine BAY K8644 show opposite effects on Ca channels. Eur J Pharmacol 114:223–226.

Freedman SB, Miller RJ (1984): Calcium channel activation: A different type of drug action. Proc Natl Acad Sci USA 81:5580–5583.

Freedman SB, Dawson G, Villereal ML, Miller RJ (1984a): Identification and characterization of voltage sensitive calcium channels in neuronal clonal cell lines. J Neurosci 4:1453–1467.

Freedman SB, Miller RJ, Miller DM, Tindall DR (1984b): Interactions of maitotoxin with voltage sensitive calcium channels in cultured neuronal cells. Proc Natl Acad Sci USA 81:4582–4588.

Freschi JE (1983): Membrane currents of cultured rat sympathetic neurons under voltage clamp. J Neurophysiol 50:1460–1480.

Freschi JE (1984): Patch clamp studies of rat sympathetic neurons in tissue culture. Soc Neurosci Abstr 10:504.

Friedman ME, Suarez-Kurtz G, Kaczorowski GJ, Katz GM, Reuben JP (1986): Two calcium currents in a smooth muscle cell line. Am J Physiol (in press).

Fukuda J, Kameyama M (1979): Enhancement of Ca spikes in nerve cells of adult mammals during neurite growth in tissue culture. Nature 279:546–548.

Fukuda J, Kameyama M (1980): Tetrodotoxin sensitive and tetrodotoxin resistant sodium channels in tissue cultured spinal ganglion neurones from adult mammals. Brain Res 182:191–197.

Fulton BP, Walton K (1981): Calcium dependent spikes in neonatal rat spinal cord in vitro. J Physiol 317: 25–26p.

Furuya S, Furuya K (1983): A quantitative analysis of intramembranous particles during the development of neuroblastoma x glioma hybrid cells. Dev Brain Res 11:235–244.

Gahwiler BH, Brown DA (1985): GABA-B-receptor activated K$^+$-current in voltage clamped CA$_3$ pyramidal cells in hippocampal cultures. Proc Natl Acad Sci USA 82:1558–1562.

Gallego R (1983): The ionic basis of action potentials in petrosal ganglion cells of the cat. J Physiol 342: 591–602.

Gallego R, Eyzaguirre (1978). Membrane and action potential characteristics of A and C nodose ganglion cells studied in whole ganglia and tissue slices. J Neurophysiol 41:1217–1232.

Galper JB, Catterall WA (1979): Inhibition of sodium channels by D-600. Mol Pharmacol 15:174–178.

Galvan M, Adams PR (1982): Control of calcium current in rat sympathetic neurons by norepinephrine. Brain Res 244:135–144.

Garcia AG, Sala F, Reig JA, Viniegra S, Friag J, Fonteriz R, Gandia L (1984a). Dihydropyridine BAY K8644 activates chromaffin cell calcium channels. Nature 309:69–71.

Garcia ML, Trumble MJ, Reuben JP, Kaczorowski GJ (1984b): Characterization of verapamil binding sites in cardiac membrane vesicles. J Biol Chem 259: 15013–15016.

Garcia ML, King VF, Reuben JP, Kaczorowski GJ (1985a): Binding of Ca^{2+} entry blockers to cardiac sarcolemmal membrane vesicles: Characterization of diltiazem binding sites. J Biol Chem (in press).

Garcia ML, King VF, Arcuri P, Siegl KS, Reuben JP, Kaczorowski GJ (1985b): Characterization of the Ca^{2+} entry blocker receptor complex in cardiac sarcolemmal membrane vesicles. J Gen Physiol 86: 21a.

Geduldig D, Junge D (1968): Sodium and calcium components of action potentials in the Aplysia giant neurone. J Physiol 199:347–365.

Geduldig D, Gruener R (1970): Voltage clamp of the

Aplysia giant neurone: Early sodium and calcium currents. J Physiol 211:217–244.

Geletyuk VI, Veprintsev BN (1972): Electrical properties of neurons of the mollusc *Lymnea stagnalis* under conditions of tissue culture. Tsitologiva 14: 1133–1139.

Gerasimov VD (1964): Effect of ion composition of medium on excitation process in giant neurons of snail. Fiziol Zh SSSR 50:457.

Gerasimov VD, Kostyuk PG, Maiskii VA (1965): The influence of divalent cations on the electrical characteristics of membranes of giant neurones. Biofizica 10:447–453.

Glossmann H, Ferry DR, Lubbecke F, Mewes R, Hofmann F (1982): Calcium channels: Direct identification with radioligand binding studies. Trends Pharm Sci 3:235–241.

Glossmann H, Ferry DR, Goll A, Rombusch M (1984): Molecular pharmacology of the Ca^{2+} channel: Evidence for subtypes; multiple drug receptor sites; channel subunits; and the development of a radioiodinated 1,4,-dihydropyridine Ca^{2+} channel label, ^{125}I-iodipine. J Cardiol Pharmacol 6:S608–S621.

Glossmann H, Ferry DR, Goll A, Striessnig J, Schober M (1985): Calcium channels: Basic properties as revealed by radioligand binding studies. J Cardiol Pharmacol 6:S608–S621.

Godfraind JM, Jessell TM, Kelly JS, McBurney RN, Mudge AW, Yamamoto M (1981): Capsaicin prolongs action potential duration in cultured sensory neurones. J Physiol 312:32p.

Gola M, Ducreux C (1985): D-600 as a direct blocker of Ca-dependent K^+-currents in Helix neurones. Eur J Pharmacol 117:311–322.

Goodman CS, Heitler WJ (1979): Electrical properties of insect neurones with spiking and non-spiking somata: Normal, axotomized and colchicine treated neurones. J Exp Biol 83:95–121.

Goodman CS, Spitzer NC (1981a): The mature electrical properties of identified neurones in grasshopper embryos. J Physiol 313:369–384.

Goodman CS, Spitzer NC (1981b): The development of electrical properties of identified neurones in grasshopper embryos. J Physiol 313:385–403.

Gopalkrishnan V, Triggle CR (1984): Specific high affinity binding of the calcium antagonist ^3H-nitrendipine to rat liver microsomes. Can J Pharmacol Physiol 62:1249–1252.

Gorke K, Pierall F-K (1980): Spike potentials and membrane properties of dorsal root ganglion cells in pigeons. Pflug Arch 386:21–28.

Gorman ALF, Thomas MV (1980): Intracellular calcium accumulation during depolarization in a molluscan neurone. J Physiol 308:259–285.

Gorman ALF, Hermann A, Thomas MV (1982): Ionic requirements for membrane oscillations and their dependence on the calcium concentration in a molluscan pacemaker neurone. J Physiol 327:185–217.

Gorman ALF, Levy S, Nasi E, Tillotson D (1984): Intracellular calcium measured with calcium sensitive microelectrodes and arsenazo III in voltage clamped Aplysia neurones. J Physiol 353:127–142.

Gotgil'f IM, Magazanick LG (1977): Effects of substances blocking calcium channels (verapamil, D-600, manganese ions) on transmitter release from motor nerve endings in frog muscle. Neirofiziologiva 9:415–422.

Gothert M, Nawroth P, Neumeyer H (1979): Inhibitory effects of verapamil, prenylamine and D-600 on Ca^{2+} dependent noradrenaline release from sympathetic nerves in isolated rabbit hearts. Naunyn-Schmiedeberg's Arch Pharmacol 310:11–19.

Gould RJ, Murphy KMM, Snyder SH (1982): ^3H-nitrendipine labeled calcium channels discriminate inorganic calcium agonists and antagonists. Proc Natl Acad Sci USA 79:3656–3660.

Gould RJ, Murphy KMM, Snyder SH (1983a): Tissue heterogeneity of calcium antagonist binding sites labelled by ^3H-nitrendipine. Mol Pharmacol 25: 235–241.

Gould RJ, Murphy KMM, Reynolds IJ, Snyder SH (1983b): Antischizophrenic drugs of the diphenylbutylpiperidine type act as calcium channel antagonists. Proc Natl Acad Sci USA 80:5122–5125.

Gould RJ, Murphy KMM, Snyder SH (1985): Autoradiographic localization of calcium channel antagonist receptors in rat brain with ^3H-nitrendipine. Brain Res 330:217–223.

Govoni S, Rius RA, Battaini F, Bianchi A, Trabucchi M (1985): Age-related reduced affinity in $[^3H]$-nitrendipine labeling of brain voltage dependent calcium channels. Brain Res 333:374–377.

Graubard K, Ross WN (1985): Regional distribution of calcium influx into bursting neurons detected with arsenazo III. Proc Natl Acad Sci USA 82:5565–5569.

Gray R, Johnston D (1985a): Macroscopic calcium currents in acutely exposed neurons from adult hippocampal slices. Biophys J 47:66a.

Gray R, Johnston D (1985b): Macroscopic Ca^{2+}-currents in acutely exposed granule cells from adult hippocampus. Soc Neurosci Abstr 11:792.

Grebb JP, Shelton RC, Freed WJ (1985): Calcium channel inhibitors prevent neuroleptic induced apomorphine supersensitivity in mice. Soc Neurosci Abstr 11:925.

Green FJ, Farmer BB, Wiseman GL, Jose MJL, Watanabe AM (1985): Effect of membrane depolarization on binding of ^3H-nitrendipine to rat cardiac myocytes. Circ Res 56:576–585.

Greenberg DA, Cooper EC, Carpenter CL (1984): Calcium channel agonist BAY K8644 inhibits calcium antagonist binding to brain and PC12 cell membranes. Brain Res 305:365–368.

Greenberg DA, Cooper EC, Carpenter CL (1985): Stimulation of calcium uptake in PC12 cells by the dihydropyridine agonist BAY K8644. J Neurochem 45:990–993.

Greene LA, Tischler AS (1982): PC12 Pheochromocytoma cultures in neurobiological research. Adv Cell Neurobiol 3:374–413.

Greengard P, Straub RW (1959): Restoration by barium of action potentials in sodium deprived mammalian B and C fibers. J Physiol 145:562–569.

Griffiths PJ, Rudel R, Taylor SR, Zite-Ferenczy F (1985): Agonist effects of taloromycin toxin and myocardial Ca^{2+} channel blockers in frog skeletal muscle fibers. J Physiol (in press).

Grinvald A, Farber IC (1981): Optical recording of calcium action potentials from growth cones of cultured neurons with a laser microbeam. Science 212:1164–1166.

Grynkiewicz G, Poenie M, Tsien RY (1985): A new generation of Ca^{2+} indicators with greatly improved fluorescence properties. J Biol Chem 260:3440–3450.

Hablitz JJ, Johnston D (1981): Endogenous nature of spontaneous bursting in hippocampal pyramidal neurones. Cell Mol Neurobiol 1:325–333.

Hablitz JJ, Heinemann U, Lux HD (1985): Activation of inward current in dorsal root ganglion cells by transient reductions in extracellular calcium. Biophys J 47:434a.

Haeusler G (1972): Differential effect of verapamil on excitation/contraction coupling in smooth muscle and on excitation/secretion coupling in adrenergic nerve terminals. J Pharmacol Exp Ther 180:672–682.

Hagiwara S (1983): Membrane potential dependent ion channels in cell membranes. Phylogenetic and developmental approaches. NY: Raven Press.

Hagiwara S, Saito S (1959): Voltage/current relations in nerve cell membrane of Fonchidium verruculatum. J Physiol 148:161–177.

Hagiwara S, Byerly L (1981): Calcium channel. Ann Rev Neuroscoi 4:69–125.

Halliwell JV (1983): Caesium loading reveals two distinct Ca-currents in voltage clamped guinea-pig hippocampal neurones in vitro. J Physiol 341:10–11p.

Halliwell JV, Scholfield CN (1984a): Somatically recorded Ca^{2+}-currents in guinea pig hippocampal and olfactory cortex neurones are resistant to adenosine actions. Neurosci Lett 50:13–18.

Halliwell JV, Scholfield CN (1984b): Adenosine resistant Ca^{2+}-currents in mammalian central nervous system. J Physiol 349:52p.

Hamilton SL, Yatani A, Hawkes MJ, Redding K, Brown AM (1985): Atrotoxin: A specific agonist for calcium currents in heart. Science 229:182–184.

Hammerschlag R, Dravid AR, Chiu AY (1975): Mechanism of axonal transport: A proposed role for calcium ions. Science 188:273–275.

Hammerschlag R, Bahkit C, Chiu AY, Dravid AR (1977): Role of calcium in the initiation of fast transport of protein: Effects of divalent cations. J Neurobiol 8:439–451.

Hanada S, Tanaka C (1985): Regional distribution of ^{3}H-nitrendipine binding in human brain. Neurosci Lett 58:375–380.

Hanada Y (1977): Morphological and electrophysiological changes in cultured spinal ganglion cells during development. Tohoku J Exp Med 121:13–25.

Harada Y, Takahashi T (1983): The calcium component of the action potential in spinal motoneurones of the rat. J Physiol 335:89–100.

Harris KM, Kongsamut S, Miller RJ (1985a): Protein kinase C mediated regulation of calcium channels in PC12 pheochromocytoma cells. Biochem Biophys Res Commun (in press).

Harris RA (1984): Differential effect of membrane pertubants on voltage activated sodium and calcium channels and calcium dependent potassium channels. Biophys J 45:132–134.

Harris RA, Bruno P (1985): Membrane disordering by anesthetic drugs: Relationship to synaptosomal sodium and calcium fluxes. J Neurochem 44:1274–1281.

Harris RA, Hood WF (1980): Inhibition of synaptosomal calcium uptake by ethanol. J Pharmacol Exp Ther 213:562–568.

Harris RA, Jones SB, Bruno P, Bylund DB (1985b): Effects of dihydropyridine derivatives and anticonvulsant drugs on ^{3}H-nitrendipine binding and calcium and sodium fluxes in brain. Biochem Pharmacol 34:2187–2191.

Hashiguchi T (1979): The calcium dependent components of action potentials of the rabbit superior cervical ganglion cells. J Tokyo Med Cell 37:533–544.

Haylock JW, White WF, Cotman CW (1978): Differences in alkaline earth stimulation of neurotransmitter release from isolated brain synaptosomes. Naunyn-Schmiedeberg's Arch Pharmacol 301:175–179.

Hedlund B, Owen DG, Barker JL (1985): Non-muscarinic effects of atropine on calcium conductances in cultured mouse spinal cord neurones. Neurosci Lett 55:355–359.

Heinonen E, Akerman KEO, Kaila K, Scott IG (1985): Dependence of cytoplasmic calcium transients on the membrane potential in isolated nerve endings of the guinea-pig. Biochem Biophys Acta 815:203–208.

Henon B, McAfee DA (1983): The ionic basis of adenosine receptor actions on post ganglionic neurones in the rat. J Physiol 336:607–620.

Hermsmeyer K, Sturek M (1985): Nitrendipine differentially blocks two types of Ca^{2+} channels in cultured vascular muscle cells. J Gen Physiol 86:24a.

Herring S, Bodewei R, Schubert B, Rohde K, Wollenberger A (1985): A kinetic analysis of the inward calcium current in 108 CC15 neuroblastoma x glioma hybrid cells. Gen Physiol Biophys 4:129–141.

Hess P, Tsien RW (1984): Mechanisms of ion permeation through calcium channels. Nature 309:453–456.

Hess P, Lansman JB, Tsien RW (1984): Different modes of calcium channel gating favored by Ca agonists and antagonists. Nature 311:338–344.

Hess P, Lansman JB, Tsien RW (1986): Calcium channel selectivity for divalent and monovalent cations: Voltage and concentration dependence of single channel current in guinea-pig ventricular heart cells. J Gen Physiol (in press).

Heyer EJ, MacDonald RL (1982): Calcium and sodium dependent action potentials of mouse spinal cord and dorsal root ganglion neurons in culture. J Neurophysiol 47:641–655.

Heyer EJ, MacDonald RL, Bergey GK, Nelson PG (1981): Calcium dependent action potentials in mouse spinal cord neurons in cell culture. Brain Res 220:408–415.

Hill DR (1985): GABA-B receptor modulation of adenylate cyclase activity in rat brain slices. Br J Pharmacol 84:249–257.

Himori N, Ono H, Taira N (1975): Dual effects of a new coronary vasodilator, diltiazem, on the contractile force of the blood perfused papillary muscle of the dog. Jpn J Pharmacol 25:350–352.

Himori N, Ono H, Taira N (1976): Simultaneous assessment of effects of coronary vasodilators on coronory blood flow and myocardial contractility by using the blood perfused canine papillary muscle. Jpn J Pharmacol 26:427–435.

Hirst GDS, Spence I (1973): Calcium action potentials in mammalian peripheral neurons. Nature New Biol 243:54–56.

Hirst GDS, Johnson SM, van Helden DF (1985): The calcium current in a myenteric neurone of the guinea-pig ileum. J Physiol 361:297–314.

Hockberger P, Connor JA (1984): Alteration of calcium conductances and outward current by cyclic adenosine monophosphate (cAMP) in neurons of Limax maximus. Cell Mol Neurobiol 4:319–338.

Hockberger P, Connor JA (1985): Properties of cultured cerebellar granule cells measured with whole cell patch recordings and imaging of Ca^{2+} indicator fluorescence. Soc Neurosci Abstr 11:155.

Hodgkin AL, Keynes RD (1957): Movements of labelled calcium in squid giant axons. J Physiol 138:253–281.

Hof RP, Reugg VT, Hof A, Vogel A (1985): Stereoselectivity at the calcium channel: Opposite actions of the enantiomers of a 1,4-dihydropyridine. J Cardiovasc Pharmacol 7:689–693.

Hoffmeister F, Benz V, Heise H, Krause P, Neuser U (1982): Behavioural effects of nimodipine in animals. Arzneim Forsch 32:347–360.

Hogestatt ED, Andersson RE, Edvinsson L (1982): Effects of nifedipine on potassium induced contraction and noradrenaline release in cerebral and extracranial arteries from rabbit. Acta Physiol Scand 114:283–292.

Holden DP, Knight DE (1984): Does the dihydropyridine CPG 28392 activate bovine chromaffin cell calcium channels. J Physiol 358:64p.

Holz GG, Rane SG, Dunlap K (1985): G-proteins mediate transmitter inhibition of neuronal calcium channels. Cornell Symposium: Ca^{2+} and Cell Regulation 23 (abstract).

Horn JP, McAfee DA (1980): Alpha-adrenergic inhibition of calcium dependent potentials in rat sympathetic neurons. J Physiol 301:191–204.

Horn R (1977): Tetrodotoxin resistent divalent action potentials in an axon of Aplysia. Brain Res 133:177–182.

Horn R (1978): Propagating calcium spikes in an axon of Aplysia. J Physiol 218:513–534.

Horn R, Miller JL (1977): A prolonged voltage dependent calcium permeability revealed by TEA in the soma and axon of Aplysia giant neuron. J Neurobiol 8:399–415.

Horne P, Triggle DJ, Venter JC (1984): Nitrendipine and isoproterenol induce phosphorylation of a 42,000 dalton protein that co-migrates with the affinity labelled calcium channel regulatory subunit. Biochem Biophys Res Commun 121:890–898.

Hoshi T, Rothlein J, Smith SJ (1984): Facilitation of Ca^{2+}-channel currents in bovine adrenal chromaffin cells. Proc Natl Acad Sci USA 81:5871–5875.

Hoss W, Formaniak M (1983): Effects of opiates on synaptosomal calmodulin and calcium uptake. Neurochem Res 8:219–229.

Hoss W, Formaniak M (1984): Calcium channel activity in the rat brain synaptosomes. Effects of neuroleptics and other factors regulating phosphorylation and transmitter release. Neurochem Res 9:109–120.

Hotson JR, Prince DA (1981): Penicillin and barium induced epileptiform bursting in hippocampal neurones. Actions on Ca^{2+} and K^+ potentials. Ann Neurol 10:11–17.

Hudspeth AJ, Corey DP (1977): Sensitivity polarity and conductance change in the response of vertebrate hair cells to controlled mechanical stimuli. Proc Natl Acad Sci USA 74:2407–2411.

Hume JR (1985): Comparative interactions of organic Ca^{2+} channel antagonists with myocardial Ca^{2+} and K^+ channels. J Pharmacol Exp Ther 234:134–140.

Ishii K, Kano T, Kurobe Y, Ando J (1983): Binding of ^{3}H-nitrendipine to heart and brain membranes from nomotensive and spontaneous hypertensive rats. Eur J Pharmacol 88:277–278.

Ishizuka S, Hattori K, Akaike N (1984): Separation of ionic currents in the somatic membrane of frog sensory neurons. J Memb Biol 78:19–28.

Ito H (1982): Evidence for initiation of calcium spikes

in C-cells of rabbit nodose ganglion. Pflug Arch 394:106–112.

Ito F, Komatsu Y (1979): Calcium dependent regenerative responses in the afferent nerve terminal of the frog muscle spindle. Brain Res 175:161–165.

Ito H, Nishi K (1982): Frequency dependent depression of ganglionic transmission by propanolol and diltiazem in the superior cervical ganglion of the guinea-pig. Br J Pharmacol 77:359–363.

Ito F, Komatsu Y, Fujitsuka N (1981): Calcium spike induced by electrical stimulation to the sensory nerve terminal of the frog muscle spindle. Neurosci Lett 27:135–137.

Ito F, Komatsu Y, Fujitsuka N (1982a): Effects of anions on calcium component in sensory nerve terminal of frog muscle spindles. Brain Res 252:197–200.

Ito F, Komatsu Y, Fujitsuka N (1982b): $G_{K(Ca)}$-dependent cyclic potential changes in the sensory nerve terminal of frog muscle spindle. Brain Res 252:39–50.

Ito F, Komatsu Y, Kaneko N (1980c): Site of origin of calcium spike in frog muscle spindle. Brain Res 202:459–463.

Ito H, Sakanashi M, Kawamura T, Nishi K (1984): Effects of organic Ca^{2+}-antagonists on membrane characteristics of nodose ganglion cells in the rabbit. Arch Int Pharmacol 271:53–63.

Iwasaki S, Sato Y (1971): Sodium and calcium dependent spike potentials in the secretory neuron soma of the x-organ of the crayfish. J Gen Physiol 57:216–238.

Jahnsen H, Llinas R (1984a): Electrophysiological properties of guinea-pig thalamic neurones: An in vitro study. J Physiol 349:205–226.

Jahnsen H, Llinas R (1984b): Ionic basis for the electroresponsiveness and oscillatory properties of guinea pig thalamic neurones in vitro. J Physiol 349:227–247.

Jahr CE, Nicoll RA (1980): Dendrodendritic inhibition: Demonstration with intracellular recording. Science 207:1473–1475.

Janis RA, Triggle DJ (1984): 1,4-Dihydropyridine Ca^{2+} channel antagonists and agonists: A comparison of binding characteristics with pharmacology. Drug Dev Res 4:257–274.

Janis RA, Bellemann P, Sarmiento JG, Triggle DJ (1985): The dihydropyridine receptors. In Fleckenstein A, van Breemen C (eds): In XI Bayer Symposium, "Cardiovascular Effects of Dihydropyridine Ca^{2+} Channel Antagonists and Agonists." Berlin: Springer-Verlag (in press).

Janis RA, Sarmiento JG, Maurer SG, Bolger GT, Triggle DJ (1984): Characteristics of the binding of ^{3}H-nitrendipine to rabbit ventricular membranes. Modification by other Ca^{2+} channel antagonists and by the Ca^{2+} agonist BAY K8644. J Pharmacol Exp Ther 231:8–15.

Jia M, Litzinger MJ (1985): Dihydropyridine effects on mammalian voltage sensitive calcium channels. Soc Neurosci Abstr 11, 519.

Johansen J, Taft WC, Yang J, Kleinhaus A, De Lorenzo RJ (1985): Inhibition of the Ca^{2+}-conductance in identified leech neurones by benzodiazepines. Proc Natl Acad Sci USA 82:3935–3939.

Johnston D, Hablitz JJ, Wilson WA (1980): Voltage clamp discloses slow inward current in hippocampal burst firing neurones. Nature 286:391–393.

Junge D (1967): Multionic action potentials in molluscan giant neurone. Nature 215:546–548.

Junge D, Miller J (1974): Different spike mechanisms in axon and soma of molluscan neurone. Nature 252:155–156.

Kaczmarek LK, Jennings HR, Strumwasser F, Nairn AC, Walter V, Wilson ED, Greengard P (1980): Microinjection of catalytic subunits of cyclic AMP dependent protein kinase enhances Ca^{2+} action potentials of bag cell neurones in cell culture. Proc Natl Acad Sci USA 77:7427–7431.

Kado RT (1973): Aplysia giant cell: Soma-axon voltage clamp current differences. Science 182:843–845.

Kajiwara M, Casteels R (1983): Effects of Ca antagonists on neuromuscular transmission in the rabbit ear artery. Pflug Arch 396:1–7.

Kalman D, Eckert R (1985): Injection of catalytic and regulatory subunits of protein kinase into Aplysia neurones alters calcium current inactivation. J Gen Physiol 86:26a.

Kamikubo K, Niwa M, Fujimura H, Miura K (1983): Morphine inhibits depolarization dependent calcium uptake by synaptosomes. Eur J Pharmacol 95:149–150.

Kaneko A, Tachibana M (1985): A voltage clamp analysis of membrane currents in solitary bipolar cells dissociated from Carassius auratus. J Physiol 358:131–152.

Kaplita PV, Triggle DJ (1983): Actions of Ca^{2+}-antagonist on the guinea-pig ileal myenteric plexus preparation. Biochem Pharmacol 32:65–68.

Karaki H, Nakagawa H, Urakawa N (1984): Effects of calcium antagonists on release of ^{3}H-noradrenaline in rabbit aorta. Eur J Pharmacol 101:177–183.

Katz B, Miledi R (1969): Tetrodotoxin resistant electrical activity in presynaptic terminals. J Physiol 203:459–487.

Katz B, Miledi R (1971): The effects of prolonged depolarization on synaptic transfer in the stellate ganglion of the squid. J Physiol 216:503–512

Kawa K (1979): Zinc dependent action potentials in giant neurones of the snail Euhadra quaestia. J Memb Biol 49:325–344.

Kazazoglou T, Schmid A, Renaud JF, Lazdunski M (1983): Ontogenic appearance of Ca^{2+} channels characterized as binding sites for nitrendipine during development of nervous, skeletal and cardiac muscle systems in the rat. FEBS Lett 164:75–79.

Kazazoglou T, Schackmann RW, Fosset M, Shapiro B (1985): Calcium channel antagonists inhibit the acrosome reaction and bind to plasma membranes of sea urchin sperm. Proc Natl Acad Sci U.S.A. 82:1460–1464.

Kendall DA, Nahorski SR (1985): Dihydropyridine calcium channel activators and antagonists influence depolarization evoked inositol phospholipid hydrolysis in brain. Eur J Pharmacol 115:31–36.

Kenessey A, Cantor EH, Spector S (1984): Low affinity dihydropyridine binding site in rat heart membranes. Fed Proc 43;1548.

Kerkut GA, Gardner DR (1967): The role of Ca ions in the action potentials of helix aspersa neurones. Comp Biochem Physiol 20:147–162.

Kerr LM, Yoshikami DC (1984): A venom peptide with a novel presynaptic blocking action. Nature 308;282-284.

Kidokoro Y, Ritchie AK (1980): Chromaffin cell action potentials and their possible role in adrenaline secretion from adrenal medulla. J Physiol 307:199–216.

Kim YI, Login IS, Yasumoto T (1985): Maitotoxin activates quantal transmitter release at the neuromuscular junction: Evidence for elevated intraterminal Ca^{2+} in the motor nerve terminal. Brain Res 346:357–362.

Klee MR, Lee MC, Matsuda Y (1973): Interaction of D-600 and cobalt with the inward and outward current systems in Aplysia neurones. Pflug Arch 343:R60.

Klein M, Shapiro E, Kandel ER (1980): Synaptic plasticity and modulation of the Ca^{2+} current. J Exp Biol 89:117–157.

Kleinhaus AL (1976): Divalent cations and the action potential of Leech Retzius cells. Pflug Arch 363:97–104.

Kleinhaus AL, Prichard JWC (1975): Calcium dependent action potentials produced in Leech Retzius cells by tetraethylammonium chloride. J Physiol 246:351–361.

Kleinhaus AL, Prichard JW (1977): Close relation between TEA responses and Ca-dependent membrane phenomena of four identified leech neurones. J Physiol 270:181–194.

Kobayashi H, Ohizumi Y, Yasimoto T(1985a): The mechanism of action of maitotoxin in relation to Ca^{2+} movements in guinea pig and rat cardiac muscles. Br J Pharmacol 86:385–391.

Kobayashi S, Kanaide H, Nakamura M (1985b): K^+ depolarization induces a direct release of Ca^{2+} from the intracellular storage sites in cultured vascular smooth muscle cells from rat aorta. Biochem Biophys Res Commun 129:877–884.

Koketsu K, Akasu T (1982): Modulation of slow inward Ca^{2+} current by adrenaline in bullfrog sympathetic ganglion cells. Jpn J Physiol 32:137–140.

Koketsu K, Nishi S (1968): Calcium spikes of nerve cell membrane: Role of Ca in the production of action potentials. Nature 217:468–470.

Koketsu K, Nishi S (1969): Calcium and action potentials of bullfrog sympathetic ganglion cells. J Gen Physiol 53:608–623.

Koketsu K, Cerf JA, Nishi S (1959): Effect of quarternary ammonium ions on electrical activity of spinal ganglion cells in frogs. J Neurophysiol 22:177–194.

Koketsu K, Nishi S, Soeda HC (1963): Effects of calcium ions on prolonged action potentials and hyperpolarizing responses. Nature 200:786–787.

Kongsamut S, Miller RJ (1986): Nerve growth factor modulates the drug sensitivity of neurotransmitter release from PC12 cells. Proc Natl Acad Sci USA (in press).

Kongsamut S, Freedman SB, Simon BE, Miller RJ (1985b): Interaction of steroidal alkaloid toxins with calcium channels in neuronal cell lines. Life Sci 36:1493–1501.

Kongsamut S, Kamp TJ, Miller RJ, Sanguinetti MC (1985a): Calcium channel agonist and antagonist effects of the stereoisomers of the dihydropyridines 202-791. Biochem Biophys Res Commun 130:141–148.

Kostyuk PG (1981): Calcium channels in the neuronal membrane. Biochem Biophys Acta 650;128-150.

Kostyuk PG (1983): Interaction of toxins and divalent cations in calcium channels of the neuronal membrane: In "Toxins as Tools in Neurochemistry." Hucho F, Ovchinnikov YA, Berlin: W. de Gryter, pp 259-265.

Kostyuk PG (1984): Intracellular perfusion of nerve cells and its effects on membrane currents. Physiol Rev 64:435–454.

Kostyuk PG, Krishtal OA (1977a): Separation of sodium and calcium currents in the somatic membrane of mollusc neurones. J Physiol 270:545–568.

Kostyuk PG, Krishtal OA (1977b): Effects of calcium and calcium chelating agents on inward and outward currents in the membrane of mollusc neurones. J Physiol 270:569–580.

Kostyuk PG, Shuba YM (1982): Selectivity of EDTA modified calcium channels to monovalent cations. Neirofiziologiya 14:491–498.

Kostyuk PG, Doroshenko PA, Martynyuk AR (1985): Fast decrease of the peak current carried by barium ions through calcium channels in the somatic membrane of mollusc neurones. Pflug Arch 404:88–90.

Kostyuk PG, Krishtal OA, Doroshenko PA (1975): Outward currents in isolated snail neurones. III. Effect of verapamil. Comp Biol Physiol 51C: 269-275.

Kostyuk PG, Krishtal OA, Pidoplichro LU, Veselovsky WS (1978): Ionic currents in the neuroblastoma cell membrane. Neuroscience 3:327–335.

Kostyuk PG, Mironov SL, Shuba YM (1983): Two ion selecting filters in the calcium channel of the somatic membrane of mollusc neurones. J Memb Biol 76:83–93.

Kostyuk PG, Veselovsky NS, Fedulova SA (1981a): Ionic currents in the somatic membranes of rat dorsal root ganglion neurones. II. Calcium currents. Neuroscience 6:2431–2437.

Kostyuk PG, Veselovsky NS, Fedulova SA (1981b): Ionic currents in the somatic membranes of rat dorsal root ganglion neurones. III. Potassium currents. Neuroscience 6:2439–2444.

Kostyuk PG, Veselovsky NS, Tsyndrenko AY (1981c): Ionic currents in the somatic membrane of rat dorsal root ganglion neurones. I. Sodium currents. Neuroscience 6:2423–2430.

Kramer RH, Zucker RS (1985a): Calcium dependent inward current in Aplysia bursting pacemaker neurones. J Physiol 362:107–130.

Kramer RH, Zucker RS (1985b): Calcium induced inactivation of calcium currents causes the interburst hyperpolarizations of Aplysia bursting neurones. J Physiol 362:131–160.

Krishtal OA, Magura IS (1970): Calcium ions as inward current carriers in mollusc neurones. Comp Biochem Physiol 35:857–866.

Krnjevic K, Puil E, Werman R (1978): EGTA and motoneural afterpotentials. J Physiol 275;199–223.

Krnjevic K, Pumain R, Renaurd L (1971): Effects of Ba^{2+} and tetraethylammonium on cortical neurones. J Physiol 215;223-245.

Krnjevic K, Lamour Y, MacDonald JF, Nistri A (1979): Effect of some divalent cations on motoneurons in cats. Can J Phys Pharmacol 57:944–956.

Kuan YF, Scholfield CN, Steel LC (1985): Effect of Ca antagonists on axonal Ba/Ca spikes in slices of guinea pig brain. J Physiol 362;35p.

Kubota M, Nakamura M, Tsukahara N (1985): Ionic conductance associated with electrical activity of guinea-pig red nucleus neurones in vitro. J Physiol:161–171.

Kunze DL, Hawkes MJ, Hamilton SL, Brown AM (1985): Binding and pharmacological studies of nitrendipine in PC12 cells. Biophys J 47:264a.

Landfield PW, Pilter TA (1984): Prolonged Ca^{2+}-dependent afterhyperpolarizations in hippocampal neurones of aged rats. Science 226:1089–1091.

Lansman JB, Hess P, Tsien RW (1986): Blockade of calcium current through single calcium channels by Cd^{2+}, Mg^2 and Ca^{2+}. Voltage and concentration dependence of Ca entry into the pore. J Gen Physiol (in press).

Larsson B, Hogestatt ED, Mattiasson A, Andersson KE (1984): Differential effects of nifedipine, verapamil and diltiazem on noradrenaline induced contractions, adrenergic transmitter release and alpha adrenoceptor binding in the female rabbit urethra. Naunyn-Schmiedeberg's Arch Pharm 326:14–21.

Latorre R, Miller C (1983): Conduction and selectivity in potassium channels. J Memb Biol 71:11–30.

Lee HR, Watson M, Yamamura HI, Roeske WR, (1985): Decreased [^{3}H]-nitrendipine binding in the brainstem of deoxycorticosterone-NaCl hypertensive rats. Life Sci 37:971–977.

Legendre P, Cooke IM, Vincent J (1982): Regenerative responses of long duration recorded intracellularly from dispersed cell cultures of foetal mouse hypothalmus. J Neurophys 48:1126–1141.

Legrand AM, Bagnis R (1984): Effects of highly purified maitotoxin extracted from dinoflagellate *Gambierdiscus toxicus* on action potential of isolated rat heart. J Mol Cell Cardiol 16:663–666.

Lemos JR, Stuenkel EL, Nordmann JJ, Cooke IM (1985): Ionic currents and channels in peptidergic neurosecretory terminals. Biophys J 47:446a.

Leng G, Mason WT (1984): Isolation of the calcium and sodium components of rat supraoptic (S.O.M.) and paraventricular (PVN) neurone action potentials recorded in vitro and in vivo. J Physiol 346:131p.

Leonard JP, Wickelgren WO (1984): Calcium action potentials in primary sensory neurones of lamprey. Soc Neurosci Abstr 10:871.

Leslie SW, Barr E, Chandler LJ (1983a): Comparison of voltage dependent ^{45}Ca^{2+} uptake rates by synaptosomes isolated from rat brain regions. J Neurochem 41:1602–1605.

Leslie SW, Friedman MB, Coleman RR (1980a): Effects of chlordiazepoxide on depolarization induced calcium influx into synaptosomes. Biochem Pharmacol 29:2439–2443.

Leslie SW, Woodward JT, Wilcox RE (1985): Correlation of rates of Ca entry and endogenous dopamine release in mouse striatal synaptosomes. Brain Res 325:99–105.

Leslie SW, Barr E, Chandler LJ, Farrar RP (1983b): Inhibition of fast and slow phase depolarization dependent synaptosomal calcium uptake by ethanol. J Pharmacol Exp Ther 225:571–575.

Leslie SW, Elrod SV, Coleman R, Belknap JK (1979): Tolerance to barbiturate and chlorpromazine induced central nervous system sedation. Involvement of calcium mediated stimulus/secretion coupling. Biochem Pharmacol 28:1437–1440.

Leslie SW, Friedman MB, Wilcox RE, Elrod SU (1980b): Acute and chronic effects of barbiturates on depolarization induced calcium influx into rat synaptosomes. Brain Res 185:409–417.

Leslie SW, McCormack J, Gonzales R, Friedman MM (1982): Lack of morphine effect on potassium stimulated calcium uptake by whole brain synaptosomes. Biochem Pharmacol 31:2697–2698.

Levitan I (1985): Phosphorylation of ion channels. J Memb Biol 87:177–190.

Lewis RS, Hudspeth AJ (1983): Voltage and time dependent conductances in solitary vertebrate hair cells. Nature 304:538–541.

Limbird LE, Buhrow SA, Speck JL, Staros JV (1983): 5-Fluorosulfonylbenzoylguanosine as a probe for the GTP binding protein α_2-receptor adenylate cyclase systems. J Biol Chem 258:10289–10293.

Litzinger MJ, Brenneman DE (1985): ^{3}H-Nitrendipine binding in non-neuronal cells from mouse spinal cord cultures. Soc Neurosci Abstr 11:86.

Litzinger MJ, Nelson PG, Pun PYK (1985): Effects of nitrendipine on the voltage sensitive calcium channel in mammalian sensory neurones. J Neurosci Res 14:415–422.

Llinas R (1984): Comparative electrobiology of mammalian central neurones. In: Dingledine R (ed): "Brain Slices." New York: Plenum Press, pp 7–24.

Llinas R, Hess R (1976): Tetrodotoxin resistant dendritic spikes in avian Purkinje cells. Proc Natl Acad Sci USA 73:2520–2523.

Llinas R, Jahnsen H (1982): Electrophysiology of mammalian thalmic neurones in vitro. Nature. 297:406–408.

Llinas R, Nicholson C (1975): Calcium role in depolarization-release coupling: An aequorin study in squid giant synapse. Proc Natl Acad Sci USA 72:188-190.

Llinas R, Sugimori M (1979): Calcium conductances in Purkinje cell dendrites: Their role in development and integration. In "Development and Chemical Specificity of Neurons", Progress in Brain Research, Vol 51. Elsevier-North Holland, pp 323–334.

Llinas R, Sugimori M (1980a): Electrophysiological properties of in vitro Purkinje cell somata in mammalian cerebellar slices. J Physiol 305:171–195.

Llinas R, Sugimori M (1980b): Electrophysiological properties of in vitro Purkinje cell dendrites in mammalian cerebellar slices. J Physiol 305:197–213.

Llinas R, Walton K (1980): Voltage dependent calcium conductances in neurones. In Cotman CW, Poste G, (eds): Elsevier-North Holland, pp 87–118.

Llinas R, Yarom Y, (1981a): Electrophysiology of mammalian inferior olivary neurones in vitro: Different types of voltage dependent ionic conductances. J Physiol 315:549–567.

Llinas R, Yarom Y (1981b): Properties and distribution of ionic conductances generating electroesponsiveness of mammalian inferior olivary neurones in vitro. J. Physiol 315:569–584.

Llinas R, Blinks JR, Nicolson C (1972): Calcium transient in presynaptic terminal of squid giant synapse: Detection with aequorin. Science 176:1127–1129.

Llinas R, Greenfield SA, Jahnsen H (1984): Electrophysiology of pars compacta cells in the in vitro substantia nigra. A possible mechanism for dendritic release. Brain Res 294: 127–132.

Llinas R, Steinberg IZ, Walton K (1976a): Presynaptic calcium currents and their relation to synaptic transmission: Voltage clamp study in squid giant synapse and theoretical model for the calcium gate. Proc

Natl Acad Sci USA 73:2918–2922.

Llinas R, Steinberg IZ, Walton K (1981): Relationships between presynaptic calcium current and postsynaptic potential in squid giant synapse. Biophys J 33:323–352.

Llinas R, Walton K, Bohr V (1976b): Synaptic transmission in squid giant synapse after potassium conductance blockage with external 3 and 4-aminopyridine. Biophys J 19:83–86.

Login IS, Judd AM, Cronin MJ, Koike K, Schettini G, Yasumoto T, MacLeod RM (1985): The effects of maitotoxin on $^{45}Ca^{2+}$ flux and hormone release in GH$_3$ rat pituitary cells. Endocrinology, 116:622–627.

Lucchi L, Govoni S, Battaini F, Pasinetti G, Trabucchi M (1985): Ethanol administration in vivo alters calcium ion control in rat striatum. Brain Res 332:376–379.

Lux HD, Brown AM (1984a): Patch and whole cell calcium currents recorded simultaneously in snail neurons. J Gen Physiol 83:727–750.

Lux HD, Brown AM (1984b): Single channel studies on inactivation of calcium currents. Science 225:432–434.

Lynn DG, Philips NJ, Hatton WC, Shabanowitz JC, (1982): Talaromycins: Application of homonuclear spin correlation maps to structure assignment. J Am Chem Soc 104:7319–7323.

MacDonald RL, Werz MA (1985): Dynorphin A decreases voltage dependent calcium conductance of mouse dorsal root ganglion neurones. J Physiol (in press).

MacDonald RL, Skerritt JH, Werz MA (1985a): Adenosine agonists reduce voltage dependent calcium conductance of mouse sensory neurones in cell culture. J Physiol (in press).

MacDonald RL, Werz MA, Grega DS (1985b): Highly selective mu and delta opioid agonists and antagonists: Action on sensory neuron calcium dependent action potentials. Soc Neurosci Abstr 11:1069.

Mackie GO, Meech RW (1985): Separate sodium and calcium spikes in the same axon. Nature 313:791–793.

MacVicar BA (1984): Voltage dependent calcium channels in glial cells. Science 226:345–1348.

MacVicar BA, Llinas R (1985): Barium action potentials in regenerating axons of the lamprey spinal cord. J Neurosci Res 13:323–335.

Madeddu L, Saito I, Hsaio T, Meldolesi J (1985a): Leptinotoxin-h action in synaptosomes and neurosecretory cells and artificial membranes. Stimulation of neurotransmitter release. J Neurochem 45:1719–1730.

Madeddu L, Scheer H, Wanke E, Meldolesi J (1985b): Ion transport activated by α-latrotoxin and congeners at the presynaptic membrane. Br J Pharmacol (in press).

Madeddu L, Pozzan T, Robello M, Rolandi R, Hsaio T, Meldolesi J (1985c): Leptinotoxin-h action in synaptosomes, neurosecretory cells and artificial membranes. Stimulation of ion fluxes. J Neurochem 45: 708–1718.

Marangos PJ, Patel J, Miller C, Martino AM (1982): Specific Ca antagonist binding sites in the brain. Life Sci 31:1575–1585.

Marangos PJ, Sperelakis N, Patel J (1984): Ontogeny of Ca antagonist binding sites in chick brain and heart. J Neurochem 42:1338–1342.

Marom S, Dagan D (1985): Calcium current in voltage clamped isolated growth cones. Soc Neurosci Abstr. 11:1183.

Marsh JD, Loh E, Lachance D, Barry WH, Smith TW, (1983): Relationship of binding of a calcium channel blocker to inhibition of contraction on intact cultured embryonic chick ventricular cells. Circ Res 53:539–543.

Masukawa LM, Prince DA (1984): Synaptic control of excitabililty in isolated dendrites of hippocampal neurones. J Neurosci 4:217–227.

Matsuda Y, Shigeru Y, Takeshi Y (1978): TTX sensitivity and Ca component of action potentials of mouse dorsal root ganglion cells cultured in vitro. Brain Res 184:69–82.

Matsuda Y, Shigeru Y, Yanezawa T (1976): A Ca-dependent regenerative response in rodent dorsal root ganglia cells cultured in vitro. Brain Res 115:334–338.

Mayer ML (1985): A calcium activated chloride current generates the afterdepolarization of rat sensory neurones in culture. J Physiol 364:217–239.

McAfee D, Yarowsky J (1979): Calcium dependent potentials in the mammalian sympathetic neurone. J Physiol 290:507–523.

McBride M, Mukherjee A, Haghani Z, Wheeler-Clark E, Brady TJ, Gandler T, Bush L, Baja ML, Willerson JT (1984): Nitrendipine effects on vascular responses and myocardial binding. Am J Physiol 247:H775–H783.

McBurney RW, Neering IR (1985): The measurement of changes in intracellular free calcium during action potentials in mammalian neurones. J Neurosci Meth 13:65–76.

McClesky E, Almers W (1985): The calcium channel in skeletal muscle is a large pore. Proc Natl Acad Sci USA 8:27149–7153.

McClesky EW, Palade PT, Almers W (1986a): The mechanism of ion selectivity in calcium channels of skeletal muscle. In Ritchie JM (ed): "Ion Channels in Neural Membranes." New York: Alan R. Liss (in press).

McClesky EW, Fox AP, Feldman D, Oliver BM, Tsien RW, Yoshikami D (1986b): The peptide toxin ω-Conus geographus toxin blocks particular types of neuronal Ca^{2+}-channels. Biophys J (in press).

McClure WO, Abbott BC, Baxter DE, Hsaio TH, Satin LS, Siger A, Yoshino JF (1980): Leptinotarsin: A presynaptic neurotoxin that stimulates release of acetylcholine. Proc Natl Acad Sci USA 77:1219–1223.

McGraw CF, Nachshen DA, Blaustein M (1982): In "Calcium and Cell Function" Cheung WY (ed): Vol II. New York: Academic Press, pp 81–110.

McLawhon R, West R, Miller RJ, Dawson G (1981): Distinct high affinity binding sites for benzomorphan drugs and enkephalin in a neuroblastoma x brain hybrid cell line. Proc Natl Acad Sci USA 78:4309–4314.

McLean MJ, MacDonald RL (1983): Multiple actions of phenytoin on mouse spinal cord neurons in cell culture. J Pharmacol Exp Ther 227:779–789.

Meiri H, Spira ME, Parnas I (1981): Membrane conductance and action potential of a regenerating axonal tip. Science 211:709–712.

Meldolesi J, Huttner WB, Tsien RY, Pozzan T (1984): Free cytoplasmic Ca^{2+} and neurotransmitter release: Studies on PC12 cells and synaptosomes exposed to α-latrotoxin. Proc Natl Acad Sci USA 81:620–624.

Meech RW, Standen NB (1975): Potassium activation in Helix aspersa neurones under voltage clamp: A component mediated by calcium influx. J Physiol 249:211–239.

Mendelson WB, Owen C, Skolnick P, Paul SM, Martin JV, Ko G, Wagner R (1984a): Nifedipine blocks sleep induction by flurazepam in the rat. Sleep 7:64–68.

Mendelson WB, Skolnick P, Martin JV, Wagner R, Paul SM (1984b): Diazepam stimulated increases in the synaptosomal uptake of ^{45}Ca^{2+}: Reversal by the dihydropyridine calcium channel antagonists. Eur J Pharmacol 104:181–183.

Messing RO, Carpenter CL, Greenberg DA (1985): Mechanism of Ca channel inhibition by phenytoin: Comparison with classical calcium channel antagonists. J Pharmacol Exp Ther 235:407–411.

Mestre M, Carriot T, Belin C, Uzan A, Renault C. Dubroeucq MC, Gueremy C, Doble A, LeFur G (1985): Electrophysiological evidence that peripheral type benzodiazepine receptors are coupled to calcium channels in the heart. Life Sci 36:391–400.

Meves H (1966): Das Aktions potential der Riesernervzellen der Weinbergschnecke Helix pomatia. Pflug Arch 204:215–241.

Meves H (1968): The ionic requirements for the production of action potentials in Helix pomatia neurones. Pflug Arch 204;214-241.

Middlemiss DN (1985): The calcium activator, BAY K8644, enhances K$^+$ evoked efflux of acetylcholine and noradrenaline from rat brain slices. Naunyn-Schmiedeberg's Arch Pharmacol 331:114–116.

Middlemiss DN, Spedding M (1985): A functional correlate for the dihydropyridine binding site in rat brain. Nature 314;94-96.

Miledi R, Parker I (1984): Chloride current induced by injection of calcium into xenopus oocytes. J Physiol 357:173-183.

Miller C, Moczydlowski E, Latorre R, Phillips M (1985): Charybdotoxin, a protein inhibitor of single Ca^{2+}-activated K^+-channels from mammalian skeletal muscle. Nature 313:316-318.

Miller RJ (1984a): How do opiates act? Trends in Neurosci 7:184-185.

Miller RJ (1984b): Toxin probes for voltage sensitive calcium channels. Trends Neurosci 7:309.

Miller RJ (1985): How many types of calcium channels exist in neurones? Trends Neurosci 8:45-47.

Miller, RJ, Freedman SB (1984): Are dihydropyridine binding sites voltage sensitive calcium channels? *Life Sci 34*:1205-1221.

Minota S, Koketsu K (1977): Effects of adrenaline on the action potential of sympathetic ganglion cells in bullfrogs. Jpn J Physiol 27:353-366.

Mishina M, Kurosaki T, Tobimatsu T, Morimoto Y, Noda M, Yamamoto T, Terao M, Lindstrom J, Takahashi T, Kuno M, Numa S (1984): Expression of functional acetylcholine receptor from cloned cDNAs. Nature 307:604-608.

Mishina M, Tobimatsu T, Imoto K, Tanaka K, Fujita Y, Fukuda K, Kurasaki M, Takahashi H, Morimoto Y, Hirose T, Inayama S, Takahashi T, Kuno M, Numa S (1985): Location of functional regions of acetylcholine receptor α-subunit by site directed mutagenesis. *Nature 313*: 364-369.

Miyake M (1978): The development of action potential mechanism in a mouse neuronal cell line in vitro. Brain Res *143*:349-354.

Miyamoto T, Ohizumi Y, Washio H, Yasumoto Y (1984): Potent excitatory effects of maitotoxin on Ca channels in the insect skeletal muscle. Pflug Arch *400*:439-441.

Mo N, Ammari R, Dun NJ (1985): Prostaglandin E_1 inhibits calcium dependent potentials in mammalian sympathetic neurons. Brain Res *334*:325-329.

Montiel C, Artalejo AR, Garcia AG (1984): Effects of the novel dihydropyridine BAY K8644 on adrenomedullary catecholamine release evoked by calcium reintroduction. Biochem Biophys Res Commun *120*:851-857.

Moolenaar WH, Spector I (1978): Ionic currents in cultured mouse neuroblastoma cells under voltage clamp conditions. J Physiol 278:265-286.

Moolenaar WH, Spector I (1979a): The calcium action potential and prolonged calcium dependent afterhyperpolarization in mouse neuroblastoma cells. J Physiol 292:297-306.

Moolenaar WH, Spector I (1979b): The calcium current and the activation of a slow potassium conductance in voltage clamped mouse neuroblastoma cells . J

Physiol 292:307-323.

Moreton RB (1968): Ionic mechanisms of the action potentials of giant neurones of Helix aspersa. Nature 219:70-71.

Mori J, Ashida H, Moru E, Tatsuno J (1982): Effects of Ca ions on action potentials in immature cultured neurons from chick cerebral cortex. J Cell Physiol *110*:241-244.

Mori K, Nowycky MC, Shepherd GM (1981): Electrophysiological analysis of mitral cells in the isolated turtle olfactory bulb. J Physiol *314*:281-294.

Mori-Okamoto J, Ashida H, Maru E, Tatsaro J (1983): Combined spikes induced by Ca and Na currents in cultured cerebellar neurones from the chick embryo. Brain Res *258*:318-322.

Mudge AW, Leeman SF, Fischbach GD (1979): Enkephalin inhibits release of substance P from sensory neurons in culture and decreases action potential duration. Proc Natl Acad Sci USA 76:527-532.

Murase K, Randic MC (1983): Electrophysiological properties of rat spinal dorsal horn neurone in vitro calcium dependent action potentials. J Physiol *334*:141-153.

Murphy KMM, Gould J, Snyder SH (1982): Autoradiographic visualization of ^{3}H-nitrendipine binding sites in rat brain: Localization to synaptic zones. Eur J Pharmacol *81*:517-519.

Murphy KMM, Gould RJ, Largent BL, Snyder SH (1983): A unitary mechanism of calcium antagonist drug action. Proc Natl Acad Sci USA 80:860-864.

Nachshen DA (1984): Selectivity of the Ca binding site in synaptosome Ca channels. J Gen Physiol 83:941-967.

Nachshen DA (1985): The early time course of potassium stimulated calcium uptake in presynaptic nerve terminals isolated from rat brain. J Physiol *361*:251-268.

Nachshen DA, Blaustein MP (1979a): Regulation of nerve terminal calcium channel selectivity by a weak acid site. Biophys J 26:329-334.

Nachshen DA, Blaustein MP (1979b): The effects of some organic "calcium antagonists" on calcium influx in presynaptic nerve terminals. Molec Pharmacol *16*:579-586.

Nachshen DA, Blaustein MP (1980): Some properties of potassium stimulated calcium influx in presynaptic nerve endings. J Gen Physiol 76:709-728.

Nachshen DA, Blaustein MP (1982): Influx of calcium strontium and barium in presynaptic nerve endings. J Gen Physiol 79:1065-1087.

Neering IR, McBurney RW (1984): Role for microsomal Ca storage in mammalian neurones. Nature *309*:158-160.

Nelson MT, French RJ, Krueger BK (1984): Voltage dependent calcium channels from brain incorporated into planar lipid bilayers. Nature *308*:77-81.

Nelson MT (1985): Single calcium channels incorporated into planar bilayers. J Gen Physiol *86*:6a.

Nerbonne JM, Gurney AM (1985): Blockade of Ca^{2+} and K$^+$ *currents* in bag cell neurones of *Aplysia californica* by dihydropyridine Ca^{2+} antagonists. J Neurosci (in press):

Nerbonne JM, Burkhalter A, Huettner JE (1985): Electrophysiological characterization of identified intrinsic cortical neurones in dissociated cell culture. Soc Neurosci Abstr 11:149.

Newberry NR, Nicoll RA (1984): Direct hyperpolarizing action of baclogen on hippocampal pyramidal cells. Nature *308*:450–452.

Newman EA (1985): Voltage dependent calcium and potassium channels in retinal glial cells. Nature *317*:809–811.

Nilius B, Hess P, Lansman JB, Tsien RW (1985): A novel type of cardiac calcium channel in ventricular cells. Nature *316*:443–446.

Nirenberg M, Wilson S, Higashida H, Rotter A, Krueger K, Basis N, Ray R, Kenimer JG, Adler M (1983): Modulation of synapse formation by cyclic adenosine monophosphate. Science *222*; 794–799.

Nishi S, North RA (1973b): Intracellular recording from the myenteric plexus of the guinea-pig ileum. J Physiol *231*:471–491.

Nishi K, Akaike N, Oyama Y, Ito H (1983): Actions of calcium antagonists on calcium currents in Helix neurones, specificity and potency. Circ Res *52(S1):* 53–59.

Nishi S, North RA (1973a): Presynaptic action of noradrenaline in the myenteric plexus. J Physiol 231:29P.

Noda M, Shimizu S, Tanabe T, Takai T, Kayano T, Ikeda T, Takahashi H, Nakayama H, Kanaoka Y, Minamino N, Kangawa K, Matsuo H, Raftery MA, Hirose T, Inayama S, Hayashida H, Miyata T, Numa A (1984): Primary structure of Electrophorus electricus sodium channel deduced from cDNA sequence. Nature *312*:121–127.

Nordstrom O, Braesch-Andersen S, Bartfai T (1986): Dopamine release is enhanced while acetylcholine release is inhibited by nimodipine (Bay e 9736) (submitted).

Norris DK, Bradford HF (1985): On the specificity of verapamil as a calcium channel blocker. Biochem Pharmacol *34*:1953–1956.

Norris DK, Dhaliwal PJ, Druce DP, Bradford HF (1983): The suppression of stimulus evoked release of amino acid neurotransmitters from synaptosomes by verapamil. J Neurochem *40*:514–521.

North, RA (1973). The calcium dependent slow afterhyperpolarization in myenteric plexus neurones with TTX resistant action potentials. Brit. J. Pharmacol., *49*:709–711.

North RA, Surprenant AM (1985) Inhibitory Synaptic potentials resulting from α_2 adrenoceptor activation in guinea-pig submucous plexus neurones. J Physiol

358:17–33.

Nowycky MC, Fox AP, Tsien RW (1985b): Long opening mode of gating of neuronal calcium channels and its promotion by the dihydropyridine calcium agonist BAY K8644. Proc Natl Acad Sci USA *82*:2178–2182.

Obaid AL, Orkand RK, Gainer H, Salzberg BM (1985): Active calcium responses recorded optically from nerve terminals of the frog neurohypophysis. J Gen Physiol *85*:481–489.

Ogura A, Takahashi M (1984): Differential effects of a dihydropyridine derivative on Ca^{2+}-entry pathways in neuronal preparations. Brain Res *301*:323–330.

Ogura A, Ohizumi Y, Yasumoto T (1984): Calcium dependent depolarization induced by a marine toxin maitotoxin in a neuronal cell. Proc Jpn Physiol Soc 34:.

Ohizumi Y, Yasumoto T (1983): Contractile response of the rabbit aorta to maitotoxin, the most potent marine toxin. J Physiol *337*:711–721. Sci USA 77:1701–1705.

O'Lague PH, Huttner SL (1980): Physiological and morphological studies of rat phemochromocytoma cells (PCIZ) chemically fused and grown in culture. Proc Natl Acad Sci USA 77:1701–1705.

O'Lague PH, Huttner SL, Vandenberg CA, Morrison-Graham K, and Horn R (1985): Morphological properties and membrane channels of the growth cones induced in PC12 cells by nerve growth factor. J Neurosci Res *13*:301–321.

O'Lague PH, Potter DD, Furshpan EJ (1978): Studies on rat sympathetic neurons developing in cell culture. Devel Biol *67*:384–403.

O'Leary ME, Suszkiw JB (1983): Effect of colchicine on ^{45}Ca^{2+} and choline uptake and acetylcholine release in rat brain synaptosomes. J Neurochem *40*:1192–1195.

Olivera BM, McIntosh JM, Cruz LJ, Luque FA, Gray WR (1984): Purification and sequence of a presynaptic peptide toxin from Conus geographus venom. Biochemistry *23*:5087–5090.

Oomura Y, Ozaki S, Maeno T (1961): Electrical activity of a giant nerve cell under abnormal conditions. Nature *191*:1265–1267.

Orchard I (1976): Ca dependent action potentials in a peripheral neurosecretory cell of the stick insect. J Comp Physiol *122*:95–102.

Owen DA, Segal M, Barker JL (1984): A Ca^{2+} dependent Cl- conductance in cultured spinal cord neurones. Nature *311*:567–570.

Paupardin-Tritsc D, Colombaioni L, Deterre P, Gerschenfeld H. (1985a): Two different mechanisms of calcium spike modulation by dopamine. J Neurosci 5:2522–2532.

Paupardin-Tritsch D, Hammonde C, Gerschenfeld H (1985b): A serotonin induced increase of calcium current in identified molluscan neurones mimicked by cGMP, not cAMP. Soc Neurosci Abstr 11; 466.

Peacock JH, Walker CR (1983): Development of calcium action potentials in mouse hippocampal cell cultures. Devel Brain Res 8:39–52.

Pellmar TC (1981): Ionic mechanism of a voltage dependent current elicited by cyclic AMP. Cell Mol Neurobiol 1:87–97.

Pellmar TC (1984): Enhancement of inward current by serotonin in neurones of Aplysia. J Neurosci 15:13–25.

Pellmar TC, Carpenter DO (1980): Serotonin induces a voltage sensitive calcium current in neurones of Aplysia californica. J Neurophysiol 44:423–439.

Pennefather P, Lancaster B, Adams PR, Nicoll RA (1985): Two distinct K^+-currents in bullfrog sympathetic ganglion cells. Proc Natl Acad Sci USA 82:3040–3045.

Penner R, Dreyer F (1984): Two different presynaptic calcium currents in mouse motor nerve terminal. Naunyn-Schmiedeberg's Arch Pharmacol 325(S): R61.

Perney TM, Dinerstein R, Miller RF (1984): Depolarization-induced increases in intracellular free calcium detected in single cultured neuronal cells. Neurosci Lett 51:165–170.

Perney TM, Hirning LD, Miller RJ (1986): Different calcium channels mediate neurotransmitter release from sensory and sympathetic neurones. Biophys J (in press).

Peroutka SF, Allen GS (1983): Calcium channel antagonist binding sites labeled by ^{3}H-nimodipine in human brain. J Neurosurg 59:933–937.

Pincus JH, Hsaio K (1981): Calcium uptake mechanisms affected by some convulsant and anticonvulsant drugs. Brain Res 217:119–127.

Pitman R (1979): Intracellular citrate or externally applied TEA ions produce calcium dependent action potentials in an insect motoneurone cell body. J Physiol 291:327–337.

Platika D, Boulos MH, Baizer L, Fishman MC (1985): Neuronal traits of clonal cell lines derived by fusion of dorsal root ganglion neurones with neuroblastoma cells. Proc Natl Acad Sci USA 82:3499–3503.

Porter ID, Gardiner IM, de Belleroche J (1985): Nimodipine has an inhibitory action on neurotransmitter release from human cerebral arteries. J Cerebral Blood Flow Metab 5:338–342.

Powers RE, Colucci NS (1985): An increase in putative voltage dependent calcium channel number following reserpine treatment. Biochem Biophys Res Commun 132:844–849.

Proctor WR, Dunwiddie TW (1983): Adenosine inhibits calcium spikes in hippocampal pyramidal neurones in vitro. Neurosci Lett 35:197–201.

Pumplin DW, Reese TS, Llinas R (1981): Are presynaptic membrane particles the Ca^{2+} channels. Proc Natl Acad Sci USA 78:7210–7213.

Pun RYK, Litzinger MJ (1984): Does nitrendipine block calcium channels in neuronal preparations? Soc Neurosci Abstr 10:157.

Quirion R (1983): Autoradiographic localization of a calcium channel antagonist ^{3}H-nitrendipine binding site in rat brain. Neurosci Lett 36:267–271.

Quirion R (1985): Characterization of binding sites for two classes of calcium channel antagonists in human forebrain. Eur J Pharmacol 113:139–142.

Quirion R, Lafaille F, Nair NPV (1985): Comparative potencies of calcium channel antagonists and antischizophrenic drugs on central and peripheral calcium channel binding sites. J Pharm Pharmacol 37:437–440.

Ramkumar V, El-Fakahany EE (1984): Increase in ^{3}H-nitrendipine binding sites in the brain of morphine tolerant mice. Eur J Pharmacol 102:371–372.

Ramkumar V, El-Fakahany EE (1985): Changes in the affinity of [^{3}H]-nimodipine binding sites in the brain upon chlorpromazine treatment and subsequent withdrawal. Res Commun Chem Pathol Pharmacol 48:463–466.

Rampe D, Janis RA, Triggle DJ (1984): BAY K8644, A 1,4-dihydropyridine Ca^{2+} channel activator: Dissociation of binding and functional effects in brain synaptosomes. J Neurochem: 43:1688–1692.

Rane SG, Dunlap K (1985a): The kinase C activator 1,2,oleoylacetylglycerol mimics norepinephrine's effects on the voltage dependent Ca^{2+}-current of embryonic chick dorsal root ganglion neurones. Soc Neurosci Abstr 11:748.

Rane SG, Dunlap K (1985b): The kinase C activator 1,2,oleoylacetylglycerol mimics norepinephrine effects on the voltage dependent calcium current of embryonic chick DRG neurones. Cornell Symp Ca^{2+} and Cell Reg 22:(abstract).

Ransom BR, Holz RW (1977): Ionic determinants of excitability in cultured mouse dorsal root ganglion and spinal cord cells. Brain Res 136:445–453.

Ransom BR, Neale E, Henkart M, Bullock PN, Nelson PG (1977): Mouse spinal cord cell culture. I. Morphology and intrinsic neuronal electrophysiologic properties. J Neurophysiol 40:1132–1150.

Reiser G, Heumann R, Kemper D, Lautenschlager E, Hamprecht B (1977): Influence of cations on the electrical activity of neuroblastoma x glioma hybrid cells. Brain Res 130:495–504.

Rengasamy A, Ptusienski J, Hosey MM (1985): Purification of the cardiac 1,4,dihydropyridine receptor/ calcium channel complex. Biochem Biophys Res Commun 1261-7.

Reuter H (1983): Calcium channel modulation by neurotransmitters, enzymes and drugs. Nature 301:569–574.

Reuter H, Porzig H, Kokubun S, Prod'hom B (1985a): 1,4,Dihydropyridines as tools in the study of Ca^{2+} channels. Trends Neurosci 8: 396–400.

Reuter H, Porzig H, Kokubun S, Prod'hom B (1985b): Voltage dependence of dihydropyridine ligand binding and action in intact cardiac cells. J Gen Physiol 86:5a.

Reynolds IJ, Gould RJ, Snyder SH (1983): ^{3}H-Verapamil binding sites in brain and skeletal muscle: Regulation by calcium. Eur J Pharmacol 95:319–321.

Reynolds IJ, Gould RF, Snyder SH (1984): Loperamide blockade of calcium channels as a mechanism for antidiarrheal effects. J Pharmacol Exp Ther 231:628–638.

Reynolds IJ, Snowman AM, Snyder SH (1985): ^{3}H-Methoxyverapamil (^{3}H-D600) and ^{3}H-desmethoxy-verapamil (^{3}H-D888) label multiple receptors in brain skeletal muscle. Soc Neurosci Abstr 11:516.

Rezvani A, Huidobro-Toro JP, Way EL (1983): Effect of 4-aminopyridine and verapamil on the inhibitory action of normorphine on the guinea-pig ileum. Eur J Pharmacol 86:111–115.

Ribares RG, Miller RJ (1985): Phenytoin inhibits voltage dependent and dihydropyridine stimulated Ca^{2+} uptake by NG108-15 cells. Soc Neurosci Abstr 11:596.

Ribeiro JD, Sa-Almeida AM, Namarado JM (1979): Adenosine and adenosine triphosphate decrease ^{45}Ca^{2+} uptake by synaptosomes stimulated by potassium. Biochem Pharmacol 28:1297–1300.

Riker WK, Matsamoto M, Takashima K (1985): Synaptic facilitation by 3-aminopyridine and its antagonism by verapamil and diltiazem. J Pharmacol Exp Ther 235:431–435.

Rogart RB, Kops AD, Dzau VJ (1986): Identification of two calcium channel receptor sites for labeled nitrendipine in mammalian cardiac and smooth muscle membrane. Proc Natl Acad Sci USA (in press).

Rogawski MA, Barker JL (1983): Effects of 4-aminopyridine on calcium action potentials and calcium current under voltage clamp in spinal neurones. Brain Res 280:180–185.

Rojas E, Taylor RE (1975): Simultaneous measurements of magnesium, calcium and sodium influxes in perfused squid giant axons under membrane potential control. J. Physiol 252:1–27.

Romey G, Lazdunski M (1982): Lipid soluble toxins thought to be specific for Na$^+$ channels block Ca^{2+} channels in neuronal cells. Nature 297:79–80.

Rosenberg RL, Hess P, Smilowitz H, Reeves JP, Tsien RW (1986): Permeation and gating of cardiac and skeletal muscle Ca^{2+} channels in lipid bilayers. Biophys J (in press).

Ross WN, Stuart AE (1978): Voltage sensitive calcium channels in the presynaptic terminals of a decrementally conducting photoreceptor. J Physiol 274:173–191.

Rotter A, Ray R, Nirenberg M (1979): Regulation of calcium uptake in neuroblastoma or hybrid cells. A possible mechanism for synaptic plasticity. Fed Proc 38:470.

Sah P, French CR, Gage PW (1985): Effects of noradrenaline on some potassium currents in CA neurones in rat hippocampal slices. Neurosci Lett 60:295–300.

Salzberg BM, Obaid AL, Senseman DM, Gainer H (1983): Optical recording of action potentials from vertebrate nerve terminals using potentiometric probes provides evidence for sodium and calcium components. Nature 306:36–40.

Salzberg BM, Obaid AL, Gainer H (1985): Large and rapid changes in light scattering accompanying secretion by nerve terminals in the mammalian neurohypophysis. J Gen Physiol 86:395–411.

Sanguinetti MC, Kass RS (1984a): Voltage dependent block of calcium channel current in calf cardiac Purkinje fibers by dihydropyridine calcium channel antagonists. Circ Res 55:336–348.

Sanguinetti MC, Kass RS (1984b): Regulation of cardiac calcium channel current and contractile activity by the dihydropyridine BAY K8644 is voltage dependent. J Mol Cell Cardiol 16:667–670.

Sarmiento JG, Epstein PM, Smilowitz H, Chester DW, Wehinger E, Janis RA (1985): Photoaffinity labeling of the 1,4-dihydropyridine Ca^{2+} channel binding site in cardiac, skeletal and smooth muscle membranes. Fed Proc 44:1640.

Sasakawa N, Kumakura K, Yasumoto S, Kato R (1983): Effects of W-7 on catecholamine release and ^{45}Ca^{2+} uptake in cultured adrenal chromaffin cells. Life Sci 33:2017–2024.

Sasakawa N, Yamamoto S, Kato R (1984): Effects of inhibitors of arachidonic acid metabolism on calm uptake and catecholamine release in cultured adrenal chromaffin cells. Biochem Pharmacol 33:2733–2738.

Schettini G, Koike K, Login IS, Judd AM, Cronin MJ, Yasumoto T, MacLeod RMC (1984): Maitotoxin stimulates hormonal release and calcium flux in rat anterior pituitary cells in vitro. Am J Physiol 247:E520–E525.

Schilling WP, Drewe JA (1985): Voltage sensitive nitrendipine binding in an isolated cardiac sarcolemma preparation. J Biol Chem (in press).

Schlichter R, Bossu J-L, Feltz A, Desarmenien M, Feltz P (1984): Characterization of the multiple currents underlying spike activity in sensory neurones: An attempt to determine the physiological role of GABA-B receptor activation on slow conducting primary afferents. Neuropharmacology 23:869–872.

Schoemaker H, Langer SZ (1985): ^{3}H-Diltiazem binding to calcium channel antagonist recognition sites in rat cerebral cortex. Eur J Pharmacol 111:273–277.

Schoemaker H, Lee HR, Roeske WR, Yamamura HI (1983): In vivo identification of calcium antagonist binding sites using ^{3}H-nitrendipine. Eur J Pharmacol *88*:275–276.

Scholfield GG, Weight FF (1984): Voltage dependent calcium current in PC12 cells. Soc Neurosci Abstr *10*:527.

Schwartz LM, McClesky EW, Almers W (1985): Dihydropyridine receptors in muscle are voltage dependent but most are not functional calcium channels. Nature *314*:747–749.

Schwartzkroin DA, Prince DA (1978): Cellular and field potential properties of epileptogenic hippocampal slices. Brain Res *147*:117–130.

Schwartzkroin DA, Slawsky MA (1977): Probable calcium spikes in hippocampal neurones. Brain Res *135*:157–161.

Schwindt P, Crill W (1980a): Role of persistent inward current in motoneurones bursting during spinal seizures. J Neurophysiol *43*:1296–1316.

Schwindt P, Crill WE (1980b): Properties of a persistent inward current in normal and TEA injected motoneurones. J Neurophysiol *43*:1700–1728.

Schwindt P, Crill W (1980c): Effects of barium on cat spinal motoneurones studied by voltage clamp. J Neurophysiol *44*:827–846.

Schwindt P, Crill W (1982): Factors influencing motoneuron rhythmic firing: Results from a voltage clamp study. J Neurophysiol *48*:875–890.

Scott BS, Edwards BAV (1980): Electrical membrane properties of adult mouse DRG neurones and the effect of culture duration. J Neurobiol *11*:291–301.

Segal M, Barker JL (1985): Rat hippocampal neurons in culture: Ca and Ca dependent conductances. J Neurophysiol (in press).

Selzer ME (1979): The effect of phenytoin on the action potential of a vertebrate spinal neurone. Brain Res *171*:511–521.

Shalaby IA, Kongsamut S, Freedman SB, Miller RJ (1984): The effects of dihydropyridines on neurotransmitter release from cultured neuronal cells. Life Sci *35*:1289–1295.

Shelton RC, Grebb JA, Freed WJ (1985): Calcium channel agonist induced murine seizures. Soc Neurosci Abstr *11*:924.

Shibanuma T, Iwanani M, Okuda K, Takenaka T, Murakami M (1980): Synthesis of optically active nicardipine. Chem Pharm Bull *28*:2809–2812.

Shrikande AU, Sarmiento JG, Janis RA, Rutledge E, Triggle DJ (1985): Characteristics of binding of BAY K8644 to high and low affinity sites on cardiac membranes. Biophys J *47*:265a.

Siegelbaum SA, Tsien RW (1983): Modulation of gated ion channels as a mode of transmitter action. Trends Neurosci *6*:307–313.

Siegelbaum SA, Camardo JS, Kandel ER (1982): Serotonin and cyclic AMP close single K$^+$-channels in Aplysia sensory neurones. Nature *299*:413–417.

Sihra TS, Scott IG, Nicholls DG (1984): Ionophore A23187, verapamil, protonophores and veratradine influence the release of GABA from synaptosomes by modulation of the plasma membrane potential rather than the cytosolic calcium. J Neurochem *43*:1624–1630.

Simon SM, Llinas RR (1985): Compartmentalization of the submembrane calcium activity during calcium influx and its significance in transmitter release. Biophys J *48*:485–498.

Slack BF (1985): Pre- and postsynaptic actions of noradrenaline and clonidine on myenteric neurones. J Neurosci (in press).

Smith SJ, Augustine GJ, Charlton MP (1985): Evidence for cooperative calcium action in secretion of synaptic transmitter. Proc Natl Acad Sci USA (in press).

Sohn RS, Ferendelli JA (1973): Inhibition of Ca^{2+} transport into rat brain synaptosomes by diphenylhydantoin. J Pharmacol Exp Ther *185*:272–275.

Sohn RS, Ferendelli JA (1976): Anticonvulsant drug mechanisms: Phenytoin, phenobarbital and ethosuximide and calcium flux in isolated presynaptic nerve endings. Arch Neurol *33*:626–629.

Spector I, Kimhi Y, Nelson PG (1973): Tetrodotoxin and cobalt blockade of neuroblastoma action potentials. Nature *246*:124–126.

Spedding M, Middlemiss DN (1985): Central effects of Ca^{2+} antagonists. Trends Pharm Sci *6*;309–310.

Spitzer NC (1979): Ion channels in development. Ann Rev Neurosci *2*:363–397.

Spitzer NC (1984): The differentiation of membrane properties of spinal neurons. In Black IB (ed): "Cellular and Molecular Biology of Neuronal Development." New York: Plenum Press, pp 95–106.

Spitzer NC, Baccaglini PI (1976): Development of the action potential in embryo amphibian neurones in vivo. Brain Res *107*:610–616.

Spitzer NC, Lamborghini JE (1976): The development of the action potential mechanism of amphibian neurones isolated in culture. Proc Natl Acad Sci USA *73*:1641–1645.

Stallcup WB (1979): Sodium and calcium fluxes in a clonal nerve cell line. J Physiol *286*:525–540.

Standen NB (1975): Ca and Na ions as charge carriers in the action potential of an identified snail neurone. J Physiol *249*:241–252.

Starke KU, Spath L, Wichmann T (1984): Effects of verapamil, diltiazem and ryosidine on the release of dopamine and acetylcholine in rabbit caudate nucleus slices. Naunyn-Schmiedeberg's Arch Pharmacol *325*:124–130.

Steinsland, OS, Johnson CE, Scriabine A (1985): Comparative effects of nitrendipine and verapamil on neuroeffector transmission in the rabbit ear artery. J Cardiol Pharmacol *7*:990–995.

Stinnakre J, Tauc L (1973): Ca influx in active Aplysia neurones detected in injected aequorin. Nature New Biol *242*:113–115.

Strichartz G, Small R, Nicholson C, Pfenninger KH,

Llinas R (1980): Ionic mechanisms for impulse propagation in growing myelinated axons: Saxitoxin binding and electrophysiology. Soc Neurosci Abstr 6:660.

Striessnig J, Zernig G, Glossmann H (1985a): Human red cell Ca^{2+} antagonist binding sites. Eur J Biochem 150:67–77.

Striessnig J, Zernig G, Glossmann H (1985b): Ca^{2+} antagonist receptor sites on human red blood cell membranes. Eur J Pharmacol 108:329–330.

Strong JA, Fox AP, Tsien RW, Kaczmarek LK (1986): Phorbol ester promotes a large conductance Ca channel in Aplysia bag cell neurones. Biophys J (in press).

Strumwasser F, Kaczmarek LK, Jennings KR, Chiu AY (1981): Studies of a model peptidergic neuronal system, the bag cells of Aplysia. In Famer DS, Lederis K (eds): "Neurosecretion—Molecules, Cells, Systems." New York: Plenum Press, pp 249–268.

Stuart AE, Oertel D (1978): Neuronal properties underlying processing of visual information in the barnacle. Nature 275:287–290.

Study RE, Breakfield XO, Bartfai T, Greengard P (1978): Voltage sensitive calcium channels regulate guanosine 3′5′ cyclic monophosphate levels in neuroblastoma cells. Proc Natl Acad Sci USA 75:6295–6299.

Stuenkel E, Lemos J, Cooke I, Nordmann JJ (1985): Cation channels of isolated peptidergic nerve terminals. J Gen Physiol 86:24(a).

Sturek M, Hermsmeyer K (1985): Two different types of Ca channels in spontaneously contracting vascular smooth muscle cells. J Gen Physiol 86:23a.

Suarez-Isla BA, Pelto DJ, Thompson JM, Rapoport SI (1984): Blockers of Ca permeability inhibit neurite extension and formation of neuromuscular synapses in cell culture. Dev Brain Res 14:263–270.

Suetake K, Kojima H, Inanaga K, Koketsa K (1981): Catecholamine is released from nonsynaptic cell soma membrane: Histochemical evidence in bullfrog sympathetic ganglion cells. Brain Res 205:436–440.

Supavilai P, Karobath M (1984): The interaction of [^{3}H] PY108068 and [^{3}H] PN200110 with calcium channels in rat brain. J Neural Trans 60:149.

Surprenant AM (1984): Two types of neurones lacking synaptic input in submucous plexus of guinea-pig small intestine. J Physiol 351:363–378.

Suzuki J (1976): Ca activation in the giant axon of the crayfish. In Reuben JP, Purpura DP, Bennett M, Kandel ER (eds): "Electrobiology of Nerve, Synapse and Muscle." New York: Raven Press, pp 27–35.

Swandulla D, Carbone E, Schafer K, Lux HD (1985): Menthol modulates calcium inactivation in neurones. Pflug Arch 405(S2):R39.

Taft WC, DeLorenzo RJ (1984): Micromolar affinity benzodiazepine receptors regulate voltage sensitive calcium channels in nerve terminal preparations. Proc Natl Acad Sci USA 81:3118–3122.

Takahashi M, Ogura A (1983): Dihydropyridines as potent calcium channel blockers in neuronal cells. FEBS Lett 152:191–194.

Takahashi M, Ohizumi Y, Hatanaka H (1985): Neuronal differentiation of Ca^{2+} channel by nerve growth factor. Brain Res 341:381–384.

Takahashi M, Ohizumi Y, Yasumoto T (1982): Maitotoxin: A Ca^{2+} channel activator candidate. J Biol Chem 257:7287–7289.

Takahashi M, Tatsumi M, Ohizumi Y, Yasumoto T (1983): Ca^{2+} channel activating function of maitotoxin, the most potent marine toxin known, in clonal rat pheochromocytoma cells. J Biol Chem 258:10944–10949.

Takata Y, Kato H (1985): Effects of Ca antagonists on the norepinephrine release and contractile responses of isolated canine saphenous veins to high KCl. Jpn J Pharmacol 37:381–384.

Talvenheimo JA (1985): The purification of channels from excitable cells. J Memb Biol 87:77–91.

Tank DW, Miller C, Webb W: (1982): Isolated patch recording from liposomes containing functionally reconstituted chloride channels from Torpedo electroplax. Proc Natl Acad Sci USA 79:7749–7753.

Tashiro N, Nishi S (1972): Effects of alkali earth cations on sympathetic ganglion cells of the rabbit. Life Sci 11(S20):941–948.

Tazaki K, Cooke IM (1970): Ionic bursts of slow depolarizing responses of cardiac ganglion neurones in the crab Partunus sanguinolentus. J. Neurophysiol 42:1022–1047.

Thayer SA, Stein L, Fairhurst AS (1984): Endogenous modulator of calcium channels. IUPHAR 9th International Congress of Pharmacology.

Thayer SA, Welcome M, Chabra A, Fairhurst AS (1985): Effect of dihydropyridine Ca^{2+} channel blocking drugs on rat brain muscarinic and α-adrenergic receptors. Biochem Pharmacol 34:175–180.

Theodosis DT, Legendre P, Vincent JD, Cooke I: (1983): Immunocytochemically identified vasopressin neurones in culture show slow calcium dependent electrical responses. Science 221:1052–1054.

Thompson SH, Aldrich RW (1980): Membrane potassium channels. In Cotman CW, Poste G, Nicolson GL (eds): "The Cell Surface and Neuronal Function." Elsevier/North-Holland, pp 49–85.

Thompson SM, Masukawa LM, Prince DA (1985): Temperature dependence of intrinsic membrane properties and synaptic potentials in hippocampal CA1 neurons in vitro. J Neurosci 5:817–824.

Thorgeirsson G, Rudolph SA (1984): Diltiazem like effect of thioridazine on the dihydropyridine binding site of the calcium channel of rat myocardial membranes. Biochem Biophys Res Commun 121:657–

663.

Titeler M, DeSousza EB, Kuhar MJ (1985): ^{3}H-Nitrendipine binding to calcium channels in bovine and rat pituitary. J Neurochem 44:1955–1958.

Toll L (1982): Calcium antagonists: High affinity binding and inhibition of calcium transport in a clonal cell line. J Biol Chem 257:13189–13192.

Towert R, Wehinger E, Meyer H, Kazda S (1982): The effects of nimodipine, its optical isomers and metabolites on isolated vascular smooth muscle. Arzneim-Forsch 32:338–346.

Triggle DJ (1981): Calcium antagonists: Basic chemical and pharmacological aspects. In Weiss GB (ed): "New Perspectives on Ca^{2+} Antagonists." American Physiology Society, pp 1–18.

Trimmer JS, Trowbridge IS, Vacquier VD (1985): Monoclonal antibody to membrane glycoprotein inhibits the acrosome reaction and associated Ca^{2+} and K$^+$ fluxes of sea urchin sperm. Cell 40:697–703.

Tsien RW (1983): Calcium channels in excitable cell membranes. Ann Rev Physiol 45:341–358.

Tsien RY, Pozzan T, Rink TJ (1982): Calcium homeostasis in intact lymphocytes: Cytoplasmic free calcium monitored with a new, intracellularly trapped fluorescent indicator. J Cell Biol 94:325–334.

Tsunoo A, Yoshii M, Narahashi (1984): Two types of calcium channels in neuroblastoma cells and their sensitivities to cAMP. Soc Neurosci Abstr 10:527.

Tsunoo A, Yoshii M, Narahashi T (1985a): Differential block of two types of calcium channels in neuroblastoma cells. Biophys J 47:433.

Tsunoo A, Yoshii M, Narahashi T (1985b): Enkephalin and somatostatin block of calcium channels in neuroblastoma cells. Soc Neurosci Abstr 11:517.

Tucker JF (1984): Effect of pertussis toxin on normorphine dependence and on acute inhibitory effects of normorphine and clonidine in guinea-pig isolated ileum. Br J Pharmacol 83:326–328.

Turner TJ, Goldin SM (1985a): Calcium channels in rat brain synaptosomes: Identification and pharmacological characterization. J Neurosci 5:841–849.

Turner TJ, Goldin SM (1985b): Effects of dihydropyridine a agonists and antagonists on Ca^{2+} uptake and neurotransmitter release by rat brain synaptosomes. Soc Neurosci Abstr 11:579.

Tuttle JB, Richelson E (1979): Phenytoin action on the excitable membrane of mouse neuroblastoma. J Pharmacol Exp Ther 211:632–637.

Twombly D, Narahashi T (1985): Phenytoin suppresses calcium channel currents in neuroblastoma cells. Soc Neurosci Abstr 11:518.

Umbach JA, Gundersen CB, Baker PF (1984): Giant synaptosomes. Nature 311:474–477.

Vacus MI, Sarmiento MIK, Cardinali DP (1984): Pineal methoxyindoles depress Ca^{2+} uptake by rat brain synaptosomes. Brain Res 294:166–168.

Van der Kloot W, Kita H (1975): The effects of the "calcium antagonist" verapamil on muscle action potentials in the frog and crayfish and on neuromuscular transmission in the crayfish. Comp Biochem Physiol 50C:121–125.

Vargas O, Del Carmen M, Soldate ML, Orrego F (1977): Potassium induced release of ^{3}H-GABA and ^{3}H-noradrenaline from normal and reserpinized rat brain cortex slices. Differences in calcium dependency and in sensitivity to potassium ions. J Neurochem 28:165–170.

Venter JC, Fraser JC, Schaber JS, Juang CY, Bolger G, Triggle DJ (1983): Molecular properties of the slow inward calcium channel. J Biol Chem 258:9344–9348.

Veraga J, Tsien RY, Delay M (1985): Inositol-1,4,5-triphosphate: A possible chemical link in excitation-contraction coupling in muscle. Proc Natl Acad Sci USA 82:6352–6356.

Vycklicky L, Michl J, Vlachova V, Vycklicky L, Vyskocil F (1985): Ionic currents in neuroblastoma clone E-7 cells. Neurosci Lett 55:197–201.

Wagner JA, Reynolds IS, Weisman HF, Dudeck P, Weisfeldt ML, Snyder SH (1986): Calcium antagonist receptors in the cardiomyopathic hamster: Selective increases in heart and brain. Science (in press).

Wakade AR, Wakade TD (1978): Inhibition of noradrenaline release by adenosine. J. Physiol 282:35–49.

Wald F (1972): Ionic differences between somatic and axonal action potentials in snail giant neurones. J Physiol 220:267–281.

Walden J, Pockberger H, Speckmann EJ, Petsche H (1985): Calcium current in identified snail neurones: Effects of the calcium agonist BAY K8644 on the calcium antagonist nifedipine. Pflug Arch 405(S2):R8.

Walz W, MacVicar BA (1985): Barium induced rhythmic depolarization of glial cells in brain slices. Soc Neurosci Abstr 11:87.

Watanabe A, Tasaki T, Lerman L (1976a): Bi-ionic action potentials in squid giant axons internally perfused with sodium salts. Proc Natl Acad Sci USA 58:2246–2252.

Watanabe A, Tasaki I, Singer I, Lerman L (1976b): Effects of tetrodotoxin on excitability of squid giant axons in sodium free media. Science 155:95–97.

Weiland GA, Oswald RE (1985): The mechanism of binding of dihydropyridine calcium channel blockers to rat brain membranes. J Biol Chem 260:8456–8464.

Werz MA, MacDonald RL (1984a): Dynorphin reduces calcium dependent action potential duration by decreasing voltage dependent calcium conductance. Neurosci Lett 46:185–190.

Werz MA, MacDonald RL (1984b): Dynorphin reduces

voltage dependent calcium conductance of mouse dorsal root ganglion Neuropeptide 5:253–256.

Werz MA MacDonald RL (1985a): Dynorphin and neoendorphin peptides decrease dorsal root ganglion neuron calcium dependent action potential duration. J Pharmacol Exp Ther 234:49–56.

Werz MA, MacDonald RL (1985b): Barbiturates decrease voltage dependent calcium conductance of mouse neurons in dissociated cell culture. Molec Pharmacol 28:269–277.

Werz MA, MacDonald RL (1985c): Phorbol esters: Opposing effects on calcium dependent action potentials of dorsal root ganglion neurones. Soc Neurosci Abstr 11:747.

West RE, Freedman SB, Dawson G, Miller RJ, Villereal ML (1982): Delta and sigma sites of clonal NCB-20 cells do not modulate calcium uptake. Life Sci 31:1335–1340.

West RE, McLawhon RW, Dawson G, Miller RJ (1983): ^{3}H-Ethylketocyclazocine binding to NCB-20 hybrid neurotumor cells. Molec Pharmacol 23:489–499.

Westfall TC, Kitay D, Wahl G (1976): The effect of cyclic nucleotides on the release of ^{3}H-dopamine from rat striatal slices. J Pharmacol Exp Ther 199:149–157.

White EJ, Bradford HF (1985): Sites of action of Ca^{2+} channel blockers in rat cortical synaptosomes. Biochem Soc Trans 13:1985–1987.

Wibo M, Delfosse I, Godfraind T (1983): Action of flunarizine and cinnarizine on calcium fluxes in synaptosomal preparations from cerebral cortex. Arch Int Pharmacol 263:333–334.

Willard AL (1980): Electrical excitability of outgrowing neurites of embryonic neurones in cultures of dissociated neural plate of Xenopus laevis. J Physiol 301:115–118.

Willard AL, Nishi R (1985): Neurons dissociated form rat myenteric plexus retain differentiated properties when grown in cell culture. Neuroscience 16:201–211.

Williams JS, Grupp IL, Grupp G, Vaghy PL, Dumont L, Schwartz A (1985): Profile of the oppositely acting enantiomers of the dihydropyridine 202791 in cardiac preparations: Receptor binding, electrophysiological and pharmacological studies. Biochem Biophys Res Commun 131:13–21.

Williams JT, North RA (1985): Catecholamine inhibition of calcium action potentials in rat locus coeruleus neurones. Neuroscience 14:102–109.

Williams JT, Henderson G, North RA (1985): Characterization of α_2-adrenoceptors which increase potassium conductance in rat locus coeruleus neurons. Neuroscience 14:95–101.

Williams JT, North RA, Shefner SA, Nishi S, Egan TM (1984): Membrane properties of rat locus coeruleus neurones. Neuroscience 13:137–156.

Wong RKS, Prince DA (1978): Participation of calcium spikes during intrinsic burst firing in hippocampal neurones. Brain Res 159:385–390.

Wong RKS, Prince DA (1979): Dendritic mechanisms underlying penicillin-induced epileptiform activity. Science 204:1228–1231.

Wong RKS, Prince DA (1981): After potential generation in hippocampal pyramidal cells. J Neurophysiol 45:87–97.

Wong RKS, Prince DA, Basbaum AL (1979): Intradendritic recordings from hippocampal neurones. Proc Natl Acad Sci USA 76:986–990.

Woodward JJ, Leslie SW (1985): Inhibition by nimodipine of BAY K8644 and KCl stimulated calcium entry into and endogenous dopamine release from striatal synaptosomes. Soc Neurosci Abstr 11;1002.

Wu PH, Phillis JW, Theirry DL (1982): Adenosine receptor agonists inhibit K$^+$ evoked Ca^{2+} uptake by rat brain cortical synaptosomes. J Neurochem 39:700–708.

Yamamoto HA, McCain HW, Isami K, Misawa S, Way EL (1981): Effects of amino acids, especially taurine and γ-aminobutyric acid (GABA), an analysis and calcium depletion induced by morphine in mice. Eur J. Pharmacol 71:177–184.

Yatani A, Brown AM (1985): The Ca^{2+} channel blocker nitrendipine blocks sodium channels in neonatal rat cardiac myocytes. Circ Res 57: 868–875.

Yellen G (1982): Single Ca^{2+}-activated nonselective cation channels in neuroblastoma. Nature 296:357–359.

Yoshida S, Matsuda Y (1979): Studies on sensory neurones of the mouse with intracellular recording and horseradish peroxidase injection techniques. J Neurophysiol 42:1134–1145.

Yoshida S, Matsuda Y (1980): Responses dependent on alkaline earth cations (Ca, Sr, Ba) in dorsal root ganglion cells of the adult mouse. Brain Res 188:593–597.

Yoshida S, Matsuda Y, Samejima A (1978): Tetrodotoxin resistant sodium and calcium components of action potentials in dorsal root ganglion cells of the adult mouse. J Neurophysiol 41:1096–1106.

Yoshii M, Tsunoo A, Narahashi T (1985a): Different properties of two types of calcium channels in neuroblastoma cells. Biophys J 47:433.

Yoshii M, Tsunoo A, Narahashi T (1985b): Effects of pyrethroids and veratradine on two types of Ca channels in neuroblastoma cells. Soc Neurosci Abstr 11:518.

Yoshii M, Tsunoo A, Kuroda Y, Wu CH, Narahashi T (1984): Maitotoxin induces steady current which is inhibited by calcium channel blockers. Soc Neurosci Abstr 10:527.

Yoshii M, Tsunoo A, Kuroda Y, Wu CH, Narahashi T (1986): Maitotoxin induced membrane current in neuroblastoma cells. Brain Res (in press).

Yoshino JE, Baxter DE, Hsaio TH; McClure W (1980):

Release of acetylcholine from rat brain synaptosomes stimulated by leptinotarsin, a new neurotoxin. J Neurochem 34:635–642.

Zelar E, Sperelkis N (1981): Ionic dependence of electrical activity in small mesenteric arteries of guineapigs. Pflug Arch 392:72–78.

Zelis R, Wichmann T, Starke K (1982): Inhibition of vascular noradrenaline release by diltiazem. Circulation 66:139.

Zipser B, Bennett MVL (1973): Tetrodotoxin resistant electrically excitable responses of receptor cells. Brain Res 62:253–260.

Zsoter TT, Wolchinsky C, Endrenyi C (1984): Effects of verapamil on ^{3}H-norepinephrine release. J Cardiovasc Pharm 6:1060–1066.

Zurgil N, Zisapel N (1983): Calcium dependent protein phosphorylation and dephosphorylation in intact brain neurons in culture. FEBS Lett 156:257–261.

Structure and Physiology of the Slow Inward Calcium Channel, pages 247–265
© 1987 Alan R. Liss, Inc.

10

Calcium Channels and Other Devices for Effecting Stimulus-Exocytosis Coupling

P.F. Baker

MRC Secretory Mechanisms Group, Department of Physiology, King's College London, Strand, London WC2R 2LS

INTRODUCTION: STRATEGIES FOR Ca COUPLING

Many aspects of cellular function are sensitive to the free Ca concentration and the term "calcium coupling" is used to describe any process by which a stimulus evokes a specific cellular response through the mediation of calcium. The key features of control by intracellular Ca are summarized in Figure 1. They are 1) maintenance of a very low cytosolic free Ca concentration, 2) the existence of pools of Ca at much higher concentrations, 3) mechanisms for transferring Ca from these pools into the cytosol, and 4) receptors for Ca in the cytosol. The resulting response is often enhanced by a dependence on $[Ca^{2+}]^n$ where $n > 1$ and normally between 2 and 4.

A sine qua non for effective coupling is that any change in cytosolic Ca must have access to the relevant receptors; but the achievement of this goal poses problems because the same mechanisms that ensure a low cytosolic free Ca will also tend to limit the spread of a Ca signal. At least two quite different solutions can be recognised: spatial proximity of Ca sources and Ca receptors, and modulation of the Ca sensitivity of specific receptors. In the limit, this latter strategy may completely shift the coupling process from calcium—the concentration of which may remain constant—to some other molecule that alters the sensitivity of a specific process for calcium. This process remains Ca-dependent and a certain "background" level of Ca is essential; but coupling is now achieved by changes in the concentration of another molecule.

The evoked, exocytotic release of prepackaged transmitter substances and hormones provide many good examples of Ca coupling [Katz, 1969; Douglas, 1968; Baker, 1974; Baker and Knight, 1984, 1986]. In what follows, I will examine a number of aspects of stimulus-exocytosis coupling; but as all Ca coupling occurs against a background of intracellular Ca buffers, I shall begin with a brief account of cytosolic Ca buffering.

THE PROBLEM OF CYTOPLASMIC Ca BUFFERING

There is general agreement that the bulk of Ca inside cells is bound. Measurement of total Ca by atomic absorption rarely reveals less than 0.1 mmol Ca/kg wet weight—and often more than 1 mmole Ca/kg wet weight—yet direct determination of cytosolic free Ca by means of aequorin, arsenazo III, Quin 2 or Ca-selective electrodes rarely give values far from 100 nM.

Intracellular Ca buffering involves a number of different processes, the relative importance of which vary from tissue to tissue. Experimentally, they can be divided into energy-dependent and energy-independent buffers. The energy-dependent group comprises mitochondria and endoplasmic reticulum (ER), including its various derivatives such as sarcoplasmic reticulum and secretory vesicles. The energy-independent group encompasses the sum of Ca binding to phospholipids and various Ca-binding proteins, some of which have no known function other than to act as Ca buffers while others have a dual role serving both to buffer Ca and by binding Ca to function as receptors that transduce changes in free Ca into changes in protein conformation and enzyme activity. Parvalbumin and the vitamin D-dependent Ca-binding proteins are good examples of the first category and troponin C and calmodulin of the second [see Siegel, 1980; Watterson and Vincenzi, 1980].

An appreciation of the extent to which a Ca transient will be damped in any particular cell or part of a cell requires a knowledge of the *quantity* of Ca that can be bound at different levels of free Ca and the *rate* at which this buffering can take place. With the possible exception of skeletal muscle, such detailed information is not generally available. A major problem in examining cytoplasmic Ca buffering is to find ways to monitor buffering under conditions as near physiological as possible. Isolated organelles, or even organelles within permeabilized cells, may behave quite differently from undisturbed organelles in situ. This is well illustrated in Figure 2 which summarizes data on Ca binding in relatively undisturbed axoplasm extruded from a squid giant axon. Free Ca was monitored by a Ca-selective electrode and Ca buffering was titrated by microinjection of aliquots of $CaCl_2$ into the axoplasm. The striking feature is the large amount of Ca that can be taken up by a high-affinity, ruthenium red-sensitive system which is almost certainly the mitochondria. Isolated mitochondria exhibit the same large capacity; but are not able to lower free Ca to the same extent as in intact axoplasm [Baker

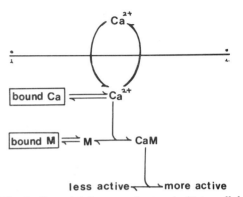

Fig. 1. *Essential features of control of intracellular reactions by calcium. M is a calcium-receptor protein such as calmodulin.*

and Schlaepfer, 1978]. The difference may be that intact cytoplasm contains factors that modify mitochondrial function. Support for this view comes from recent work of Nicchita and Williamson [1984] who showed that low concentrations of spermine can improve the efficiency of mitochondrial Ca binding permitting the stabilization of a lower free calcium. The effectiveness of other cytoplasmic Ca buffers may also be subject to analogous, but as yet unknown, factors.

The net effect of these Ca-binding systems is to limit the diffusional spread of a pulse of calcium. This has been demonstrated in a variety of ways from the limited diffusion of ^{45}Ca to direct determination using Ca-sensitive microelectrodes and visualization using image intensification [Rose and Loewenstein, 1976]. In large cells such as the squid axon and snail neurone, Ca entering at the periphery—for instance during nervous activity—is virtually undetectable at the centre of the cell, and it is possible to define a space constant for Ca diffusion equal to D/k, where D is the diffusion coefficient of free Ca and k is the rate constant for Ca binding [Baker et al., 1971; Gorman et al., 1984].

Conversely, anything that impairs cytoplasmic Ca binding should augment the transient rise in free Ca associated with a Ca pulse. If specific inhibitors of the various binding systems were available, the relative effectiveness of the systems as buffers could be examined by monitoring the change in free Ca in response to a constant Ca challenge in the absence and presence of the inhibitor. One such experiment is illustrated in Figure 3 which shows the effect of ruthenium red on Ca buffering in the squid axon. The Ca challenge was provided by exposing the axon to

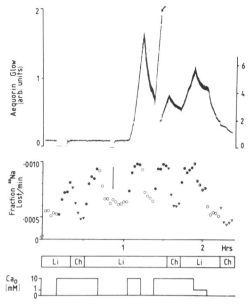

Fig. 3. *Effect of injecting ruthenium red (final concentration 50 μM) on the increase in intracellular free Ca caused by transfer of a squid axon from Na to Li sea water. Upper trace, aequorin light output—note scale change at arrow. Lower trace, ^{22}Na efflux in the presence of 10^{-5}M ouabain. Solution changes are indicated at the bottom of the figure. Ruthenium red was injected at the vertical line (lower trace). Note that although Ca_o-dependent Na efflux [Baker, 1972] is apparently unaffected by ruthenium red, the resulting rise in intracellular free Ca is much increased. Temperature 20°C (unpublished data of Allen and Baker).*

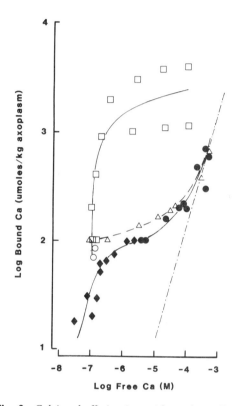

Fig. 2. *Calcium buffering in squid axoplasm. Data obtained by monitoring free Ca in extruded axoplasm with a Ca-selective microelectrode and injecting either CaCl$_2$ to add Ca or EGTA to sequester Ca. □, binding determined by injection of Ca into fresh axoplasm; △, binding determined by injection of Ca into fresh axoplasm preinjected with ruthenium red to give a final concentration of 640 μM; ●, binding determined by injection of Ca into fully poisoned axoplasm; ○, binding determined by injection of EGTA into fresh axoplasm; ◆, binding determined after injection of EGTA into fully poisoned axoplasm. Temperature 18°C. The dotted line has a slope of unity. The difference between it and the solid line through the points in fully poisoned axoplasm reveals a saturable, energy-independent component of binding with an apparent affinity for Ca about 150 nM. [From Baker and Umbach, in press.]*

Na-free sea water which stimulates Ca entry in exchange for internal Na (Ca$_o$-Na$_i$ exchange). Stimulation of this exchange reaction raises free Ca by a small amount and this can normally be detected by intracellular aequorin. In the experiment illustrated, this change was barely detectable before injection of ruthenium red but became very pronounced after injection, showing that ruthenium red-sensitive processes play an important part in restricting the rise in free Ca due to activation of Ca$_o$-Na$_i$ exchange. So far, no equivalent selective inhibitor of Ca binding by endoplasmic reticulum has been found although the effectiveness of this system at lowering free Ca can be strongly enhanced by injection of oxalate.

Whatever the processes responsible for cytoplasmic Ca binding, their loading with Ca is ultimately controlled by the Ca made available to them by the plasma membrane through which Ca both enters and leaves the cell [see Baker 1972; 1976].

Ca COUPLING: THE CLOSE PROXIMITY SOLUTION
The Generation of Ca Transients

In order to change cytosolic free Ca there must be sources of Ca at high concentration from which Ca can be transferred into the cytosol where the size of the Ca transient generated will be determined by the quantity of Ca transferred and the various Ca buffer systems present. Such sources can be either extracellular, where free Ca is at least 10^4 times higher than in the cytosol, or intracellular, where any of the systems that bind Ca under physiological conditions can, under appropriate conditions, release calcium. The former mechanisms permit extracellular Ca to enter a cell, while the latter redistribute intracellular Ca. It follows that aspects of cell function that depend on Ca entry across the plasma membrane will be absolutely dependent on extracellular Ca, whereas those that depend on intracellular sources may persist in the complete absence of external calcium. Because of the Ca-sequestering properties of cytoplasm, extracellular Ca is likely to have rapid access only to receptors located close to the plasma membrane, whereas intracellular stores can be located anywhere in a cell, and their release of Ca can be used to trigger Ca-dependent processes located deep within the cell.

Ca Channels at the Extracellular Intracellular Interface

The steepest Ca gradient is to be found at the plasma membrane. Here the chemical and electrical gradients strongly favour the inward leak of calcium; but whether or not such movement takes place is under the control of a variety of voltage-sensitive and chemically controlled channels. Net changes in intracellular free Ca can be monitoried by aequorin, arsenazo III, Quin 2 or Ca-selective microelectrodes and the mean free Ca seems to increase into the micromolar range.

The best characterized chemically controlled channel is the nicotinic acetylcholine receptor, the ionophore of which permits a variety of cations including Ca to permeate [see Katz, 1969; Miledi et al., 1980].

It seems likely that other physiological agonists such as glutamate acting on NMDA receptors also act directly to open Ca channels; but clear proof is still lacking. At the present time, far and away the best characterized route for increased Ca entry is via voltage-sensitive Ca channels. Although the tetrodotoxin-sensitive sodium channels permit some Ca to enter [Baker et al., 1971], of far greater significance is the Ca entry that takes place via a separate family of voltage-sensitive channels—the so-called Ca channels [Baker, 1972; Baker and Glitsch, 1975; Hagiwara and Byerly, 1981; Kostyuk, 1981 and this volume]. These are insensitive to tetrodotoxin but can usually be blocked by a variety of divalent and trivalent cations as well as organic calcium antagonists such as the phenylalkylamines, verapamil and D600. One major subset of these channels can also be blocked by the dihydropyridines, nifedipine and nitrendipine. The underlying unit conductances tend to be small and difficult to resolve and have mainly been studied using Ba as the permeant cation [Fenwick et al, 1982b; Nowycky et al., 1985].

From the viewpoint of my topic, this particular source of Ca current is restricted to the plasma membrane or extensions of it, and the Ca that enters the cell may only have access to Ca receptors located close to the mouth of the Ca channels. We have already seen that binding severely restricts the diffusion of a steady influx of Ca at the cell surface, and a further limitation in coupling Ca-dependent processes to channel activity will be the distance that a Ca ion can diffuse in the relatively short period of time that normally elapses between channel opening and activation of the Ca-dependent process: a period of the order of 1 msec in the case of Ca-activated exocytosis at the neuromuscular junction but possibly appreciably longer in other secretory tissues. Following the analysis of Baker et al. [1971], Ca entering through a channel—effectively a point source—is unlikely to diffuse more than 500 Å in 1 msec, limiting the possibility of rapid coupling to receptors located within this distance of the Ca channels. This limitation may explain the existence at the neuromuscular junction of regions, termed active zones, that are apparently specialized for effecting release (Fig. 4). The salient feature of these active zones is that exocytosis takes place in regions characterized by the presence of parallel arrays of intramembranous particles [Dreyer et al., 1973; Pumplin and Reese, 1977; Venezin et al., 1977; Haeuser et al., 1979]. One speculative hypothesis is that the particles represent Ca channels, and the special morphology serves to ensure that Ca inflow is directed at the sites where exocytosis takes place. In this context, it is of particular interest that the severe disruption of the active zones of the neuromuscular junction seen in patients with the Eaton-Lambert syndrome is associated with impairment of the quantal release of acetylcholine [Lang et al., 1983].

Release from Intracellular Sites

If Ca entering at the cell surface can only reach receptors located close to the entry sites, a different strategy is needed to ensure exposure of other sites to Ca transients. Skeletal muscle is an excellent example where the inward spread of an electrical signal via infoldings of the surface membrane causes release of Ca from a membrane-bound store, the sarcoplasmic reticulum, that is located throughout the cross-section of the muscle and always within a very short distance of the myofilaments. Something analogous though much less well developed may exist in many cells. Thus, a Ca store can be located anywhere in a cell and, provided a suitable messenger exists, release its Ca in response to a specific signal. Cytosolic Ca-buffering will ensure that the released Ca will also remain

spatially restricted; but provided the store is located close to a cohort of Ca receptors, the stimulus-store-receptor set can provide a very specific and effective system for control by intracellular Ca of various aspects of cell function.

In principle, any of the various intracellular Ca stores could function in this way: but the only one for which clear evidence exists so far is the endoplasmic reticulum. The demonstration that inositol 1,4,5 *tris* phosphate (IP_3)—a product of the hydrolysis of phosphatidylinositol-*bis*-phosphate (PIP_2) (Fig. 5)—can mobilise cell calcium [Streb et al., 1983], apparently from the endoplasmic reticulum has, at one blow, provided a possible mechanism for Ca release from the endoplasmic reticulum and also linked this to events occurring at the plasma membrane where the phosphodiesterase (phospholipase C), which hydrolyses PIP_2, can be activated by a variety of extracellular signals including transmitter substances, neuromodulators, and hormones [Hokin and Hokin, 1953; Michell, 1975; Berridge, 1984; Berridge and Irvine, 1984]. There seems every likelihood that this route of Ca mobilization will prove to be widespread; but it is still too early to assess its full significance. It is of interest that very recently it has been suggested that IP_3 may be involved in excitation-contraction coupling in skeletal muscle, which had previously been thought to be controlled electrically [Vergara and Tsien, 1985; Volpe et al., 1985].

The mechanism by which IP_3 releases Ca from the ER is unknown, but it is presumably some sort of IP_3-activated Ca channel. The importance of the IP_3 system for calcium coupling is that it can provide a link between plasma membrane events and calcium release deep within the cell, the water soluble IP_3 molecule serving as second messenger. The nature of the receptor with which IP_3 interacts and the mechanism by which Ca is released have yet to be elucidated. Speculating a little, there is a very real possibility that IP_3 may prove to be only one of a family of intracellular Ca-mobilizing messengers–each associated with a particular class of Ca store, thereby permitting selective control over spe-

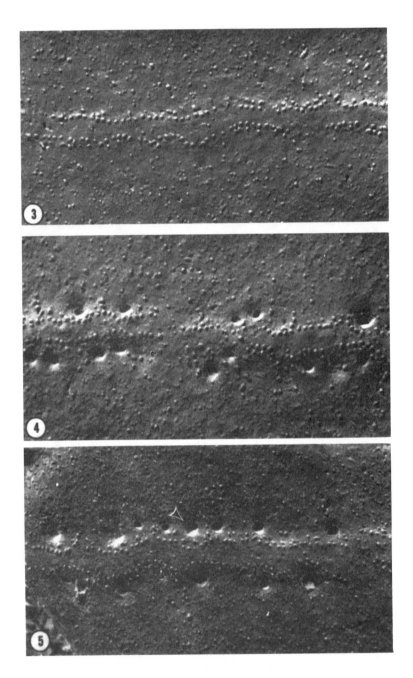

Fig. 4. *Freeze fracture replicas of exocytosis at an active zone in a frog motor neurone terminal. Exocytosis captured by fast freezing. Upper picture before and lower ones after stimulation. Note the parallel rows of intramembranous particles and appearance of exocytotic stomata in the lower pictures. [From Haeuser et al., 1979.]*

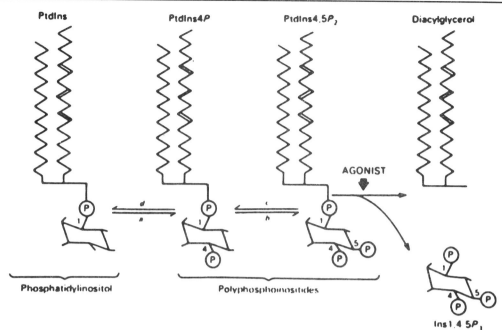

Fig. 5. *Phosphatidylinositol as source of diacylgly-cerol and inositol* tris *phosphate. Diacylglycerol presumably remains in the membrane where it can* *activate the enzyme protein kinase C, and inositol* tris *phosphate passes into the cytosol where it can mobilize bound calcium. [From Berridge, 1984.]*

cific Ca-sensitive aspects of cell function. The sphere of influence of the IP_3 message will depend on its stability within the cell.

Ca COUPLING: THE VARIABLE SENSITIVITY SOLUTION

Calcium receptors serve to transduce alterations in free Ca into changes in cell function. They may either be permanently fixed to an effector mechanism, for example a potassium channel, or free to diffuse to a more distant effector; but in all instances Ca binding leads to altered function, and the chain of events is always *increased* free Ca leading to *increased* receptor occupancy and altered function.

Another way to achieve the same end is to alter the sensitivity of the process for calcium. Thus, if the Ca sensitivity of a receptor effector complex is increased, Ca-dependent processes can be initiated with a smaller Ca transient or even without any change in free Ca at all. There are a number of examples of altered Ca sensitivity and perhaps many more

yet to be recognised. The four best known general mechanisms are:

1) Phosphorylation either of the Ca receptor or molecular species with which it interacts. An example of sensitivity modification by phosphorylation is the cAMP-dependent phosphorylation of phosphorylase b kinase which increases its apparent affinity for Ca [Brostrom et al, 1971]. There is also evidence that phosphorylation of Ca-activated K channels may increase their affinity for calcium (Ewald et al., 1985). The converse effect, a reduction in Ca affinity, is seen following cAMP-dependent phosphorylation of troponin-I and of myosin light chain kinase [see Ray and England, 1976; Rasmussen and Waisman, 1983].

2) Alterations in phospholipid metabolism. The best example is the dramatic alteration in Ca sensitivity of the enzyme protein kinase C by diacylglycerol (DAG) (Fig. 6) [Kishimoto et al., 1980; Kaibuchi et al., 1981]. When PI is hydrolysed, it liberates diacylglycerol plus inositol phosphates. As has already been men-

Protein kinase C activation

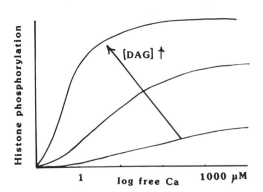

Fig. 6. *Diagrammatic representation of the increased sensitivity of protein kinase C to calcium brought about by diacylglycerol. Kinase activity is expressed in terms of histone phosphorylation. The kinetics illustrated are consistent with a reaction sequence of the following kind: E ECa ECa.DAG, where E represents the kinase.*

tioned, at least one inositol phosphate, IP_3, can mobilize Ca sequestered in the endoplasmic reticulum; but the hydrophobic diacylglycerol presumably remains trapped in the membrane where it interacts with protein kinase C. The simultaneous production in one locality of diacylglycerol, which serves to increase the sensitivity of one specific enzyme (protein kinase C) to Ca, and IP_3, which mobilises free Ca, will tend to ensure preferential activation of the C-kinase even in the presence of other enzymes sensitive to calcium. From the standpoint of stimulus-exocytosis coupling, it is of particular interest that conditions which would be expected to favour activation of protein kinase C also increase the sensitivity of exocytosis to calcium (Fig. 6) [Knight and Baker, 1983].

3) Alterations in membrane potential. Changes in membrane potential have been shown to alter the Ca sensitivity of certain Ca-activated potassium channels: depolarization increasing the channel open time at constant free Ca [Barrett *et al.*, 1982]. That the effect of voltage is mediated through altering the sensitivity of the channel to Ca is sup-

ported by the finding that at very low free Ca concentrations, depolarization has no effect (see Fig. 7). In view of the large number of channels controlled by Ca—both in terms of activation (K channels, nonselective cation channels, anion channels) and inactivation (Ca channels)—interaction between voltage and Ca sensitivity could have widespread implications.

4) Exposure to a variety of pharmacological agents. Thus caffeine seems to increase the Ca sensitivity of Ca-induced Ca release from the sarcoplasmic reticulum of skeletal muscle [Endo, 1977], and general anaesthetics increase the light emission from the Ca-sensitive photoprotein aequorin at constant free Ca [Baker and Schapira, 1980].

These four general mechanisms, acting either singly or in combination, provide ways to activate Ca-dependent processes without the need to alter cytosolic free Ca. If the production of such sensitivity-modulating factors is localized, and if only certain receptors are affected, specific sensitivity modulation provides a powerful method for achieving differential activation of Ca-dependent processes within a single cell.

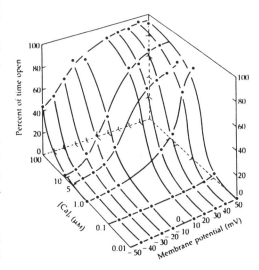

Fig. 7. *Summary of the effects of voltage and calcium on the open time of a single Ca-activated K channel in an excised membrane patch taken from a rat myotube in culture. [From Barrett et al., 1982.]*

CALCIUM AND THE TRIGGERING OF EXOCYTOSIS

Having considered various ways in which Ca receptors may be activated, I now wish to look in some detail at one particular Ca-dependent process—the initiation of exocytosis. At its simplest, a rise in free Ca leads to activation of exocytosis; but there are instances when exocytosis is activated with little or no rise in free Ca—or even in response to a fall in free Ca. I will begin by examining exocytosis in adrenal medullary cells where the major factor triggering exocytosis appears to be a rise in free calcium.

Adrenal Medullary Cells

Bovine adrenal medullary cells are a very convenient preparation because enzyme digestion of thin slices of the bovine adrenal releases a large number of viable cells. These can be studied immediately or maintained for many weeks in culture. Figure 8 summarizes the major factors involved in excitation-exocytosis coupling in these cells [Baker and Knight, 1984]. The cell membrane contains nicotinic acetylcholine receptors, tetrodotoxin-sensitive Na channels, D600-sensitive Ca channels, and a variety of potassium channels. As acetylcholine can evoke secretion in the presence of TTX, it is unlikely that the Na channels form an essential element in the coupling process. Rather, interaction of acetylcholine with the nicotinic receptor leads to a transient depolarization which opens the Ca channels directly [Fenwick et al., 1982a]. In addition, under experimental conditions, the Ca channel can be opened by direct depolarization with high K or indirectly by veratridine which brings about depolarization by opening the sodium channels. In all instances, Quin 2 reveals that secretion is associated with a Ca transient: intracellular free Ca rising from close to 100 nM into the micromolar range [Knight and Kesteven, 1983].

A very convenient feature of secretion in these cells is that, in addition to catecholamines, the secretory vesicles contain a number of other molecules including proteins (dopamine-β-hydroxylase, chromogranins, and enkephalins), and the simultaneous release of all these very different vesicular molecules, but not cytosolic molecules of similar size, provides a set of characteristic chemical markers for exocytosis.

A major problem in the study of exocytosis is that it is controlled by events occurring at the inner face of the plasma membrane, which is relatively inaccessible to experimental manipulation. An electrical technique has recently been developed that permits the plasma membrane barrier to be by-passed without impairing exocytosis and endocytosis [Baker and Knight, 1978; Knight and Baker, 1982]. This is achieved by exposing a suspension of cells to one or more brief high-voltage pulses. The externally applied field required to effect dielectric breakdown of the surface membrane of a sphere increases as the diameter of the sphere decreases. It follows that by suitable choice of field it is easy to cause localized breakdown of the plasma membrane without affecting intracellular organelles. By exposing cells to a series of brief high-voltage pulses it is possible to create 10–20 pores, each of effective diameter 4 nm, as judged by permeation of probes of different sizes. The resulting "leaky" cells equilibrate rapidly with substances of low molecular mass placed in the external solution. Such substances include catecholamines, EGTA and ATP. The "leaky" bovine adrenal medullary cells do not reseal, but remain fully accessible for up to 1 hour. Permeable cells can also be produced by exposure to low concentrations of detergents which generate quite large holes in the plasma membrane [Brooks and Treml, 1983; Dunn and Holz, 1983; Wilson and Kirshner, 1983]. The main drawback to the use of detergents is that they also exert inhibitory effects on exocytosis [Baker and Knight, 1981]. For this reason, electrical permeabilization is to be preferred, as it is both quick and clean.

The nature of the solution to which the cell interior is exposed is important. We have found a well-buffered medium based on potassium glutamate to be most satisfactory. Se-

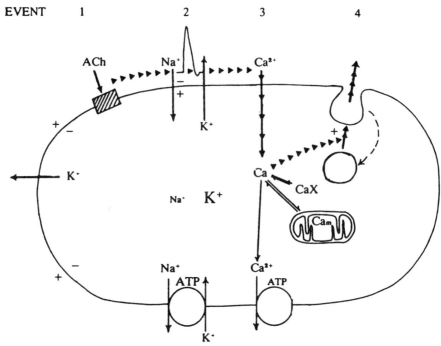

Fig. 8. *Schematic diagram of the adrenal medullary cell showing the possible sequence of events (1–4) from stimulus to secretion. 1) Acetylcholine interacts with receptors and leads to 2) a train of action potentials. Calcium enters 3) as a result of the depolarization and 4) promotes exocytosis.*

cretion proves to have a very specific requirement for Mg-ATP and to be sensitive to the nature of the major anion. Provided these constraints are met, the release of catecholamines from "leaky" cells depends entirely on the free Ca^{2+} to which they are exposed and no longer requires a cholinergic stimulus.

At a free Ca concentration of 10 nM or lower, less than 1% of the total cellular catecholamine is released on making the cells "leaky"; but if the free Ca is subsequently raised into the micromolar range, up to 30% of the cellular catecholamine appears in the external medium. The catecholamine seems to be released by exocytosis because it is accompanied by the vesicular protein dopamine-β-hydroxylase and the peptide enkephalin, but not the cytosolic enzyme lactate dehydrogenase. This rather simple experiment permits one to draw two important conclusions: 1) that there is very little free catecholamine in the cytosol; and 2) that the

Ca concentration required to evoke exocytosis from "leaky" cells is about three orders of magnitude lower than in intact cells (see Table I). It should be noted that release is no longer inhibited by D600, showing that Ca channels have been by-passed, and the vesicles are reacting with a plasma membrane that is presumably depolarized since it has the same solution on both sides.

The suggestion has often been made that the concentration of Ca immediately beneath the plasma membrane of secretory cells may rise to levels in excess of micromolar, perhaps reaching millimolar, and it might be argued that even in "leaky" cells, the weakly buffered micromolar concentrations of Ca that evoke secretion are effecting the release of much higher concentrations of CA locally. This seems highly unlikely because in "leaky" cells the Ca activation curve shows no change over a wide range of Ca-EGTA buffer concentrations. In addition, the Ca concentration required to effect secretion in "leaky" cells is compatible with the Ca transient observed with Quin 2 in intact cells. The data on activation of catecholamine release from "leaky" cells suggest that two Ca ions may cooperate to effect secretion.

Table I summarizes a number of properties of catecholamine secretion from "leaky" bovine adrenal medullary cells and the effects of a variety of potential inhibitors. So far we have only found relatively few interventions that affect catecholamine release, and most of these are unlikely to be of importance physiologically although they may throw light on the underlying mechanism. Of particular interest is the finding that secretion is unaffected by a number of agents that should interfere with the cytoskeleton. From the viewpoint of mechanism, the dependence of secretion on Mg-ATP is perhaps the most significant clue and worthy of close scrutiny.

In order to observe activation of catecholamine secretion by micromolar concentrations of Ca, it is essential that Mg-ATP is also present. In the absence of Mg, ATP alone is ineffective, and Mg-ATP cannot be replaced by a variety of other nucleotides both hydrolysable and nonhydrolysable. As the concentration of Mg-ATP is reduced, the extent of exocytosis becomes less, but there is no detectable change in the apparent affinity for calcium. As "leaky" adrenal medullary cells undergo cycles of exocytosis and endocytosis following exposure to Ca, it is possible that Mg-ATP is required for endocytosis and perhaps not at all for exocytosis, although this seems rather unlikely. Bearing this caveat in mind, it is nevertheless worth exploring the possible involvement of Mg-ATP in exocytosis because ATP has been accorded a central role in a number of current hypotheses, and

TABLE I. Properties of Ca^{2+}-Dependent Catecholamine Release From "Leaky" Adrenal Medullary Cells

Activation half maximal at Ca^{2+}-concentration of 1 μM
Requirement for Mg^{2+}-ATP is very specific; half maximal activation requires 1 mM
Unaffected by:
  Agonists and antagonists of ACh receptors
  Ca^{2+}-channel blocker D600 (100 μM)
  Agents that bind to tubulin (colchicine, vinblastine, 100 μM)
  Cytochalasin B (1 mM)
  Inhibitors of anion permeability (SITS, DIDS, 100 μM)
  Protease inhibitors TLCK (1 mM); leupeptin (1mM)
  Cyclic nucleotides (cAMP, cGMP, 1 mM)
  S-adenosyl methione (5 mM)
  Phalloidin (1 mM)
  Vanadate 10^{-4} M
  Leu- and Met-enkephalins, substance P (100 μM)
  Somatostatin (1 μM)
  NH_4Cl (30 mM)
Inhibited by:
  Chaotropic anions: SCN > Br > (1)
  Detergents (complete inhibition after 10 min incubation with 10 μg ml of digitonin: Brij 58 or saponin)
  Trifluoperazine (complete inhibition with 30 μg ml^{-1})
  High Mg^{2+} concentration: small increase in apparent K_m for Ca^{2+}
  Accompanies large reduction in V_{max}
  High osmotic pressure: large reduction in V_{max} but no significant changes in the affinity for Ca^{2+}
  Carbonylcyanid p-trifluormethoxyphenylhydrazone (FCCP) (45% inhibition by 10 μM)
  N-ethyl malecimide (NEM) (100% inhibition at 10^{-3} M)
  GTP-γ-S (50% inhibition at 5 μM)
  Botulinum and tetanus toxins

the "leaky" cells provides an excellent opportunity to subject these hypotheses to experimental examination.

A particularly intriguing set of hypotheses centre on the existence in the vesicle membrane of an ATP-dependent proton pump, the activity of which maintains the interior of the vesicle at an acid pH and electrically positive with respect to the cytosol. The potential and proton gradient could both be essential for exocytosis. A related suggestion is that the trigger for exocytosis may involve an alteration in the permeability of the vesicle membrane, leading either to a gain of anions or to an exchange of vesicular H^+ ions for extravesicular cations. In either case, the proton pump would be stimulated, and the vesicles should gain osmotically active particles and swell. There is some evidence in model systems that vesicle swelling greatly facilitates membrane fusion.

In "leaky" cells it is possible to dissipate the vesicle pH gradient or potential either singly or together and examine the effects of these manoeuvres on Ca-dependent release of cathecholamine. The experiments show quite clearly that Ca-dependent release of catecholamine can persist in the absence of either factor and when the proton pump is inhibited [see Knight and Baker, 1982, 1985a]. These results strongly suggest that if ATP is directly involved in exocytosis, it is unlikely to exert its effects via the vesicular proton pump. This conclusion would also seem to exclude hypotheses in which the vesicle permeability is altered, leading to increased proton pumping. This last group of hypotheses also fails to find support in experiments in which Ca-dependent secretion in "leaky" cells can take place in a medium based largely on sucrose [see Knight and Baker, 1982]. Nevertheless, Ca-dependent secretion—both in intact and "leaky" cells—is blocked by exposure to media of osmotic pressures greater than physiological, suggesting that alterations in osmotic activity may contribute in some way to exocytosis.

If Mg-ATP does not act through the vesicular proton pump, are there any clues as to how it might function? Experiments with $[^{32}P]$ Mg-ATP have shown that a number of proteins in chromaffin cells are phosphorylated in the presence of Ca; but as yet there is no clear evidence linking any of these phosphoproteins directly with secretion. One of the most interesting clues to emerge recently is illustrated in Figure 9. The phorbol ester, 12-0-tetradecanoylphorbol-13-acetate (TPA), shifts the Ca activation curve for catecholamine secretion to the left [Knight and Baker, 1983]. This shift is only seen in response to esters which activate protein kinase C (for example TPA and phorbol-12,13-dibenzoate, but not phorbol or phorbol-13-acetate), and the concentration of TPA required to modulate the Ca sensitivity of secretion (half-maximal effect at 2 nM) is very similar to that needed to activate protein kinase C. Activation of C-kinase requires Ca, a phospholipid, and diacylglycerol, which is normally derived from the breakdown of phosphatidylinositol, and TPA appears able to replace diacylglycerol [Castagna et al., 1982]. If the action of TPA on protein kinase C proves to be specific, these results could strongly implicate protein kinase C in exocytosis.

However, at least for the bovine adrenal, there are a number of caveats to this proposal. First, TPA has rather little effect on exocytosis in intact chromaffin cells; second, the diacylglycerol analogue 1-oleoyl-2-acetyl glycerol (OAG) has no effect in either intact or "leaky" cells—although another analogue 1,2 dioctanoylglycerol acts like TPA—and, finally, GTP-γ-S, which should promote endogenous DAG production, inhibits exocytosis even in the presence of TPA (Fig. 10) [Knight and Baker, 1985].

Before discussing the possible significance of these results, it is worth looking at the effects of TPA, OAG, and GTP-γ-S, on other exocytotic systems. In general, phorbol esters that activate protein kinase C also stimulate exocytosis in a wide variety of secretory systems [see for instance Baker, 1984], including even parathyroid cells which normally secrete in response to a fall in free Ca [Brown et al., 1984] and, of the various cell types examined,

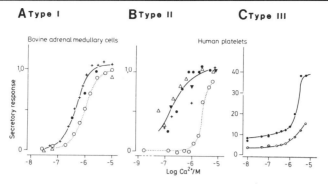

Fig. 9. *Modification of Ca-dependent secretion in "leaky" cells by exposure to the phorbol ester TPA and other agents. Examples of the three classes of response that have been observed. A) The small leftward shift seen in catecholamine secretion from bovine adrenal medullary cells in the presence of 3 nM TPA (♦), 100 μM dioctanoylglycerol (+) [from*

Knight and Baker, 1983]. B) The marked leftward shift seen in 5-HT secretion from human platelets: 30 nM TPA (▼), 20 μM OAG (●), 50 μM GTP-γ-S (△). C) The lack of any shift, only an increase in exent of exocytosis of N-acetylglucosaminidase, also from platelets: 10 μg/ml TPA (●) [from Knight et al., 1984.]

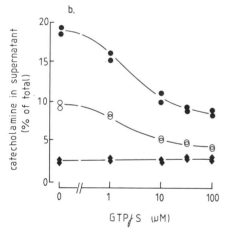

Fig. 10. *Inhibition by GTP-γ-S of Ca-dependent exocytosis from "leaky" bovine adrenal medullary cells. Cells were rendered permeable, exposed to GTP-γ S for 6 min, and challenged with Ca-BAPTA buffers generating free Ca of 6 μM (●), 0.7 μM (○) and 0.01 μM (♦). Temperature 26°C. [From Knight and Baker, 1985b.]*

adrenal medullary cells are amongst the least sensitive whilst platelets are amongst the most sensitive.

Serotonin Release from Platelets

Under physiological conditions, stimulation of platelets by agents such as thrombin, collagen or platelet activating factor leads to release of both serotonin and a variety of enzymes of lysosomal origin. Release is normally associated with a rise in intracellular free Ca; but conditions can be found where free Ca either does not rise or even falls, yet release of serotonin still occurs [Rink and Hallam, 1984; Hallam et al, 1984]. Secretion of 5-HT in the absence of any detectable alteration in free Ca is also seen following exposure of platelets to TPA or OAG. These effects are so striking that it has been suggested that TPA and OAG are activating a Ca-independent secretory pathway [see discussion in Baker, 1984]. However, experiments with platelets that have been rendered "leaky" by exposure to brief high-voltage fields do not support this view (Fig. 9B) [Knight and Scrutton, 1984a; Knight et al., 1984]. The Ca activation curve for 5-HT release is shifted markedly to the left by thrombin or by exposure to TPA or OAG; but secretion still requires Ca and can be blocked in the presence of a strong Ca buffer such as BAPTA. As thrombin activates PI breakdown in the platelet, it is very likely that the thrombin effect is mediated via DAG production which serves to activate exocytosis at the resting level of free Ca.

Two further features of exocytosis in "leaky" platelets are of considerable interest:

1) cAMP shifts the Ca activation curve for 5-HT release to the right, and 2) analogues of GTP such as GTP-γ-S shift it to the left [Knight and Scrutton, 1984b]. It seems likely that both actions are exerted, at least in part, through control of endogenous diacylglycerol production.

The picture that emerges from these experiments is that 5-HT secretion in the platelet can be activated either by a rise in free Ca, or by a rise in DAG, or a combination of the two. Kraft and Anderson [1983] have shown that exposure to TPA causes cytosolic protein kinase C to fall and membrane-associated C-kinase to rise, which suggests that one consequence of endogenous DAG production may be to facilitate association of protein kinase C with membranes. Such association might promote exocytosis.

Enzyme Release from Platelets

The release of lysosomal enzymes such as β-N-acetylneuraminidase from platelets is affected by TPA in quite a different way from serotonin. These enzymes are packaged separately from serotonin, and their release is Ca-dependent; but addition of TPA or DAG is without effect on the apparent affinity for Ca and only affects the extent of secretion (see Fig. 9C).

Mast Cells

The explosive discharge of histamine that follows exposure of mast cells to IgG is associated with a rise in free Ca [White et al., 1984], but can also be strongly potentiated at constant Ca by TPA. In a very elegant series of experiments on individual mast cells attached to a patch pipette, exocytosis was monitored as the stepwise increase in capacitance that accompanies addition of membrane to the cell surface [Fernandez et al., 1984]. Rather surprisingly, under these conditions exocytosis is apparently insensitive to Ca but can be triggered by GTP-γ-S even when the pipette contains a high concentration of EGTA. One possible explanation for these findings is that GTP-γ-S is required to promote PI breakdown and DAG production; but

a direct effect of GTP-γ-S on exocytosis must also be a strong possibility.

The Control of Exocytosis

The ultimate goal of stimulus-exocytosis coupling is to cause the secretory vesicle membrane to fuse with the plasma membrane thereby releasing into the extracellular fluid materials prepackaged within the vesicle. The nature of the fusion event remains obscure, but it is tempting to draw analogies with fusion of viral and host cell membranes which is facilitated by the exposure of a hydrophobic peptide which serves to link the two membranes [White et al., 1981; Hsu et al., 1981]. Freeze-fracture studies of fast-frozen secretory cells all suggest that the initial fusion event is very small—perhaps 10 nm in diameter—and only later expands in size [Schmidt et al., 1983]. It follows that the initial step in exocytosis might also be localized to a small, highly reactive site.

The data outlined above leave little doubt that the classical control of exocytosis by Ca must now give way to a more complex system in which at least two variables, Ca and DAG (and perhaps others), interact apparently through protein kinase C. Secretion in "leaky" cells can be divided into three classes on the basis of the effects of phorbol esters on the Ca activation curve. These are illustrated in Figure 9 and described below:

Type I: Characterized by rather little effect of phorbol esters, at most a small leftward shift in the Ca activation curve.

Type II: Characterized by a large effect of TPA or DAG increasing the apparent affinity for Ca and bringing about a small increase in the extent of exocytosis.

Type III: Characterized by a lack of effect of phorbol esters and DAG on the sensitivity to Ca. These agents only affect the extent of secretion.

It is of considerable interest that these apparently different kinetics can be generated via the same enzyme simply by specifying different preferred orders of substrate binding. Thus, considering only the two substrates, Ca and DAG, there are three possibilities:

1) $E \underset{\longleftarrow}{\overset{DAG}{\longrightarrow}} E^{DAG} \underset{\longleftarrow}{\overset{Ca}{\longrightarrow}} E^{DAG}_{Ca}$

2) $E \underset{\longleftarrow}{\overset{CA}{\longrightarrow}} E_{Ca} \underset{\longleftarrow}{\overset{DAG}{\longrightarrow}} E^{DAG}_{Ca}$

3) $E \underset{\overset{Ca}{\searrow}}{\overset{DAG}{\nearrow}} \begin{matrix} E^{DAG} \\[4pt] E_{Ca} \end{matrix} \underset{\overset{DAG}{\nwarrow}}{\overset{Ca}{\searrow}} E^{DAG}_{Ca}$

The Ca dependencies of exocytosis predicted by schemes 1, 2, and 3 above are shown in Figure 11. They are quite different. Scheme 1 shows a small, but limited, leftward shift on adding DAG; scheme 2 a much larger shift that continues to increase as the DAG concentration is increased, such that at high DAG concentrations secretion will seem to be Ca-independent; and scheme 3 shows no shift at all, only an increase in the extent of secretion.

The striking parallel between the Ca dependencies of Figure 11 and the three major types of exocytosis seen, so far, in permeable

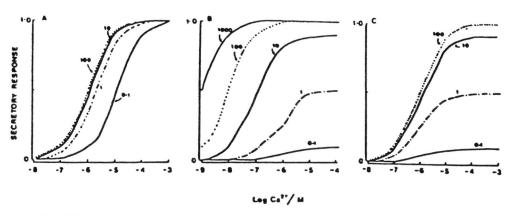

Fig. 11. *Ca-dependence of secretion calculated on the assumption of ordered binding of DAG and Ca to protein kinase C. Numbers by the curves refer to DAG concentrations (μM).*

A. $E \underset{K_D}{\overset{DAG}{\longrightarrow}} E^{DAG} \underset{K_{Ca}}{\overset{Ca}{\longrightarrow}} E^{DAG}_{Ca}$ $F_{E^{DAG}_{Ca}} = \dfrac{1}{1 + \dfrac{K_{Ca}}{Ca}\left(1 + \dfrac{K_D}{D}\right)}$

B. $E \underset{K_{Ca}}{\overset{Ca}{\longrightarrow}} E_{Ca} \underset{K_D}{\overset{DAG}{\longrightarrow}} E^{DAG}_{Ca}$ $F_{E^{DAG}_{Ca}} = \dfrac{1}{1 + \dfrac{K_D}{D}\left(1 + \dfrac{K_{Ca}}{Ca}\right)}$

C. $E \underset{\overset{Ca}{\searrow}}{\overset{DAG}{\nearrow}} \begin{matrix} E^{DAG} \\[4pt] E_{Ca} \end{matrix} \underset{\overset{DAG}{\nearrow}}{\overset{Ca}{\searrow}} E^{DAG}_{Ca}$ $F_{E^{DAG}_{Ca}} = \dfrac{1}{1 + \dfrac{K_D}{D} + \dfrac{K_{Ca}}{Ca}\left(1 + \dfrac{K_D}{D}\right)}$

For ease of calculating the curves, the affinity constants K_{Ca} and K_D for Ca and DAG, respectively, have been set at 1 μM.

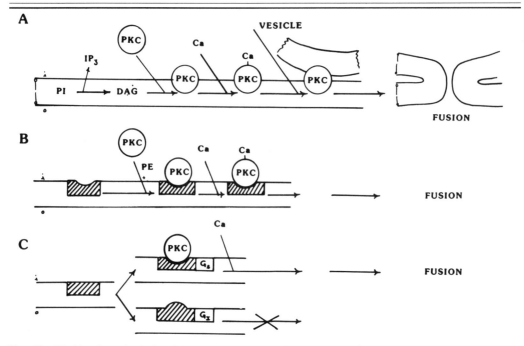

Fig. 12. *Working hypothesis involving protein kinase C (PKC) as an initiator of the membrane fusion event that underlies type I exocytosis. A,B, and C represent schemes of increasing complexity. In A) DAG (or phorbol ester, PE) facilitates a nonspecific protein kinase C-membrane interaction; in B) inter-* *action is assumed to involve a specific membrane component; and in C) the availability of this component is subject to modulation by GTP-γ-S-binding proteins that can be either stimulatory (G_s) or inhibitory (G_I). Based on data from the adrenal medullary chromaffin cell.*

cells may be more than a coincidence. Thus scheme 1 resembles type I and is remarkably similar to the behaviour of catecholamine secretion in the adrenal medulla; scheme 2 closely parallels type II and mirrors serotonin secretion in platelets; and scheme 3 resembles type III which includes enzyme secretion from platelets and insulin release from pancreatic β-cells. It is possible to combine these different classes of exocytosis in a single cell where their co-existence may help explain the differential release of stored chemicals which seems to be a feature of a number of cells. Figure 11 shows that the differential release of serotonin and lysosomal enzymes from platelets can be achieved simply by specifying scheme 2 order of binding for serotonin release (type II exocytosis) and permitting random binding (scheme 3) for enzyme secretion (type III exocytosis).

If protein kinase C is intimately involved with exocytosis, how does it act? The obvious

possibility is that it phosphorylates a substrate which helps bring about membrane fusion; but although exocytosis requires Mg-ATP and many intracellular substrates are phosphorylated in a Ca-dependent fashion, a unique substrate whose phosphorylation closely parallels exocytosis in a number of different systems has yet to emerge. This may simply reflect the fact that the relevant molecules are present in very low concentrations but in the absence of a clear substrate, an alternative idea that merits close examination is that, in the presence of Mg-ATP, protein kinase C may itself be a fusogen. It partitions strongly into membranes in the presence of TPA and seems to associate with secretory vesicles in a Ca-dependent fashion [Creutz et al., 1983]. It thus has the properties to act as a molecular bridge between secretory vesicle and plasma membrane, and generation of such a bridge might be the first step towards membrane fusion. The concept of protein kinase C as a membrane fusogen is highly speculative; but certainly worthy of experimental investigation. The apparent requirement for 1 Mg-ATP could imply that one activated protein kinase C molecule effects the exocytosis of one vesicle, and the order of substrate binding to the kinase might, as discussed above, lead to the apparently different patterns of exocytosis described earlier in this paper.

Of the many possible extensions to this idea, one is that the protein kinase C-membrane association site might be subject to facilitatory or inhibitory modulation, for instance by GTP binding proteins (Fig. 12). This might be particularly important in type I exocytosis, where the direct involvement of a GTP binding site could explain the inhibitory action of GTP-γ-S on Ca and TPA-dependent exocytosis in bovine adrenal medullary cells (Fig. 10), and it might provide a target for pharmacological agents such as botulinum toxin—and other possible endogenous agents—that bring about short- and long-term alterations in secretory function [Knight et al., 1985]. In this context, it is of considerable interest that a GTP-binding protein—of as yet unknown function—has recently been extracted in large amounts from brain [Sternweiss and Robishaw, 1984].

REFERENCES

Baker PF (1972): Transport and metabolism of calcium ions in nerve. Prog Biophys Mol Biol 24:177–223.

Baker PF (1974): Excitation-secretion coupling. In "Recent Advances in Physiology," Vol 9. Edinburgh: Churchill Livingston, pp 51–86.

Baker PF (1976) The regulation of intracellular calcium. SEB Symposium XXX:67–88.

Baker PF (1984): Multiple controls for secretion: Nature (Lond) 310:629–630.

Baker PF, Glitsch HG (1975): Voltage-dependent changes in the permeability of nerve membranes to calcium and other divalent cations. Phil Trans Roy Soc Lond B 270:389–409.

Baker PF, Hodgkin AL, Ridgway EB (1971): Depolarization and Ca entry in squid giant axons. J Physiol Lond 218:709–755.

Baker PF, Knight DE (1978): Calcium-dependent exocytosis in bovine adrenal medullary cells with leaky plasma membranes. Nature (Lond) 276:620–622.

Baker PF, Knight DE (1981): Calcium control of exocytosis and endocytosis in bovine adrenal medullary cells. Phil Trans Roy Soc Lond B 296:83–103.

Baker PF, Knight DE (1984): Calcium control of exocytosis in bovine adrenal medullary cells. TINS 7:120–126.

Baker PF, Knight DE (1986): Exocytosis: control by calcium and other factors. British Medical Bulletin 42:399–404.

Baker PF, Schapira AHV (1980): Anaesthetics increased light emission from aequorin at constant ionized calcium. Nature (Lond) 284:168–169.

Baker PF, Schlaepfer WW (1978): Uptake and binding of calcium by axoplasm isolated from giant axons of Loligo and Myxicola. J Physiol Lond 276:103–125.

Barrett JN, Magelby KL, Pallotta BS (1982): Properties of single calcium-activated potassium channels in cultured rat muscle. J Physiol Lond 331:211–230.

Berridge MJ (1984): Inositol trisphosphate and diacylglycerol as second messengers. Biochem J 220:345–360.

Berridge MJ, Irvine RF (1984): Inositol trisphosphate, a novel second messenger in cellular signal transduction. Nature (Lond.) 312:315–321.

Brooks JC, Treml S (1983): Catecholamine secretion by chemically skinned cultured chromaffin cells. J Neurochem 40:468–473.

Brostrom CO, Hunkeler FL, Krebs EG (1971): The regulation of skeletal muscle phosphorylase kinase by Ca^{2+}. J Biol Chem 246:1961–1967.

Brown EM, Redgrave J, Thatcher J (1984): Effect of the phorbol ester TPA on PTH secretion. FEBS Lett. 175:72–75.

Castagna M, Takai Y, Kaibuchi K, Sana K, Kikkawa U, Nishizuka Y (1982): Direct activation of calcium-activated phospholipid-dependent protein kinase by tumour-promoting phorbol esters. J Biol Chem 257:7847–7851.

Creutz CE, Dowling LG, Sando JJ, Villar-Palasi C, Whipple JH, Zaks WJ (1983): Characterization of the chromobindins. J Biol Chem 258:14664–14674.

Douglas WW (1968): Stimulus-secretion coupling: The concept and clues from chromaffin and other cells. Br J Pharmacol 34:451–474.

Dreyer F, Peper K, Akert K, Sandri L, Moor H (1973): Ultrastructure of the 'active zone' in the frog neuromuscular junction. Brain Res 62:373–380.

Dunn LA, Holz RW (1983): Catecholamine secretion by digitonin-treated adrenal medullary chromaffin cells. J Biol Chem 258:4989–4993.

Endo M (1977): Calcium release from the sarcoplasmic reticulum. Physiol Rev 57:71–108.

Ewald DA, Williams A, Levitan JB (1985): Modulation of single Ca^{2+} dependent K^+-channel activity by protein phosphorylation. Nature (Lond) 315:503–506.

Fenwick EM, Marty A, Neher E (1982a): A patch clamp study of bovine chromaffin cells and of their sensitivity to acetylcholine. J Physiol Lond 331:577–597

Fenwick EM, Marty A, Neher E (1982b): Sodium and calcium channels in bovine chromaffin cells. J Physiol Lond 331:599–635.

Fernandez JM, Neher E, Gomperts BD (1984): Capacitance measurements reveal stepwise fusion events in degranulating mast cells. Nature (Lond) 312:453–455.

Gorman ALF, Levy S, Nasi E, Tillotson D (1984): Intracellular calcium measured with calcium-sensitive microelectrodes and arsenazo III in voltage-clamped Aplysia neurones. J Physiol Lond 353:127–142.

Haeuser JE, Reese TS, Dennis MJ, Jan Y, Evans L (1973) Synaptic vesicle exocytosis captured by quick freezing and correlated with quantal transmitter release. J Cell biol. 81:275–300.

Hagiwara S, Byerly L (1981): Calcium channel. Ann Rev Neurosci 4:69–125.

Hallam TJ, Sanchez A, Rink TJ (1984): Stimulus response coupling in human platelets. Biochem J 218:819–827.

Hokin MR, Hokin LE (1953): Enzyme secretion and the incorporation of ^{32}P into phospholipids of pancreas slices. J Biol Chem 203:967–977.

Hsu M-C, Scheid A, Choppin PW (1981): Activation of the Sendai virus fusion protein (F) involves a conformational change with exposure of a new hydrophobic region. J Biol Chem 256:3557–3563.

Kaibuchi K, Takai Y, Nishizuka Y (1981): Co-operative roles of various membrane phospholipids in the activation of calcium-activated, phospholipid-dependent protein kinase. J Biol Chem 256:7146–7149.

Katz B (1969): "The Release of Neural Transmitter Substances." Liverpool Univesity Press.

Kishimoto A, Takai Y, Mori T, Kikkawa U, Nishizuka Y (1980): Activation of calcium and phospholipid-dependent protein kinase by diacylglycerol: Its possible relation to phosphatidylinositol turnover. J Biol Chem 255:2273–2276.

Knight DE, Baker PF (1982): Calcium-dependence of catecholamine release from bovine adrenal medullary cells after exposure to intense electric fields. J Membrane Biol 68:107–140.

Knight DE, Baker PF (1983): The phorbol ester TPA increases the affinity of exocytosis for calcium in 'leaky' adrenal medullary cells. FEBS Lett 160:98–100.

Knight DE, Baker PF (1985a): The chromaffin granule proton pump and calcium-dependent exocytosis in bovine adrenal medullary cells. J Membrane Biol 83:147–156.

Knight DE, Baker PF (1985b): Guanine nucleotides and Ca-dependent exocytosis: Studies on two adrenal cell preparations. FEBS. Lett. 189:345–349.

Knight DE, Kesteven NT (1983): Evoked transient intracellular free Ca^{2+} changes and secretion in isolated bovine adrenal medullary cells. Proc Roy Soc Lond B 218:177–199.

Knight DE, Niggli V, Scrutton MC (1984): Thrombin and activators of protein kinase C modulate secretory responses of permeabilised human platelets induced by Ca^{2+}. Eur J Biochem 143:437–446.

Knight DE, Scrutton MC (1984a): The relationship between intracellular second messengers and platelet secretion. Biochem Soc Trans 12:969–972.

Knight DE, Scrutton MC (1984b): Cyclic nucleotides control a system which regulates Ca^{2+}-sensitivity of platelet secretion. Nature (Lond) 309:66–68.

Knight DE, Tonge DA, Baker PF (1985): Inhibition of exocytosis in bovine adrenal medullary cells by Botulinum toxin type D. Nature (Lond) 317:719–721.

Kostyuk PG (1981): Calcium channels in the neuronal membrane. Biochem Biophys Acta 650:128–150.

Kraft AS, Anderson WB (1983): Phorbol esters increase the amount of Ca^{2+} phospholipid-dependent protein kinase associated with plasma membrane. Nature (Lond) 301:621–623.

Lang B, Newsom-Davis J, Prior C, Wray D (1983): Antibodies to motor nerve terminals: An electrophysiological study of a human myasthenic syndrome transferred to mouse. J Physiol Lond 344:335–345.

Michell RH (1975): Inositol phospholipids and cell surface receptor function. Biochim Biophys Acta 415:81–147.

Miledi R, Parker I, Schalow G (1980): Transmitter induced calcium entry across the postsynaptic membrane at frog end plates measured using arsenazo III. J Physiol Lond 300:197–212.

Nicchita CV, Williamson JR (1984): Spermine: A regulator of mitochondrial calcium cycling. J Biol Chem 259:12978–12983.

Nowycky MC, Fox AP, Tsien RW (1985): Three types of neuronal calcium channel with different calcium agonist sensitivity. Nature (Lond) 316:440–443.

Pumplin DW, Reese TS (1977): Action of brown widow spider venom and Botulinum toxin on frog neuromuscular junction examined with the freeze fracture technique. J Physiol Lond 273:443–457.

Rasmussen H, Waisman DM (1983): Modulation of cell function in the calcium messenger system. Rev Physiol Biochem Pharmacol 95:111–149.

Ray KP, England PJ (1976): Phosphorylation of the inhibitory sub-unit of troponin and its effect on the calcium-dependence of cardiac myofibril adenosine triphosphatase. FEBS Lett 70:11–16.

Rink TJ, Hallam T (1984): What turns platelets on? TIBS 12:215–219.

Rose B, Loewenstein WR (1976): Permeability of a cell junction and the local cytoplasmic free ionized calcium concentration: A study with aequorin. J Membrane Biol 28:87–119.

Schmidt W, Patzak A, Lingg G, Winkler H, Plattner H (1983): Membrane events in adrenal chromaffin cells during exocytosis: A freeze-etching analysis after rapid cryofixation. Eur J Cell Biol 32:31–37.

Siegel FL (1980): Calcium-binding proteins: Structure and function. "Developments in Biochemistry," Vol 14. Elsevier/North Holland, pp 1–511.

Streb H, Irvine RF, Berridge MJ, Schultz I (1983): Release of Ca^{2+} from a non-mitochondrial intracellular store in pancreatic acinar cells by inositol-1,4,5-triphosphate. Nature (Lond) 306:67–69.

Sternweis PC, Robishaw JD (1984): Isolation of two proteins with high affinity for guanine nucleotides from membranes of bovine brain. J Biol Chem 259:13806–13813.

Venezin M, Sandri C, Akert K, Wyss UR (1977): Membrane-associated particles of the presynaptic active zone in rat spinal cord. A morphometric analysis. Brain Res 130:393–404.

Vergara J, Tsien RY (1985): Biophys J 47:351a.

Volpe P, Salviati G, DiVirgilio F, Pozzan T (1985): Inositol 1,4,5-tris phosphate induces calcium release from sarcoplasmic reticulum of skeletal muscle. Nature (Lond) 316:347–349.

Watterson DM, Vincenzi FF (1980): Calmodulin and cell functions. Ann NY Acad Sci 356:1–446.

White J, Matlin K, Helenius A (1981): Cell fusion by Semliki Forest, influenza and vesicular stomatitis viruses. J Cell Biol 89:674–679.

White JR, Ishizaka T, Ishizaka K, Sha'afi RI (1984): Direct demonstration of increased intracellular concentration of free calcium as measured by Quin 2 in stimulated rat peritoneal mast cells. Proc Nat Acad Sci USA 81:3978–3982.

Wilson SP, Kirschner N (1983): Calcium-evoked secretion from digitonin-permeabilized adrenal medullary chromaffin cells. J Biol Chem 258:4994–5000.

Index

Contents of Previous Volumes

Volume 8: Dopamine Receptors